W. Käfer ∎ B. Cakir ∎ T. Mattes ∎ H. Reichel ∎ (Eds.)

Orthopaedic Spine Surgery – An Instructional Course Textbook

W. Käfer   B. Cakir   T. Mattes
H. Reichel   (Eds.)

Orthopaedic Spine Surgery
– An Instructional Course Textbook

With 134 Figures in 280 Separate Illustrations
and 24 Tables

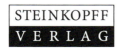

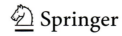

Dr. med. WOLFRAM KÄFER
Attending Orthopaedic Surgeon

Priv.-Doz. Dr. med. BALKAN CAKIR
Attending Orthopaedic Surgeon

Dr. med. THOMAS MATTES
Deputy Head of the Department of Orthopaedics

Prof. Dr. med. HEIKO REICHEL
Professor of Orthopaedic Surgery
and Head of the Department of Orthopaedics

Department of Orthopaedics
University of Ulm
Oberer Eselsberg 45
89081 Ulm, Germany

ISBN 978-3-7985-1828-5 Steinkopff Verlag

Bibliographic information published by Die Deutsche Nationalbibliothek
Die Deutsche Bibliothek lists this publication in the Deutsche Nationalbibliografie;
detailed bibliographic data is available in the Internet at http://dnb.d-nb.de.

This work is subject to copyright. All rights are reserved, whether the whole or part of the material is concerned, specifically the rights of translation, reprinting, reuse of illustrations, recitation, broadcasting, reproduction on microfilm or in any other way, and storage in data banks. Duplication of this publication or parts thereof is permitted only under the provisions of the German Copyright Law of September 9, 1965, in its current version, and permission for use must always be obtained from Steinkopff Verlag. Violations are liable for prosecution under the German Copyright Law.

Steinkopff Verlag
a member of Springer Science+Business Media

www.steinkopff.com

© Steinkopff-Verlag 2008
Printed in Germany

The use of general descriptive names, registered names, trademarks, etc. in this publication does not imply, even in the absence of a specific statement, that such names are exempt from the relevant protective laws and regulations and therefore free for general use.

Product liability: The publishers cannot guarantee the accuracy of any information about the application of operative techniques and medications contained in this book. In every individual case the user must check such information by consulting the relevant literature.

Production: Klemens Schwind
Cover design: Erich Kirchner, Heidelberg – Illustration: Rose Baumann, Schriesheim
Typesetting: K+V Fotosatz GmbH, Beerfelden
Printing and binding: Stürtz GmbH, Würzburg

SPIN 12242962   105/7231 – 5 4 3 2 1 0 – Printed on acid-free paper

Preface

A dramatic increase of technology in spine surgery has been witnessed over the past two decades. Concepts such as total disc replacement, posterior dynamic stabilization, kyphoplasty, and minimal-invasive procedures have been introduced, leading to an enormous rise in the number of spinal surgeries.

Generally, the application of any new surgical technique demands more skills than the use of established techniques does. Therefore, theoretical and practical training for example in the setting of an instructional course of orthopaedic spine surgery are of prime importance.

Based on the instructional course of orthopaedic spine surgery, the "Ulm Spine Week", which is held annually at the Department of Orthopaedics in collaboration with the Department of Anatomy and Cellular Neurobiology of the University of Ulm and the Department of Neurosurgery of the Military Hospital Ulm, the idea of this textbook evolved and was realized with the support of Steinkopff, Heidelberg. A panel of experts in the field of spine surgery presents established techniques and promising trends in their articles.

Three chapters of this book cover a variety of issues related to the treatment of degenerative, rheumatic, deformity-related, traumatic, and tumorous/infectious disorders of the cervical, thoracic, and lumbar spine. Another chapter addresses lumbar non-fusion technologies, since we believe that this novel technology deserves specific clarification.

This book is not only meant to be a practical guide for the participants of our instructional course, but also to be a manual of great value for all surgeons dealing with spinal pathologies.

The editors would like to sincerely thank all contributors and Dr. G. Volkert from Steinkopff, Heidelberg.

Ulm, February 2008

Wolfram Käfer
Balkan Cakir
Thomas Mattes
Heiko Reichel

Contents

Degenerative/rheumatic disorders and deformities

1 Posterior instrumentation of the cervical spine using the neon occipito-cervical system 3
MARCUS RICHTER and MICHAEL REITH

- Introduction 3
- Principles and objectives of the neon occipito-cervical system 3
- Surgical instruments and implants 5
- Anaesthesia and positioning 6
- Surgical technique 7
- Postoperative management 14
- Errors, hazards, and complications 14
- References 14

2 Treatment principles in rheumatoid instability of the cervical spine ... 17
TUGRUL KOCAK and KLAUS HUCH

- Introduction 17
- Morphologic variations of rheumatic instability 17
- Clinical picture 18
- Imaging 19
- Non-surgical therapy of the rheumatoid cervical spine 19
- Surgical treatment 20
- Summary 23
- References 23

3 Surgical techniques in cervical spinal canal stenosis 27
ULRICH KUNZ and CHRIS SCHULZ

- Introduction 27
- Conservative treatment options 28
- Indications for surgical treatment 28
- Anterior procedures 28
- Posterior procedures 31
- References 33

4 Techniques of thoracic and lumbar pedicle screws, lumbosacral fixation, and costotransversectomy ... 35
BENJAMIN ULMAR

- Historical development of pedicle screw instrumentation 35
- Anatomical background 35
- Implant components of the internal fixateur 40
- Indications for pedicle screws and transpedicular instrumentation 41
- Surgical approach and handling of the transpedicular instrumentation 41
- Costotransversectomy (postero-lateral approach to the thoracic spine) . 42
- References 42

5 Fusion procedures for degenerative disorders of the lumbar spine – indications, techniques, and results 45
WOLFRAM KÄFER, BALKAN CAKIR, and HEIKO REICHEL

- Introduction 45
- Low back pain – definition and epidemiology 45
- Surgical techniques 46
- Indications for lumbar fusion procedures 52
- Outcome 57
- Trends 58
- Summary 59
- References 59

6 Herniation of the lumbar intervertebral disc – when is surgery required? 63
BALKAN CAKIR, HEIKO REICHEL, and WOLFRAM KÄFER

- Background 63
- Paresis 64
- Pain 66
- Type of disc herniation 67
- Conclusion 69
- References 69

7 Lumbar spinal canal stenosis – decompression with or without stabilization? 73
ULRICH KUNZ and CHRIS SCHULZ

- Introduction 73
- Conservative treatment options 74
- Indications for surgical treatment 75
- Surgical technique 75
- Summary 77
- References 78

8 Spondylolisthesis – diagnosis and therapy 79
THOMAS MATTES and HEIKO REICHEL

- Introduction 79
- Classification and grading 79
- Etiology 79
- Prevalence and localization 80
- Diagnosis 80

- Conservative treatment ... 81
- Surgical treatment ... 82
- Summary ... 83
- References ... 84

9 Current concepts in scoliosis surgery ... 85
JENS SEIFERT and PETER BERNSTEIN

- Indications for surgery ... 85
- Surgical approaches ... 85
- Implants and fixation techniques ... 86
- Correction principles ... 87
- Combination of different techniques ... 89
- Spondylodesis ... 90
- New concepts in scoliosis surgery ... 90
- References ... 91

10 Syringomyelia – causes and treatment ... 93
UWE MAX MAUER

- Definition ... 93
- Pathophysiology ... 93
- Clinical history of posttraumatic syringomyelia ... 94
- Diagnostics ... 94
- Surgical management ... 95
- References ... 96

11 Computer navigation in spine surgery ... 97
THOMAS MATTES

- Introduction ... 97
- Computed tomography (CT)-based navigation ... 98
- Fluoroscopy-based navigation ... 99
- Fluoroscopic 3-D navigation ... 99
- Summary ... 100
- References ... 100

Trauma

12 Treatment of cervical spine injuries ... 105
CHRISTOPH ULRICH

- Introduction ... 105
- Diagnostics ... 105
- Conservative treatment ... 107
- Surgical treatment ... 107
- Stabilization techniques ... 107
- Upper cervical spine injuries ... 111
- Lower cervical spine injuries ... 116
- References ... 119

13 Thoracic spine injuries – open versus endoscopic procedures 121
MARKUS ARAND and MARKUS SCHULTHEISS

- Introduction 121
- Instrumentation system 121
- Operative technique 122
- Special considerations 125
- Summary 126
- References 126

14 Surgical treatment of fractures of the lumbar spine 129
FLORIAN GEBHARD and MARKUS SCHULTHEISS

- Introduction 129
- Anatomy, pathophysiology and fracture classification 129
- Clinical findings 129
- Spinal stabilization techniques 130
- Clinical pathway 130
- Operative technique 131
- Treatment modalities of osteoporotic fractures 132
- Evidence-based spine surgery 134
- Critical evaluation 135
- Summary 135
- References 135

15 The role of vertebroplasty and kyphoplasty in the management of osteoporotic vertebral compression fractures 137
RENÉ SCHMIDT

- Introduction 137
- Diagnostical work-up 137
- Indication 139
- Technique 142
- Conclusion 143
- References 143

Tumor and infection

16 Tumor lesions of the cervical spine – pitfalls and their solution 149
KLAUS HUCH
                                                                    149

- Introduction 149
- Imaging 149
- Treatment options 150
- Pitfalls 150
- Conclusion 153
- References 155

17 Tumorous diseases of the thoracic and lumbar spine 157
Jürgen Nothwang and Christoph Ulrich

- Introduction 157
- Incidence 157
- Localization 157
- Classification 158
- Biomechanics 158
- Differential diagnosis 158
- Diagnostic work-up 158
- Surgical management 159
- Summary 163
- References 163

18 Epidemiology and prognosis in spinal metastasis 165
Klaus Huch

- Introduction 165
- Results of our retrospective cohort study 166
- Discussion 167
- References 168

19 Spondylitis and spondylodiscitis 169
Rolf Sobottke and Peer Eysel

- Introduction 169
- Infection path 169
- Pathogen spectrum 170
- Epidemiology 171
- Predisposition 171
- Differential diagnoses 171
- Diagnostics 171
- Therapy 179
- Prognosis 184
- Conclusions for practise 185
- References 185

Non-fusion technology

20 Biomechanical characteristics of different non-fusion implants 191
Hans-Joachim Wilke

- Introduction 191
- Methods of the performed in-vitro tests 191
- Dynamic stabilization system (Dynesys) versus rigid fixators 192
- Interspinous implants (X-Stop, Coflex, Wallis, Diam) 193
- Total posterior-element replacement system (TOPS) 194
- Total disc prostheses 195
- Prosthetic disc nucleus (PDN) 196
- Tissue engineered collagen matrix nucleus replacement 196
- Summary 197
- Limitations and conclusion 198
- References 198

21 Interspinous devices – implants, indications and results 201
RENÉ SCHMIDT and BALKAN CAKIR

- Introduction 201
- Implants 201
- Mode of action 203
- Indications 204
- Results 205
- Conclusion 206
- References 206

22 Lumbar total disc replacement – implants, indications, and results ... 209
BALKAN CAKIR, RENÉ SCHMIDT, WOLFRAM KÄFER, and HEIKO REICHEL

- Background 209
- Postulated goals of TDR 209
- Implants and biomechanical concepts 209
- Inclusion and exclusion criteria for TDR 211
- Diagnostics 212
- Operative technique 212
- Clinical and radiological results 212
- Summary 213
- References 214

Authors

MARKUS ARAND
Department of Trauma
and Orthopaedic Surgery
Klinikum Ludwigsburg
Posilipostrasse 4
D-71640 Ludwigsburg
Germany

PETER BERNSTEIN
Department of Orthopaedics
University of Dresden "Carl Gustav Carus"
Fetscherstrasse 74
D-01307 Dresden
Germany

BALKAN CAKIR
Department of Orthopaedics
University of Ulm
Oberer Eselsberg 45
D-89081 Ulm
Germany

PEER EYSEL
Department of Orthopaedic Surgery
University of Cologne
Joseph-Stelzmann-Strasse 9
D-50924 Köln
Germany

FLORIAN GEBHARD
Center for Surgery
Department of Trauma, Hand-, Plastic-
and Reconstructive Surgery
University of Ulm
Steinhövelstrasse 9
D-89075 Ulm
Germany

KLAUS HUCH
Department of Orthopaedics
University of Ulm
Oberer Eselsberg 45
D-89081 Ulm
Germany

WOLFRAM KÄFER
Department of Orthopaedics
University of Ulm
Oberer Eselsberg 45
D-89081 Ulm
Germany

TUGRUL KOCAK
Department of Orthopaedics
University of Ulm
Oberer Eselsberg 45
D-89081 Ulm
Germany

ULRICH KUNZ
Department of Neurosurgery
Armed Forces Hospital
D-89070 Ulm
Germany

THOMAS MATTES
Department of Orthopaedics
University of Ulm
Oberer Eselsberg 45
D-89081 Ulm
Germany

UWE MAX MAUER
Department of Neurosurgery
Armed Forces Hospital
D-89070 Ulm
Germany

JÜRGEN NOTHWANG
Department of Traumatology
Klinik am Eichert
Eichertstrasse 3
D-73035 Göppingen
Germany

HEIKO REICHEL
Department of Orthopaedics
University of Ulm
Oberer Eselsberg 45
D-89081 Ulm
Germany

MICHAEL REITH
Spine Center
St. Josefs-Hospital
Beethovenstrasse 20
D-65189 Wiesbaden
Germany

MARCUS RICHTER
Spine Center
St. Josefs-Hospital
Beethovenstrasse 20
D-65189 Wiesbaden
Germany

RENÉ SCHMIDT
Department of Orthopaedic Surgery
and Traumatology
University Hospital Mannheim
Theodor-Kutzer-Ufer 1–3
D-68135 Mannheim
Germany

MARKUS SCHULTHEISS
Center for Surgery
Department of Trauma, Hand-, Plastic-
and Reconstructive Surgery
University of Ulm
Steinhövelstrasse 9
D-89075 Ulm
Germany

CHRIS SCHULZ
Department of Neurosurgery
Armed Forces Hospital
D-89070 Ulm
Germany

JENS SEIFERT
Department of Orthopaedics
University of Dresden "Carl Gustav Carus"
Fetscherstrasse 74
D-01307 Dresden
Germany

ROLF SOBOTTKE
Department of Orthopaedic Surgery
University of Cologne
Joseph-Stelzmann-Strasse 9
D-50924 Köln
Germany

BENJAMIN ULMAR
Department of Trauma Surgery
BG Trauma Center
University of Tübingen
Schnarrenbergstrasse 95
D-72076 Tübingen
Germany

CHRISTOPH ULRICH
Department of Traumatology
Klinik am Eichert
Eichertstrasse 3
D-73035 Göppingen
Germany

HANS-JOACHIM WILKE
Institute of Orthopaedic Research
and Biomechanics
University of Ulm
Helmholtzstrasse 14
D-89081 Ulm
Germany

Degenerative/rheumatic disorders and deformities

Posterior instrumentation of the cervical spine using the neon occipito-cervical system

MARCUS RICHTER and MICHAEL REITH

Introduction

The constant further refinement of the implant systems and the increasing acceptance of pedicle screws for the cervical and upper thoracic regions have led to marked improvement of posterior instrumentation [2, 3, 13]. As in the lumbar spine, the use of computer-navigation systems can significantly reduce the rate of faulty positioning of pedicle screws in the cervical region [12, 16, 17]. The markedly improved biomechanical properties, particularly using pedicle screws with a fixed-angle implant system [18], reduce the rate of implant failure, allow instrumentation of fewer segments, obviate the need for additional anterior instrumentation and thus also reduce morbidity.

Subaxial cervical instrumentation can be performed with lateral mass screws (technique of Magerl or An) or pedicle screws. Currently, subaxial instrumentation with lateral mass screws using Magerl's technique is regarded as the gold standard [6, 19]. For some years various authors have also been recommending cervical instrumentation (C2–C7) with pedicle screws and have reported improved biomechanical properties and clinical outcomes compared with lateral mass screws [1, 2, 4, 8, 9, 11]: the pullout force for pedicle screws was more than double [10] and the biomechanical stability of the instrumentation considerably greater [11]. Pedicle screws are therefore a viable alternative particularly where there is poor bone quality or greater strain on the implant, e.g. in instances of multi-segmental instabilities, unstable injuries of the cervico-thoracic junction, fractures in ankylosing spondylitis or insufficient anterior support [10]. In addition there are reports of implant loosening after instrumentation of the lateral mass which resulted in loss of correction and subsequent nonunion [5, 7]. Pedicle screws are the technique of choice for upper thoracic instrumentation. Alternatives such as transverse process screws or laminar and pedicle hooks have distinctly inferior biomechanical properties and should therefore only be used as an exception

Principles and objectives of the neon occipito-cervical system

The neon® implant system (Ulrich medical, Ulm, Germany) is a modular, angle-stable implant system, which improves biomechanical stability, reduces surgical risk and decreases operating time in comparison with other procedures like sublaminar cerclage and cortico-cancellous bone grafts [14].

This system allows for posterior instrumentation and fusion after closed or open reduction for management of instabilities or deformities. In case of stenosis of the spinal canal with symptomatic cord compression or irreducible deformities, additional decompression may be necessary. In patients with spinal metastases and a limited life expectancy, instrumentation alone without fusion may be sufficient.

Advantages

- Improved biomechanical stability compared with other implant systems due to:
  - High angular stability of the screw-rod connection.
  - Rod diameter 4.5 mm: The increase in the rod diameter to 4.5 mm instead of the 3.5 mm usually used in the cervical spine increases the bending strength of the rod by more than 100%.
  - Cannulated 4.0 mm pedicle screws for the cervical region.

- Cannulated 5.0 mm pedicle screws for the upper thoracic region.
  - 3.5 mm lateral mass screws.
- Simple and universal applicability due to:
  - Great angular variability of the screw-rod connection.
  - Simple instrumentation through different screw-rod connectors, polyaxial connectors and two different spacers.
  - Cannulation of the cervical/thoracic screws.
  - Possibility of connecting the instruments to a computer-navigation system.
  - Reduced need for rod bending due to a number of different screw-rod connectors, polyaxial connectors and two different spacers.
  - Instruments for percutaneous instrumentation with pedicle screws.
- Percutaneous insertion of the pedicle screws allows shorter surgical incision and reduces morbidity.
- Reliable achievement of stability and fusion with elimination of pain and functional impairment.
- Occipital fixation with screws or toggle.
- Atlas claw for instrumentation C1 and lower cervical vertebrae.

Disadvantage

- In the case of multilevel stabilization contouring of the rod and securement of the rod to the screws can be difficult.

Indications

- Traumatic instabilities: Cervical and cervicothoracic fractures in patients with ankylosing spondylitis (Bechterew's disease); unstable injuries of the cervico-thoracic junction; locked and anteriorly irreducible dislocations; multisegmental fractures and instabilities (>two segments); unstable nonunion of dens; unstable Jefferson fracture; atlanto-occipital dislocation; rupture of the transverse ligament; rupture of alar ligaments; unstable rotatory dislocation C1/C2 or recurrent rotatory dislocation C1/C2 as after closed reduction and immobilization in a halo.
- Instabilities due to neoplasia with/without cord compression: Metastases or primary tumors endangering stability or compressing the cord.
- Degenerative diseases: Multisegmental cervical spondylotic myelopathy (CSM).
- Spondylodiscitis.
- Rheumatoid instability including C1/C2 and atlanto-axial instabilities.
- Postoperative instabilities, e.g. after laminectomy.
- Posttraumatic and postinfectious kyphoses.
- Congenital atlanto-axial instabilities.
- Osteoarthritis of the C1/C2 joints (very rare).

Contraindications

- Infection at the operative site.
- Inability to undergo anaesthesia.

Patient information

- General operative risks such as infection, impaired wound healing, postoperative bleeding, thrombosis, embolism.
- Injury of spinal cord, nerve roots or vertebral artery.
- Implant failure: Loss of correction, implant loosening, implant breakage, implant displacement.
- In the case of poor screw purchase instrumentation of more segments may be necessary.
- Revision surgery because of pseudarthrosis, implant failure, infection or other complications.
- Postoperative restriction of cervical spine mobility depending on the type and length of the lesion and instrumentation.

Preoperative work-up

- Clinical assessment including neurological status.
- Imaging procedures: Plain radiographs in two planes; flexion-extension radiographs and, if necessary, lateral bending radiographs; computed tomography (CT) and/or magnetic resonance imaging (MRI).
- Preoperative planning based on CT and multiplanar reconstructions: Evaluation of the course of the vertebral artery as well as planning of the direction and length of the screws.
- If necessary, preoperative shaving.

- During anesthesia induction, i.v. antibiotic prophylaxis with third generation cephalosporin, repeated after four hours in the case of longer operating time.

Surgical instruments and implants

Neon implants for cervical and upper thoracic instrumentation

- **Neon 5.0 mm screw as upper thoracic pedicle screw**
  Self-tapping, cannulated, diameter 5.0 mm, color silver, lengths 30–50 mm (in 5 mm increments); the screw can be inserted over a 1.5 mm guide wire after predrilling with a 3.5 mm drill bit; at an angle of 15° to the screw axis, the screw head contains a threaded bore for insertion of the neon easy fit (Fig. 1.1 a).

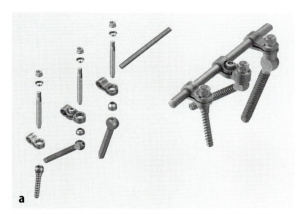

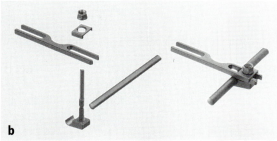

Fig. 1.1. a Neon implant components for cervical instrumentation (magnified drawing and complete instrumentation) (with permission of Urban & Vogel, Germany). **b** Neon cross-connector for cervical instrumentation (magnified drawing and complete instrumentation) (with permission of Urban & Vogel, Germany).

- **Neon 4.0 mm screw as cervical or upper thoracic pedicle screw**
  Self-tapping, cannulated, diameter 4.0 mm, color silver, lengths 22–50 mm (in 2 mm increments); the screw can be inserted over a 1.5 mm guide wire after drilling with a 3.5 mm drill bit; at an angle of 15° to the screw axis, the screw head contains a threaded bore for insertion of the neon easy fit (Fig. 1.1 a).
- **Neon 3.5 mm screw as cervical lateral mass screw**
  Self-tapping, non-cannulated, diameter 3.5 mm, color silver, lengths 10–20 mm (in 2 mm increments); the screw can be inserted after drilling with a 2.6 mm drill bit; at an angle of 45° to the screw axis, the screw head contains a threaded bore for insertion of the neon easy fit (Fig. 1.1 a).
- **Polyaxial neon connector for fixed-angle polyaxial rod/screw fitting**
  Three different lengths for easy instrumentation and to reduce the need to bend the rod in the frontal plane; color-coded: 15 mm (green), 17 mm (red) and 19 mm (blue, with additional locking screw to increase stability), consisting of connector, asymmetric washer and locking nut.
- **Cross connector**
  To increase primary stability in the case of multisegment instrumentation, severe instability or if particularly high demands are placed on the stability of the instrumentation; consists of locking clamp, washer, hex nut and neon cross connector (Fig. 1.1 b).
- **Atlas claw**
  Consisting of atlas hook and counterpart. Application: C1/C2 instrumentation in combination with transarticular screws C1/C2 to replace the three-point buttressing with bone graft and cerclage construct according to Gallie or Brooks.

Neon instruments

- **Tissue protector with adjustment for drilling depth**
  Consisting of handle, depth stop, locking nut and 3.5 mm adapter (for 5 mm screws) and adapters for a computer-assisted surgery (CAS) system.

Anaesthesia and positioning

- General endotracheal anaesthesia with muscle relaxation.
- At the start, supine position, prepping, and attachment of the Mayfield skull tongs approximately 2 cm above the external auditory meatus. Positioning on a head rest without rigid fixation of the head is also possible but is not recommended as the possibilities of reduction are limited in such a case.
- Turning into a prone position on a gel-filled mattress, support of thorax and pelvis with foam pillows, stabilization of both arms with adhesive tape, continuous arm traction via a pulley system with 2–3 kg weights (Fig. 1.2).
- Under image intensification, closed reduction if necessary. Preoperatively, the image intensifier should be positioned for optimal sagittal views for instrumentation.
- Prepping and draping with the image intensifier adjusted to the sagittal plane.

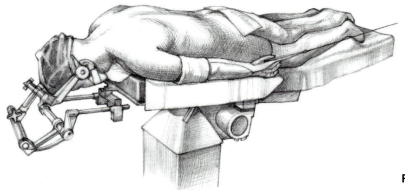

Fig. 1.2. Positioning of the patient (with permission of Urban & Vogel, Germany).

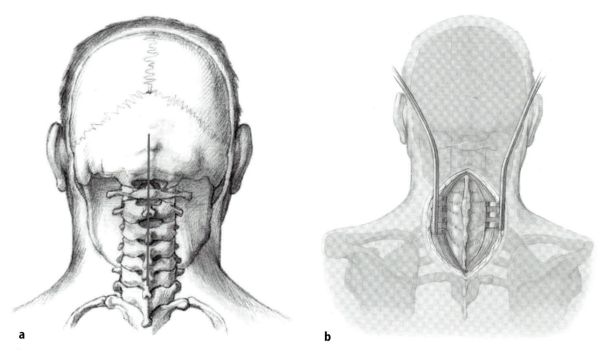

Fig. 1.3 a, b. Posterior approach to the cervical spine (with permission of Urban & Vogel, Germany).

Surgical technique

Surgical approach

After prepping, draping, and application of antibacterial, transparent adhesive film, a median skin incision is centered over the region to be instrumented (Fig. 1.3a). The fascia is divided with cautery knife or ultrasonic scalpel followed by subperiosteal exposure with an ultrasonic scalpel or Cobb elevator and unfolded compresses of the posterior aspects of the spinal segments to be instrumented (Fig. 1.3b).

At the end of the operation wound closing over a subfascial drain with single sutures, skin closure with strong single sutures 2-0.

Lateral mass screw placement using the technique described by Magerl
(Fig. 1.4)

On account of the low risk of faulty positioning of screws this technique is currently regarded as the gold standard for posterior instrumentation of the cervical spine from C3–C7 [9]. The entry point of the screw is 1–2 mm medial and cranial to the center of the lateral mass. The screw should be inserted with a lateral inclination of 20–30° and parallel to the space of the cranial intervertebral joint in the direction of the anterolateral margin of the upper articular process. This allows a maximum screw length with low risk of injury to neurovascular structures. Average screw length is 14–18 mm. The self-tapping 3.5 mm neon lateral mass screw is used as standard screw.

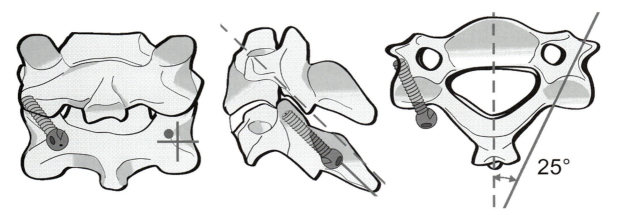

Fig. 1.4. Lateral mass screw placement using the technique described by Magerl (with permission of Urban & Vogel, Germany).

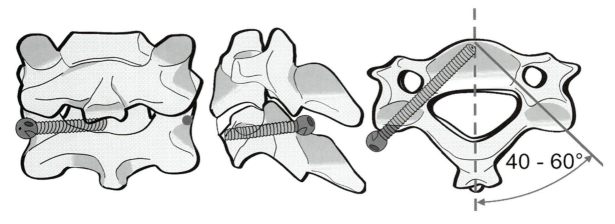

Fig. 1.5. Transpedicular screw placement C3–C7 (with permission of Urban & Vogel, Germany).

Transpedicular screw placement C3–C7
(Fig. 1.5)

Instrumentation with pedicle screws produces considerably greater primary stability compared with instrumentation with lateral mass screws. The pullout strength of pedicle screws is more than double than that of lateral mass screws. Average screw length is 26–34 mm. However, there is an increased risk of screw faulty positioning with the possibility of injury to the vertebral artery (above C7) or nerve structures. To determine the entry points of the pedicle screws, CT with multiplanar reconstructions of the pedicle of the vertebra to be instrumented should be performed preoperatively. With the help of the multiplanar reconstructions the entry point, angular orientation and length of the screw can be determined preoperatively. Pedicle screws should not be used if the pedicle width is <3.5 mm. Generally the screw entry point for C3 to C7 is very lateral and just below the caudal joint facet of the cranial vertebra. The convergence of the screws is 40–60° on average but can deviate considerably from this in individual cases. If the segment to be instrumented is short and the approach incision small, percutaneous screw insertion can be useful in order to achieve the necessary convergence. The self-tapping, cannulated 4.0 mm neon pedicle screw is used as standard screw.

Transpedicular upper thoracic screw placement (Fig. 1.6)

In the upper thoracic spine the entry point of the screw is generally at the upper margin of the transverse process at the lowest point of the concavity. In most cases the convergence is 0–30°. The screw orientation is slightly downwards in an anterior direction relative to the upper endplate of the vertebra. Although there is a lesser risk of incorrect screw positioning in the thoracic spine than in the cervical spine, preoperative CT with multiplanar reconstructions of the pedicles of the vertebrae to be instrumented is recommended in order to determine the entry points of the pedicle screws. The pedicle width in the upper thoracic spine is considerably greater than in the middle thoracic spine, T1 having a diameter of 8.1 mm, for example [20]. The self-tapping, cannulated 5.0 mm neon screw is used as standard screw. In the case of small pedicle dimensions the self-tapping, cannulated 4.0 mm neon screw may also be used.

Posterior cervical instrumentation

Using the image intensifier, identification of the entry point for the lateral mass screw, and decortication with an awl. Using the tissue protector with depth stop and exchangeable attachments the hole is started with a 2.6 mm drill bit. For lateral mass screws we recommend setting an initial drilling depth of 14 mm which can then be increased stepwise as required. De-

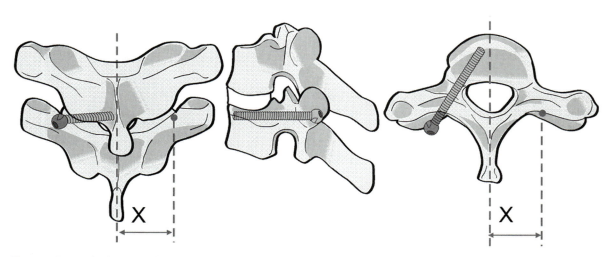

Fig. 1.6. Transpedicular upper thoracic screw placement (with permission of Urban & Vogel, Germany).

termination of screw length with a depth gauge and insertion of a 3.5 mm neon screw of appropriate length with the locking screwdriver. The screw is placed in the screwdriver in such a way that the threaded bore for the easy fit is not visible and then secured with the knurled thumb screw. The blunt guide wire can be used for the instrumentation but in the case of bicortical drilling care should be taken not to advance the wire too far anteriorly. After removal of the locking screwdriver the non-locking screwdriver can be used to align the screw head correctly, i.e. with the threaded bore facing as much as possible in a posterior direction. After all screws have been inserted the rod length and contour are determined using the neon phantom rod. The neon rod bender should be used to contour the rod to achieve the desired sagittal profile (in the cervical spine normally a lordosis). Contouring in the frontal plane is usually not necessary. If in case of multisegmental instrumentation the screws are not in line, which can be the case particularly when a combination of different screw techniques is used (e.g. pedicle screws and lateral mass screws), this can be compensated by using connectors of different lengths. Then the easy fits are inserted making sure they point as far as possible posteriorly. Next the contoured rod is mounted on the easy fits with the appropriate connectors. Additional differences in height between the screws and the rod can be compensated with the spacers. If spacers are to be used these can be placed on the respective easy fits before attaching the connectors. Now the self-aligning asymmetric washers are placed over the easy fits and then the hex nuts screwed on, thus achieving a fixed-angle screw-rod connection. When tightening the hex nuts it is important to hold the rod with the rod holder to prevent screw pullout. The use of the polyaxial connectors facilitates instrumentation since the considerably larger hole for the easy fit allows an angle of 16° between screw and rod in any direction. When all easy fit hex nuts have been tightened, the protruding parts of the easy fit must be cut off. This is done with the shear-off instrument and the shear-off hex nut. The shear-off hex nut is screwed onto the easy fit with the rounded side facing the hex nut of the easy fit using the T-handle of the shear-off instrument. Then the shear-off counterpart is mounted on the hex nut of the easy fit. The T-handled shear-off instrument is pushed through the counterpart onto the shear-off nut. By stabilizing the counterpart and turning the T-handle shear-off instrument the easy fit is cut off flush with the easy fit hex nut. Finally all easy fit hex nuts should be checked again and tightened if necessary. Easy fit hex nuts can become loose when the easy fit is trimmed if the counterpart is not sufficienctly stabilized.

If lateral mass screws only are used, the rod can be placed either laterally or medially. However, if pedicle screws are used, the rod should be placed medial to the screws on account of the very lateral position of the screw entry points. If pedicle screws are used, due to the necessary convergence of 40–60° between C3 and C6, the drilling of the pedicle and insertion of the screws should be performed percutaneously via an additional incision using the short trocar system. In this case, first the screw entry point is identified via the medial posterior incision and the cortex opened with an awl or burr. Then an additional incision 1 cm in length is made and the trocar system inserted percutaneously. Figure 1.7 shows the position of percutaneously inserted trocar sleeves. If a computer-navigation system is not being used, the pedicle angle of all pedicles to be instrumented should be measured preoperatively by CT with reconstructions in the pedicle axis. Intraoperatively, it is advisable to check the correct angle of the tissue protector with a goniometer. Through the trocar system an initial hole is then drilled with the 2.6 mm drill and the drill hole probed to detect any pedicle perforation. The depth stop of the tissue protector

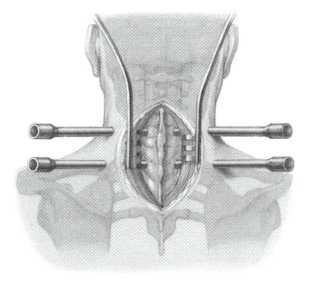

Fig. 1.7. Positioning of percutaneously inserted trocar sleeves (with permission of Urban & Vogel, Germany).

should be set to the screw length determined during preoperative planning. If no planning was performed, a setting of 26 mm is recommended. Then the blunt guide wire is inserted through the trocar system and the screw length read off the depth stop of the tissue protector with trocar system with the help of the markings on the guide wire. To determine the screw length the depth stop is set so that the marking on the blunt guide wire is flush with the depth stop. Then the screw length can be read off the adjustment scale. If a computer-navigation system is used, preoperative determination of the pedicle angle is not necessary as the angle can be checked intraoperatively using the computer-navigation system [15]. The trocar is removed from the outer sleeve and the cannulated screw of appropriate length inserted over the guide wire with the cannulated non-locking screwdriver. In case of open instrumentation the cortex is penetrated with the tissue protector with the sharp 2.6 mm drill bit, the pedicle is probed, the blunt guide wire inserted, the screw length determined with the measuring sleeve and the markings on the guide wire, the cannulated screw inserted over the guide wire with the cannulated non-locking screwdriver. For pedicle instrumentation the use of the guide wire is strongly recommended to avoid lateral perforation of the pedicle by the screw. After placement of the screws, insertion of the easy fit and instrumentation with appropriate polyaxial connectors and longitudinal rods is required.

Posterior cervico-thoracic instrumentation

For placement of C6 pedicle screws, percutaneous drilling of the pedicle with the trocar system as described above. For C7 and the upper thoracic region an open technique is recommended on account of the lesser convergence of the screws. For this, first identification of the respective pedicle entry points, decortication with an awl and drilling of the pedicle through the tissue protector with 2.6 mm adapter and 2.6 mm drill bit in C7 and with 3.5 mm adapter and 3.5 mm drill bit in the upper thoracic region is required. After drilling the initial hole, probing of the pedicle and determination of the screw length using the tissue protector the blunt guide wires are inserted and the screws placed over the guide wires. The guide wires demonstrate the different degrees of convergence in C6, C7 and the upper thoracic vertebrae. 4.0 mm screws are used for the cervical vertebrae and 5.0 mm screws for the thoracic vertebrae. The reduction of the angle between the screw axis and the easy fit bore to 15° in the case of the 5 mm screws permits a practically horizontal position of the connectors corresponding to the lesser degree of convergence of the upper thoracic pedicles. Further instrumentation with connectors and rods is performed as described above. To increase the primary stability use of a cross-link system is recommended at the cervico-thoracic junction. For this a locking clamp is hooked under the rod on each side, from medial or lateral depending on the anatomy, and a transverse bar of appropriate length is selected. It may be necessary to shorten the transverse bar with a side cutter. The cross connector is mounted from posterior and secured with one washer and easy fit hex nut on each side using the socket wrench. The extension pins of the locking clamp are broken off at the pre-determined breaking point.

Transarticular C1/C2 screw positioning according to Magerl (Fig. 1.8)

Based on the preoperative CT a decision must be taken whether a safe transarticular screw positioning is possible without injury to the vertebral artery. This is not possible in 15–20% of patients due to a variation in the course of the vertebral artery [18, 21]. The entry point for the transarticular C1/C2 screw insertion lies in a straight sagittal line in the centre of the isthmus (connection between the cranial and caudal joint facet) at the inferior border of the caudal facet of C2, 2 mm cranial and lateral to the medial border. In case of variations in the course of the vertebral artery a shorter isthmus screw not reaching the vertebral artery can be used while maintaining the described technique and direction of the screw.

Placement of transpedicular screw C2 (Fig. 1.9)

The direction of the transpedicular screw in C2 differs slightly from that of C3 to C7 as the convergence is markedly less. This convergence amounts to 25° and the screw should rise by 10° in relation to the endplate C2. Contrary to

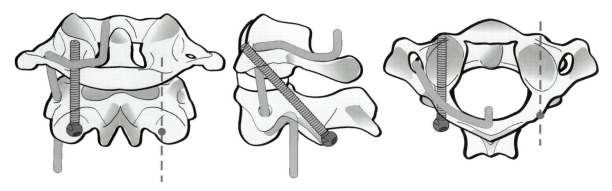

Fig. 1.8. Transarticular C1/C2 screw positioning according to Magerl (with permission of Urban & Vogel, Germany).

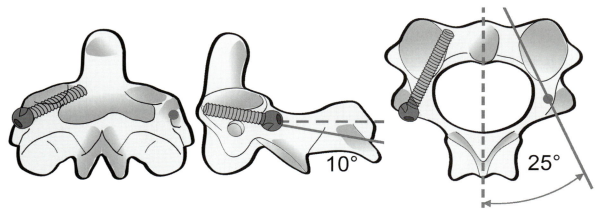

Fig. 1.9. Placement of transpedicular screw C2 (with permission of Urban & Vogel, Germany).

C3 to C7 the width of the pedicle C2 is 8 mm (5 mm in C3 to C7). The medial border of the pedicle can easily be determined with a dissector.

Massa lateralis screw C1 (Fig. 1.10)

The direction of the screw in the sagittal plane rises slightly in relation to the articular space C1/C2 and at a right angle in the frontal plane. The entry point lies distal to the posterior arch of the atlas at the transition to the lateral mass of C1. The nerve root of C2, which runs posterior to the point of insertion, is retracted caudally with a dissector before drilling and insertion of screw.

Atlanto-axial instrumentation with an atlas claw

For instrumentation extending over several levels screws and wires can be inserted through one incision. In such a case, the guide wire either is inserted with the help of a 1.6 mm tissue protector or with the wire guide. If the latter is used, a shorter incision is sufficient as it allows to bend the wire which is impossible with a rigid tissue protector (Fig. 1.11 a). The length of the screw is determined with the measurement sleeve (Fig. 1.11 b). Once the wires are in place, screws of appropriate length are inserted with the flexible or rigid screw driver (Fig. 1.11 c). Independent of the technique of screw insertion the instrumentation is performed as follows: The easy fits are inserted into the threaded bore of the screw heads. Attachment of the appropriately shortened contoured atlas claws with a 14 mm long connector. From cranial the hook is slipped over the posterior part of the arch of the atlas 1.5 mm lateral to the mid line and at a right angle to the arch. The connector is then secured with a hex nut (Fig. 1.11 d). The grub screw of the counterpart is then attached into the screw driver hex 2.5 mm. Positioning of the counterpart of the

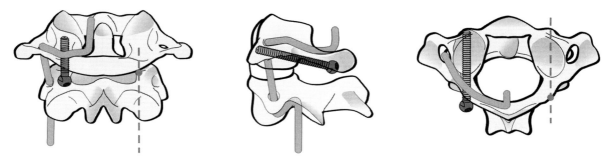

Fig. 1.10. Massa lateralis screw C1 (with permission of Urban & Vogel, Germany).

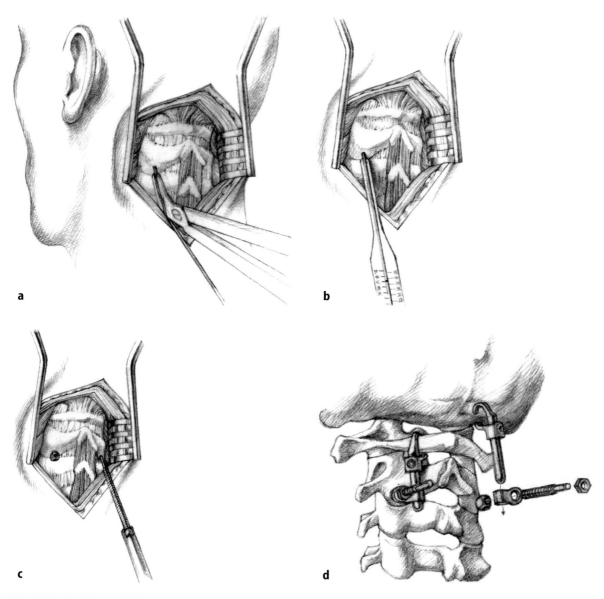

Fig. 1.11 a–d. Atlanto-axial instrumentation with atlas claw (with permission of Urban & Vogel, Germany).

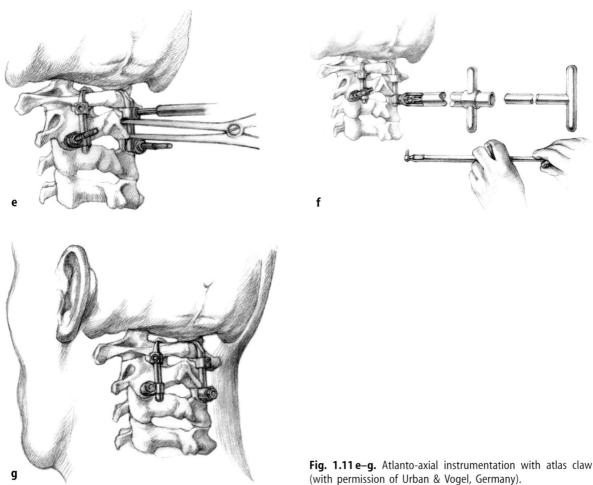

Fig. 1.11 e–g. Atlanto-axial instrumentation with atlas claw (with permission of Urban & Vogel, Germany).

atlas claw parallel to the hook of the rod. With the help of the distraction forceps that is positioned between the connector and counterpart, the counterpart is pushed under the caudal end of the arch of the atlas. Tightening of the grub screw of the counterpart (Fig. 1.11 e).

Identical procedure on the opposite site. The protruding parts of the easy fit are cut with the shear off instrument and the shear off hex nut. The shear off hex nut with its rounded part is directed to the nut of the easy fit and screwed on using the T-handle shear off instrument. The shear off counterpart is mounted on the easy fit, the T-handle shear off instrument is pushed through the T-handle on the shear off hex nut. Through stabilization of the shear off counterpart and turning of the T-handle the easy fit is cut with the shear off hex nut (Fig. 1.11 f). Finally, the tightness of all easy fit hex nuts should be checked and tightened if necessary. These nuts could loosen during cutting of the easy fits if the shear off counterpart is not sufficiently stabilized. The posterior instrumentation C1/C2 with the atlas claw is now complete (Fig. 1.11 g). If a posterior fusion is warranted, the posterior bony structures C1/C2 are freshened with a burr before instrumentation with the atlas claw but after insertion of the transarticular screws. Following instrumentation autologous cancellous bone from the posterior iliac crest can be apposed. Bone substitutes may be applied. A cortico-cancellous bone graft is not necessary.

Postoperative management

- Radiographic evaluation in two planes immediately after surgery in the operating room.
- Bedrest until the first postoperative day.
- Drain removal and first dressing change on 2nd postoperative day.
- Stitches removed on 10th to 14th postoperative day.
- Mobilization with a soft collar for four weeks postoperatively beginning on the first postoperative day.
- In the case of poor bone quality (e.g. rheumatoid patients) a rigid collar for six weeks may be necessary.
- Clinical and radiographic follow-up three, six, twelve, and 24 months postoperatively.

Errors, hazards, and complications

Iatrogenic injury to nerve roots, spinal cord or vertebral artery through incorrect screw placement:

- Lateral mass screws: The chief risk is damage to the dorsal branch of the respective posterior root (6–8%). Injury to the vertebral artery is also possible.
- Cervical pedicle screws: The main risk is injury to the vertebral artery through lateral perforation of the pedicle. The lateral cortex of the pedicle is considerably thinner than the medial cortex and the necessary convergence of the screws of between 40 and 60° is difficult to achieve on account of the soft tissues. The use of cannulated screws significantly reduces this risk. In small incisions and very muscular patients, the necessary convergence can be achieved more easily by means of percutaneous screw insertion using a trocar system. If injury to the vertebral artery occurs, the vertebral artery should be exposed and ligated or coagulated if insertion of the screw does not produce adequate hemostasis. If injury to the nerve root or the dura occurs during pedicle drilling or screw insertion, the dura leak should first be exposed and closed. If correct screw positioning is no longer possible, either lateral mass screws should be used (if possible) or the stabilization extended by one segment. Injury to the cervical cord caused by pedicle screws is unlikely and only possible if the entry point of the screw is significantly too medial.
- Upper thoracic pedicle screws: The main risk is injury to the dura through medial perforation of the pedicle. A further risk is the lateral perforation of the pedicle and the vertebral body if there is insufficient convergence resulting in a reduced holding power. The use of cannulated screws reduces this risk. In case of lateral perforation, an attempt should be made to achieve greater convergence of the drill holes in the pedicle using the same entry point. For the procedure in the case of injury to the nerve roots or spinal cord, see above. In contrast to cervical pedicle screws, injury to the dura or the spinal cord is possible in the case of upper thoracic pedicle screws even with a correct entry point if the convergence is too great.

Impaired wound healing: Early revision with debridement and, if necessary, temporary use of vacuum seal to avoid development of a deep infection.

Infection of the implant bed: Early revision with debridement, particularly of the implant bed. Removal of the implant is not usually necessary. Insertion of Septopal chains (antibiotic beads) is recommended. Intravenous antibiotics should be initiated perioperatively and optimized according to the microbiological results.

References

1. Abumi K, Itoh H, Taneichi H, Kaneda K (1994) Transpedicular screw fixation for traumatic lesions of the middle and lower cervical spine: description of the techniques and preliminary report. J Spinal Disord 7:19–28
2. Abumi K, Kaneda K, Shono Y, Fujiya M (1999) One-stage posterior decompression and reconstruction of the cervical spine by using pedicle screw fixation systems. J Neurosurg 90(Suppl): 19–26
3. Abumi K, Shono Y, Taneichi H, Ito M, Kaneda K (1999) Correction of cervical kyphosis using pedicle screw fixation systems. Spine 24:2389–2396
4. Abumi K, Takada T, Shono Y, Kaneda K, Fujiya M (1999) Posterior occipitocervical reconstruction using cervical pedicle screws and plate-rod systems. Spine 24:1425–1434

5. Fehlings MG, Errico T, Cooper P, Benjamin V, DiBartolo T (1993) Occipitocervical fusion with a five-millimeter malleable rod and segmental fixation. Neurosurgery 32:198–207
6. Heller JG, Estes BT, Zaouali M, Diop A (1996) Biomechanical study of screws in the lateral masses: variables affecting pull-out resistance. J Bone Joint Surg Am 78:1315–1321
7. Heller JG, Silcox DH 3rd, Sutterlin CE 3rd (1995) Complications of posterior cervical plating. Spine 20:2442–2448
8. Jeanneret B, Gebhard JS, Magerl F (1994) Transpedicular screw fixation of articular mass fracture-separation: results of an anatomical study and operative technique. J Spinal Disord 7:222–229
9. Jeanneret B, Schären S (2004) Dorsale Stabilisierung der Halswirbelsäule und der oberen Brustwirbelsäule mit CerviFix. Operat Orthop Traumatol 16:89–116
10. Jones EL, Heller JG, Silcox DH, Hutton WC (1997) Cervical pedicle screws versus lateral mass screws. Anatomic feasibility and biomechanical comparison. Spine 22:977–982
11. Kotani Y, Cunningham BW, Abumi K, McAfee PC (1994) Biomechanical analysis of cervical stabilization systems. An assessment of transpedicular screw fixation in the cervical spine. Spine 19:2529–2539
12. Ludwig SC, Kowalski JM, Edwards CC 2nd, Heller JG (2000) Cervical pedicle screws: comparative accuracy of two insertion techniques. Spine 25:2675–2681
13. Ludwig SC, Kramer DL, Vaccaro AR, Albert TJ (1999) Transpedicle screw fixation of the cervical spine. Clin Orthop 359:77–88
14. Richter M (2003) Dorsale Instrumentierung der Halswirbelsäule mit dem „neon occipito-cervical system". Teil 1: Atlantoaxiale Instrumentierung. Operat Orthop Traumatol 15:70–89
15. Richter M, Amiot LP, Neller S, Kluger P, Puhl W (2000) Computer Assisted Surgery in posterior instrumentation of the cervical spine – An in-vitro feasibility study. Eur Spine J 9 (Suppl):65–70
16. Richter M, Amiot LP, Puhl W (2002) Computernavigation bei der dorsalen Instrumentierung der HWS – Eine in-vitro Studie. Orthopäde 31:372–377
17. Richter M, Mattes T, Cakir B (2004) Computer assisted posterior instrumentation of the cervical and cervico-thoracic spine. Eur Spine J 13:50–59
18. Schmidt R, Wilke HJ, Claes L, Puhl W, Richter M (2003) Pedicle screws enhance primary stability in multilevel cervical corporectomies: Biomechanical in-vitro comparison of different implants including angle- and non-angle stable instrumentations. Spine 28:1821–1828
19. Seybold EA, Baker JA, Criscitiello AA, Ordway NR, Park CK, Connolly PJ (1999) Characteristics of unicortical and bicortical lateral mass screws in the cervical spine. Spine 24:2397–2403
20. Ugur HC, Attar A, Uz A, Tekdemir I, Egemen N, Genc Y (2001) Thoracic pedicle: surgical anatomic evaluation and relations. J Spinal Disord 14:39–45
21. Yonenobu K, Fuji T, Ono K, Okada K, Yamamoto T, Harada N (1985) Choice of surgical treatment for multisegmental cervical spondylotic myelopathy. Spine 10:710–716

2 Treatment principles in rheumatoid instability of the cervical spine

TUGRUL KOCAK and KLAUS HUCH

Introduction

Rheumatoid arthritis is a chronic, mostly progressive inflammatory general disease of mesenchymal tissue, manifesting mainly as synovialitis. The prevalence of rheumatoid arthritis is between 0.5 and 1%. Women are three times more often involved as men. Revealing a familiar accumulation of the disease and a proven association to HLA-antigens (HLA-DR4) in 50% to 80% of the patients, a genetic influence is very likely.

General symptoms of rheumatoid arthritis are arthralgia, morning stiffness, inappetence, fatigue, myalgia, subfebrile temperature and disposition for depression. Symmetric arthritis of peripheral joints, e.g. the metacarpophalangeal joints and the proximal interphalangeal joints, is often correlated with joint swelling, associated with warmth and pain during palpation and motion. Further extraarticular manifestations are not rare. Important pathologic appearances are tendovaginitis (especially in hand region), bursitis, pleuritis, pericarditis, ceratoconjunctivitis, hepatitis, anaemia, polyneuropathy, and vasculitis. Critical complications are amyloidosis (approximately 5% of the cases), gastrointestinal ulceration and cervical myelopathy. In an advanced phase the rheumatoid factor is detectable in 80% of the patients. Furthermore, an increase of the leukocyte count, the erythrocyte sedimentation rate and the acute phase proteins (CRP) can be observed. Radiological findings show at first osteoporosis nearby the joints, and in the further progress joint space narrowing, erosions, subluxations and more rarely ankylosis [36]. Potential differential diagnosis are ancylosing spondylitis (Bechterew's disease), infection, collagenose, gout, and arthritis of different reasons (septic, reactive, associated with psoriasis, and enterohepatic).

According to the American Rheumatism Association (ARA-criteria, revised 1987 [1]) four out of the seven following criteria must be present for the diagnosis of rheumatoid arthritis: Morning stiffness (of at least one hour duration for more than six weeks), arthritis of three or more joint regions and arthritis of hand or finger joints (for more than six weeks), symmetrical arthritis (for more than six weeks), rheumatoid nodules, positive rheumatoid factor, and typical radiological changes in the hand (erosions and/or osteoporosis nearby the joints).

Morphologic variations of rheumatic instability

In rheumatoid arthritis the cervical spine is involved in approximately 20% of the patients [7]. For hands and feet, radiological changes are described in over 50% of patients 20 years after the onset of the disease [24]. The cervical spine can be involved in the early phase of the disease; in addition, the progression correlates well with the rheumatoid activity in the upper and lower extremities [26]. As first sign of atlantoaxial involvement there is a typical pattern of instability, caused by an inflammatory synovial proliferation and increasing destruction of ligamentous (transverse, apical and alar ligaments), articular and bony structures [28]. The atlantoaxial subluxation is the most frequent manifestation of rheumatoid arthritis in the cervical spine. If the transverse ligament is solely involved, a subluxation of 3 to 4 mm may result. A greater anterior atlanto-axial subluxation or posterior atlanto-axial subluxation suggests a destruction of the apical and the alar ligaments or an erosion of the dens [26]. Frequently spontaneous ankylosis in a mildly subluxated position [11] or severe C1/C2 subluxation, which might be fixed in a kyphotic mal-position, can be seen [13].

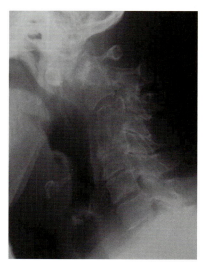

Fig. 2.1. Lateral X-ray of a high-grade instability C0–C3 and spontaneous fusion C3/C4.

The development of inflammatory soft tissue, the so called pannus, which is sometimes noted as a peridental pseudotumour, can cause an atlanto-axial instability and is very often associated with other rheumatic changes of the cervical spine [38]. As a result of chronic C1/C2 instability or massive pannus tissue a compression of the spinal cord and cervical nerve roots may occur, leading to severe myelopathy, which can cause sudden death. The progressive course of the disease frequently leads to a destruction of the lateral mass of the atlas and a consecutive reduction of the distance from the axis to the foramen magnum. This migration of the dens in relation to the atlas and the foramen magnum results in vertical instability, which might cause the radiological impression of a decrease of atlanto-axial instability and a reduction of inflammatory pannus tissue [2]. Destructive changes also can be seen at the level of C2 and the occipital condyles [2]. The incidence of vertical instability is thought to be 4% to 35% in patients with rheumatoid arthritis [22]. Lateral atlanto-axial subluxation represents a sub-group and refers to changes in the facet joints C1/C2.

After the phase of vertical instability subaxial involvement of the facet joints and the uncovertebral joints may occur if the disease progresses.

Due to an increase in laxicity of ligamentous structures, subaxial segmental instability (anterolisthesis or retrolisthesis) may occur in 7% to 29% of the patients [22, 34]. As a result of the progressive dysfunction of the subaxial segments the destruction of the discs and endplates is supported. In advanced stages of the disease an ankylosis of the cervical spine in flexion can result (Fig. 2.1).

Clinical picture

The typical clinical sign of involvement of the cervical spine in rheumatoid arthritis is neck pain, which is caused by instability, inflammation, joint arrosion, and affection of the major occipital nerve. The pain can be located cervical, occipito-cervical, temporal or in the shoulder region (C5/C6) and is frequently increased by movements of the head. Palpation of the spinous processes during passive functional testing of the cervical spine occasionally may detect atlanto-axial subluxation. The range of motion of the cervical spine usually is restricted in all directions. Asymmetrical destruction of the lateral atlanto-axial joints may lead to a mal-positioning of the head and the spine itself. The physiological lordosis of the cervical spine also can be altered to a pathological kyphosis, as well as spinal processes can become prominent due to atlanto-axial instability. Further potential clinical signs are dysphagia, speech disorder, sleep apnoea, and double imaging. Sometimes the Lhermitte-sign can be provoked, which is characterized by severe pain during passive inclination of the cervical spine. The interval between the evidence of an atlanto-axial instability and the development of neurological symptoms can vary greatly [24].

If neurological deficits are present, a remission with conservative therapy is very unlikely [37]. Monsey observed a worsening of neurological deficits in 15% to 35% of patients with rheumatoid arthritis [22]. With further progression of the disease typical signs of myelopathy can occur, such as increased reflexes, gait disturbance, raised muscle tonus, disorder of motor function or sphincter function, and dysaesthesia of upper and lower extremities. These signs of myelopathy correlate well with the width of the spinal canal. Critical values are a diameter less than 13 mm at the occipito-cervical region and a diameter less than 12 mm at the subaxial cervical spine [42]. Other symptoms of myelopathy are the scapulo-humeral reflex (cranialization of the scapula and humeral abduction after punch on the acromion or spina scapulae) according to Shimizu and co-workers [35] and the atrophy of hand muscles [27]. The diagnose of onset of myelopathy can be delayed or even missed, because clinical symptoms of myelopathy like gait disturbance or disorder of motor function are likely to be interpreted incorrectly, if peripheral joints are severely involved or if coincidental symptoms occur (e.g. the carpal-tunnel syndrome, polyneuropathy or side effects of drug therapy). Therefore neurophysiological examination (motor and sensory evoked potentials) is clearly indicated in addition to the clinical examination and the radiological work-up. In addition, vascular pathologies (leading to vertigo or syncope) apart from mechanical factors need to be considered and excluded [42]. Once a myelopathy is established, a quick worsening of the neurological situation is imminent [37].

Imaging

The first unspecific signs of an inflammatory reaction like widening of joint space, blurred joint areas, and thickness of the soft tissue shadow can be detected in the X-rays of the cervical spine in the occipito-cervical joints, the facet joints and the uncovertebral joints. With progression of the disease the intervertebral spaces become narrower and erosions of the vertebral endplates develop. Pathognomonic for the underlying condition are osteolytic changes of the dens axis and the spinal processes [4]. X-rays of the cervical spine in antero-posterior and lateral projection and a transoral view of the dens are required as the initial step in the radiological work-up. Functional X-rays of the cervical spine (in maximal flexion and extension) serve to exclude instability. With conventional lateral X-rays only, atlanto-axial instability may be missed in 50% of the cases [10].

The intervals between radiological controls are determined individually depending on the clinical course of the disease. If the patient responds well to a specific drug therapy, intervals of about six months appear to be sufficient [15]. The anterior and posterior atlanto-dental distances as measures for instability can be assessed in flexion, whereas the reduction of the dislocation is apparent in extension. If there is an anterior atlanto-dental distance greater than 5 mm (normal distance less than 3 mm in men and less than 2.5 mm in women), a relevant translational instability needs to be assumed [10]. The McGregor line, which runs from the dorsal cranial hard palate to the deepest point of the occipital squama, is helpful to detect a basilar impression. If the tip of the dens crosses this line more than 5 mm, this is considered pathological [4]. In advanced stages of disease with difficult identification of the tip of the dens in lateral X-rays, the sign of Redlund-Johnell and Pettersson may be a diagnostical alternative [2]. If the distance between the middle of the endplate of C2 and the McGregor line measures less than 34 mm in men and less than 29 mm in women, a vertical instability with dislocation can be assumed [32]. Subaxial instability is defined as mal-alignment of cervical vertebral bodies of more than 3.5 mm.

Magnetic resonance imaging (MRI) allows the visualization of spinal cord compression by pannus tissue. Functional MRI performed in flexion may detect a compression of the spinal cord due to peridental pannus [17]. In flexion a diameter of the spinal canal of less than 6 mm is indicative for a surgical intervention [5].

Computed tomography (CT) with multiplanar reconstruction also allows the assessment of pathologically altered structures (e.g. the tip of the dens). Chung and co-workers found out that the pedicles of the axis of patients with rheumatic diseases are smaller compared to those of healthy persons [3]. Therefore a CT scan of the atlanto-axial segment is recommended in case of schedule of a surgical procedure.

To identify painful segments diagnostic infiltration of the cervical facet joints may be useful.

Non-surgical therapy of the rheumatoid cervical spine

A concise patient education about this disease and its potential progress as well as about different treatment principles is of crucial importance. Physiotherapy, occupational therapy, physical therapy, cervical collars and drug therapy (non-steroidal anti-inflammatory drugs and disease-modifying drugs) are well-established treatment options, leading to a reduction of pain and inflammation and a preservation of mobility. However, a sufficient treatment of apparent atlanto-axial instability is not possible with conservative therapy. In addition, physiotherapy bears the risk of neurological deterioration in patients with cervical instability.

The choice of drug therapy depends on several factors such as drug half-life, dose range and tolerability.

One option is the use of cyclo-oxygenase-II inhibitors (e.g. Meloxicam), which belong to the NSAIDs and which are believed to be associated with a reduced gastrointestinal toxicity compared to salicylates (e.g. Aspirin).

In general, a basic medication should be chosen to reduce the inflammatory process [25]. Methotrexate (MTX) is sufficient to decrease the inflammatory activity of rheumatoid arthritis and allows long-term treatment. An oral pyrimidine inhibitor (Leflunomide) also can be used. Corticosteroids at low doses are very effective for pain reduction [39]. Toxicities of corticosteroids include hypertension, diabetes and cataracts. Tumor necrosis factor (TNF) inhibitors (Infliximab, Etanercept, Adalimumab) are alternatives, which can inhibit the inflammatory effects of TNF. However, blocking TNF increases the risk for serious infection including reactivation of tuberculosis [12]. It is well documented that the combination of Infliximab and Methotrexate is more effective than Methotrexate alone as well as IL-1 receptor antagonists (Anakinra) have also been shown to be effective in combination with Methotrexate. Combined treatment (Sulfasalazine, Methotrexate, Hydroxychloroquine, Prednisolone) generally appears to be more effective than a mono-therapy with Prednisolone in preventing cervical subluxation [14].

For further reduction of pain image-guided injections of the cervical facet joints can be applied. A cervical collar can be used to avoid cervical flexion and to reduce pain. In addition, the collar may offer some psychological support.

Surgical treatment

Instability, neurological deficits and therapy resistant pain with cervical myelopathy are indications for surgical interventions at the occipito-cervical and cervical spine [13]. The Ranawat classification can be used for the assessment of neurological deficits (Table 2.1) [29]. Patients with Ranawat II and IIIA stages are thought to benefit most from surgical interventions [21].

Advanced drug therapy often can stop the ongoing process of bony destruction, which is triggered by inflammation. However, it can't heal apparent instability. Under these circumstances it is important to consider prophylactic stabilization of cervical segments with imminent instability. In early stages of disease surgical interventions with a relatively little morbidity can be performed [7]. Therefore, risky interventions like transoral decompression or corporectomy with extended dorsal stabilization may be become unnecessary. If prophylactic surgery is planned, choosing the optimal time for the surgical treatment is important. The pain-free patient with cervical instability is often less motivated for surgery because he or she fears a limitation of head motion. Therefore, the indication for a surgical treatment has to be individually discussed with the patient. The experience of the surgeon and the stage of the disease are important for decision-making. The risks of disease progression as well as the risks of surgery have to be explained in detail. Once a cervical myelopathy is clinically apparent, the chance for recovery is significantly decreased [37]. Some authors see the indication for surgery, if electrophysiological investigations reveal pathological somato-sensory evoked potentials (SEP) and motoric evoked potentials (MEP), which are indicative for myelopathy, in combination with an increasing instability, even in the absence of clinical symptoms [32].

If the patient decides against surgery, close follow-up including a neurological, electrophysiological, and radiological assessment in inter-

Table 2.1. Ranawat classification for judging neurological deficits [29].

I.	No neurological deficit.
II.	Subjective weakness referring to hyperreflexia and dysaesthesia.
III A.	Objective weakness referring to pyramidal signs, able to walk.
III B.	Objective weakness referring to pyramidal signs, not able to walk.

vals of six to twelve months is advisable. The strategy of treatment also has to consider the general medical condition of the patient. Functional aspects also may decide about the sequence of surgical procedures. A correction of a foot deformity might facilitate ambulation before total knee arthroplasty in case of symptomatic knee joint arthritis. After multisegmental fusion of the cervical spine anaesthesiologists may have problems to intubate the patient. However, a highly unstable cervical spine should be fixed sufficiently before multiple other surgeries are conducted in order to avoid traumatic myelopathy by repetitive myelon compression during intubation.

In this context cases of death are described during perioperative manipulation of the cervical spine [23]. Laryngoscopical examinations should be performed carefully, particularly in patients with pain during extension of the cervical spine [18]. In case of posterior procedures, the head of the patient is regularly fixed with a clamp in a prone position as well as surgery should be performed with use of two image intensifiers.

Occipito-cervical fusion

In vertical instability and advanced destruction of the C0/C1 joints stabilization of C0/C1 or C0–C2 is indicated. Even in additional subaxial and atlanto-axial instability the occiput should be included in the fusion site. In patients with clinically apparent myelopathy the risk of postoperative complications is significantly increased.

At the occiput (highest bone stock in the mid-line) the fixation is performed with screws or hooks, whereas cervical screws are fixed transarticularly (facet joints), transpedicularly or in the lateral mass. If pedicle screws are used, anatomical variations of the vertebral artery at C3–C6 should be kept in mind. Wire fixation at the occipital region is disadvantageous because of the pseudarthrosis rate in combination with secondary implant failure. Wire or cable fixation increases the risk for spinal cord injury, especially in patients with a constricted spinal canal. The instrumentation should achieve a physiological position of the occipito-cervical junction to prevent accelerated subaxial instability due to mal-alignment of the cervical spine [19, 33]. Furthermore it must be considered that a fixation with the occiput significantly enlarges the mechanical lever arm leading to a decompensation of the adjacent segments in about 40% of the cases [20]. To prevent early implant loosening autologous bone should be used.

Atlanto-axial fusion

A stabilization of the segment C1/C2 using a bone graft between the posterior arch of the atlas and the spinal process of the axis can be performed in isolated atlanto-axial instability with an anterior atlanto-dental distance of more than 8 mm [40]. A halifax clamp can also be used without additional bone graft. Both methods have more a historical than a practical meaning. The advantage of these procedures is their simple technique. Risks are the wire insertion in the spinal canal, the reduced stability in rotation, frequent loosening with the necessity of a re-operation (clip technique) and a pseudarthrosis rate of up to 30%.

Transarticular screws C1/C2 (Fig. 2.2 a–c) in the technique according to Magerl [41] offer a more stable fixation after direct reposition of C1/C2, but require a minimal width of the pars interarticularis of C2 of 6 mm in CT-reconstructions.

Transarticular insertion of the C1/C2 screws in addition with a bone graft in the technique according to Gallie will result in a three-point fixation with increased stability, which lowers the rate of pseudarthrosis under 5% [6]. This surgical method is technically demanding and requires a thorough knowledge of anatomical landmarks. Lesions of the vertebral artery are considered to be a specific risk of this procedure and occur in up to 4% [41]. Computer-navigation provides a more secure screw position and thus may reduce the risk of such a lesion of the vertebral artery [40]. Some devices offer the opportunity of a supplemental fixation by combining the transarticular C1/C2 screws with an atlas claw [30, 31], which will improve the rigidity of the three-point fixation.

Instead of the placement of transarticular screws for C1/C2 fusion, screws also can be inserted in the lateral masses of the atlas and the isthmus of the axis for atlanto-axial fixation. Instrumentation of the lateral masses of C1 and the pedicles of C2 can be considered as another alternative surgical procedure for C1/C2 fusion [8].

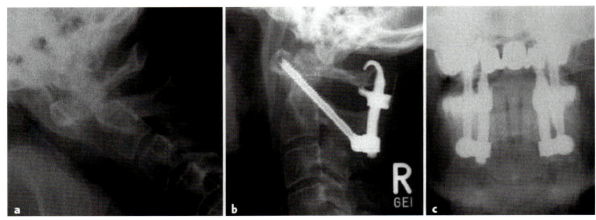

Fig. 2.2a–c. 62-year-old woman with progressive translational instability C1/C2 without basilar impression (**a** lateral X-ray); posterior instrumentation with transarticular C1/C2 screws and atlas claw (neon, Ulrich medical, Ulm, Germany), which is supplemented by autologous bone (**b** lateral X-ray and **c**: antero-posterior X-ray) (Copyright Urban & Vogel; reproduced with permission [30]).

Disadvantage might be a direct force transmission on the atlas, which can cause an early loosening of the screws with a secondary loss of reposition due to the poor bone quality of patients with rheumatic diseases. If compression of the myelon persists after posterior C1/C2 fusion, additional transoral decompression with or without anterior spondylodesis needs to be considered [13].

Transoral decompression

Posterior stabilization of the cervical spine without anterior decompression often results in a decrease of the peridental pannus, which initially compromises the myelon [16]. However, if myelon compression persists after posteriorly fused atlanto-axial instability, a transoral decompression with resection of the odontoid has to be considered [13]. The approach goes through the posterior wall of the pharynx to the base of the odontoid. If there are distinct anatomical variances, a division of the jaw or the palate may become necessary. The resection of the odontoid requires an excision of the anterior arch of C1 and thus will lead to additional instability. In cases without initial posterior stabilization, such procedure should be considered in order to create sufficient biomechanical stability.

An anterior stabilization of the anterior arch of the atlas is the surgical alternative, but inheres the risk of an increased infection rate. In severe circumferential narrowing of the spinal canal anterior decompression may be combined with additional posterior decompression via laminectomy. In such cases, the resulting instability needs to be neutralized by fusion.

Early loosening of the screws in osteoporotic bone, a lesion of the vertebral artery, pseudarthrosis and subaxial instability are the major complications of fusion in patients with rheumatic instability of the cervical spine.

Decompression and stabilization of the subaxial cervical spine

If the disease affects the subaxial cervical spine, stabilization and decompression are also indicated. Due to the inflammatory activity and the resulting destruction of bony structures, severe deformities can develop. Depending on the localization of the lesion, anterior, posterior or combined interventions might be indicated. For multilevel narrowing of the spinal canal corporectomy of the affected vertebral bodies is necessary. The resulting defect can be bridged either with an autologous bone graft or with a cage and should be stabilized additionally with an anterior plate. Potential sintering needs to be considered. Indication for laminectomy may consist of pathological cervical lordosis, dorsal pannus formation and severe segmental antelisthesis. A dorsal stabilization with fusion of the destabilized segments should be considered. Generally, anterior fusion of the cervical spine in rheumatic disorders is difficult to obtain due to osteoporosis. Transpedicular screw fixation with an angle-stable system offers a more stable alternative especially in patients with poor bone quality or in longer instrumentations [31].

A lesion of the spinal cord or the vertebral artery belongs to the typical complications of these procedures. The biomechanical stability of an instrumentation with pedicle screws is significantly higher compared to lateral mass screws as well as the pull-out strength for pedicle screws is more than doubled compared to lateral mass screws [9].

Summary

Conventional X-rays represent the basic diagnostic tool for the rheumatoid cervical spine (cervical spine in antero-posterior and lateral views and functional X-rays). Even at an early stage of the disease signs of instability can be detected in the occipito-cervical joints and at subaxial levels. However, a close correlation between clinical symptoms and pathological X-ray changes does often not exist. The MRI serves as an advanced imaging tool in such cases and in case of suspected myelopathy (e.g. due to pannus formation). The MRI should be performed in slight inclination to be able to assess a potential instability. The detection of an early stage of cervical instability is important for the decision of further treatment (e.g. advanced drug therapy vs. surgical treatment).

Currently there are no evidence-based guidelines regarding the ideal moment for a surgical intervention in patients with atlanto-axial or subaxial instability without neurological deficit. However, delaying surgery to late-stage disease can cause more extensive and more high-risk interventions. Therefore, early symptoms (disorder of fine motor skills in the upper extremity) must be looked for carefully. Evoked potentials (motoric and sensitive) represent an important additional diagnostic tool. Patients with bad responsiveness to DMARD-medication must be controlled in closer follow-ups.

Neurological dysfunction, therapy-resistant pain and a radiologically proven increase of instability with critical narrowing of the spinal canal are well-accepted indications for surgery. Using an adequate surgical technique a stable fixation and fusion can regularly be obtained, even in cases with severe osteoporosis. In cases with apparent myelopathy a neurological deterioration without surgery is likely to occur. Patients with pure C1/C2 instability should be operated on using an atlanto-axial fusion technique. If the occiput must be included in the fusion site due to pathology at the level C0/C1, one should look also for subaxial instability. Transoral decompression may be necessary in case of a vertical instability C0/C1 and destruction of the odontoid and should be combined with a dorsal stabilization. Patients with apparent myelopathy have a significant increase of perioperative morbidity. Therefore, the main goal of all conservative treatment modalities and surgical interventions is to prevent the development of myelopathy.

References

1. Arnett FC, Edworthy SM, Bloch DA, McShane DJ, Fries JF, Cooper NS, Healy LA, Kaplan SR, Liang MH, Luthra HS et al (1988) The American Rheumatism Association 1987 revised criteria for the classification of rheumatoid arthritis. Arthritis Rheum 31(3):315–324
2. Casey AT, Crockard HA, Geddes JF, Stevens J (1997) Vertical translocation: the enigma of the disappearing atlantodens interval in patients with myelopathy and rheumatoid arthritis: Part 1. Clinical, radiological and neuropathological features. J Neurosurg 87:856–862
3. Chung SS, Lee CS, Chung HW, Kang CS (2006) CT analysis of the axis for transarticular screw fixation of rheumatoid atlantoaxial instability. Skeletal Radiol 35:679–683
4. Dihlmann W (2002) Gelenke-Wirbelverbindungen: Klinische Radiologie einschließlich Computertomographie-Diagnose, Differentialdiagnosen. Thieme, Stuttgart
5. Dvorak J, Grob D, Baumgartner H, Gschwend N, Grauer W, Larsson S (1989) Functional evaluation of the spinal cord by magnetic resonance imaging in patients with rheumatoid arthritis and instability of upper cervical spine. Spine 14:1057–1064
6. Grob D (2000) Atlantoaxial immobilization in rheumatoid arthritis: a prophylactic procedure? Eur Spine J 9:404–409
7. Grob D (2004) Chirurgische Aspekte der rheumatischen Halswirbelsäule. Orthopäde 33:1201–1212
8. Harms J, Melcher RP (2001) Posterior C1-C2 fusion with polyaxial screw and rod fixation. Spine 26:2467–2471

9. Jones EL, Heller JG, Silcox DH, Hutton WC (1997) Cervical pedicle screws versus lateral mass screws. Anatomic feasibility and biomechanical comparison. Spine 22:977–982
10. Kauppi M, Neva MH (1998) Sensitivity of lateral view cervical spine radiographs taken in the neutral position in atlantoaxial subluxation in rheumatic diseases. Clin Rheumatol 17:511–514
11. Kauppi M, Sakaguchi M, Konttinen YT, Hämäläinen M, Hakala M (1996) Pathogenic mechanism and prevalence of the stable atlantoaxial subluxation in rheumatoid arthritis. J Rheumatol 23:831–834
12. Keame J, Gershon S, Wise RP, Mirabile-Levens E, Kasnica J, Schwieterman WD, Siegel JN, Braun MM (2001) Tuberculosis associated with infliximab, a tumor necrosis factor α-neutralizing agent. N Engl J Med 345:1098–1104
13. Kerschbaumer F, Kandziora F, Klein C, Mittlmeier T, Starker M (2000) Transoral decompression, anterior plate fixation, and posterior wire fusion for irreducible atlantoaxial kyphosis in rheumatoid arthritis. Spine 25:2708–2715
14. Korpela M, Laasonen L, Hannonen P, Kautiainen H, Leirisalo-Repo M, Hakala M, Paimela L, Blafield H, Puolakka K, Mottonen T; FIN-RACo Trial Group (2004) Retardation of joint damage in patients with early rheumatoid arthritis by initial aggressive treatment with disease-modifiying antirheumatic drugs: five-year experience from the FIN-RACo study. Arthritis Rheum 50:2072–2081
15. Kothe R, Wiesner L, Rüther W (2002) Die rheumatische Halswirbelsäule. Aktuelle Konzepte zur Diagnostik und Therapie. Orthopäde 31:1114–1122
16. Lagares A, Arrese I, Pascual B, Gomez PA, Ramos A, Lobato RD (2006) Pannus resolution after occipitocervical fusion in a non-rheumatoid atlanto-axial instability. Eur Spine J 15:366–369
17. Laiho K, Soini I, Kauppi M (2003) Magnetic resonance imaging of the rheumatic cervical spine. J Bone Joint Surg Am 85:2482
18. MacArthur A, Kleiman S (1993) Rheumatoid cervical joint disease – a challenge to the anaesthetist. Can J Anaesth 40:154–159
19. Matsunaga S, Onishi T, Sakou T (2001) Significance of occipitoaxial angle in subaxial lesion after occipitocervical fusion. Spine 26:161–165
20. Matsunaga S, Sakou T (2003) Prognosis of patients with upper cervical lesions caused by rheumatoid arthritis: comparison of occipitocervical fusion between C1 laminectomy and nonsurgical management. Spine 15:1581–1587
21. McRorie ER, McLoughlin P, Russell T, Beggs I, Nuki G, Hurst NP (1996) Cervical spine surgery in patients with rheumatoid arthritis: an appraisal. Ann Rheum Dis 55:99–104
22. Monsey RD (1997) Rheumatoid arthritis of the cervical spine. J Am Acad Orthop Surg 5:240–248
23. Munthe E (1987) The cervical spine in rheumatoid arthritis (Editorial). Scand J Rheum 16:7
24. Neva MH, Kaarela K, Kauppi M (2000) Prevalence of radiological changes in the cervical spine – a cross sectional study after 20 years from presentation of rheumatoid arthritis. J Rheumatol 27:90–93
25. Neva MH, Kauppi M, Kautiainen H (2000) Combination drug therapy retards the development of rheumatoid atlantoaxial subluxations. Arthritis Rheum 43:2397–2401
26. Nguyen, Ludwig SC, Silber J, Gelb DE, Anderson PA, Frank L, Vaccaro AR (2004) Contemporary concepts review rheumatoid arthritis of the cervical spine. Spine 4:329–334
27. Ono K, Ebara S, Fuji T, Yonenobu K, Fujiwara K, Yamashita K (1987) Myelopathy hand. New clinical signs of cervical cord damage. J Bone Joint Surg Br 69:215–219
28. Puttlitz CM, Goel VK, Clark CR, Traynelis VC, Scifert JL, Grosland NM (2000) Biomechanical rationale for the pathology of rheumatoid arthritis in the craniovertebral junction. Spine 25:1607–1616
29. Ranawat CS, O'Leary P, Pellicci P, Tsairis P, Marchisello P, Dorr L (1997) Cervical spine fusion in rheumatoid arthritis. J Bone Joint Surg Am 61:1003–1010
30. Richter M (2003) Posterior Instrumentation of the Cervical Spine for Instability using the "neon occipito-cervical system". Part 1: Atlanto-Axial Instrumentation. Oper Orthop Traumatol 15:70–89
31. Richter M (2005) Posterior instrumentation of the cervical spine using the neon occipito-cervical system. Part 2: Cervical and cervicothoracic instrumentation. Oper Orthop Traumatol 17:579–600
32. Riew KD, Hilibrand AS, Palumbo MA, Sethi N, Bohlmann HH (2001) Diagnosing basilar invagination in the rheumatoid patient. The reliability of radiographic criteria. J Bone Joint Surg Am 83:194–200
33. Sandhu FA, Pait TG, Benzel E, Henderson FC (2003) Occipitocervical fusion for rheumatoid arthritis using the inside-outside stabilization technique. Spine 28:414–419
34. Santavirta S, Kankaanpää U, Sandelin J, Laasonen E, Konttinen YT, Slätis P (1987) Evaluation of patients with rheumatoid cervical spine. Scand J Rheumatol 16:9–16
35. Shimizu T, Shimada H, Shirakura K (1993) Scapulohumeral reflex (Shimizu). Its clinical significance and testing maneuver. Spine 18:2182–2190
36. Steinbrocker O, Traeger CH, Batterman RT (1949) Therapeutic criteria in rheumatoid arthritis. JAMA 140:659–662

37. Sunahara N, Matsunaga S, Mori T, Ijiri K, Sakou T (1997) Clinical course of conservatively managed rheumatoid arthritis patients with myelopathy. Spine 22:2603–2608
38. Sze G, Brant-Zawadzki MN, Wilson CR, Norman D, Newton TH (1986) Pseudotumor of the craniovertebral junction associated with chronic subluxation: MR imaging studies. Radiology 161: 391–394
39. Van Everdingen AA, Jacobs JWG, Siewertsz van Reesema DRS, Bijlisma JW (2002) Low-dose prednisone therapy for patients with early active rheumatoid arthritis: Clinical efficacy, disease-modifying properties, and side effects. Ann Intern Med 136:1–12
40. Weidner A, Wahler M, Chiu ST, Ullrich CG (2000) Modification of C1-C2 transarticular screw fixation by image-guided surgery. Spine 25:2668–2673
41. Wright NM, Lauryssen C (1998) Vertebral artery injury in C1-2 transarticular screw fixation: results of a survey of the AANS/CNS section on disorders of the spine and peripheral nerves. J Neurosurg 88:634–640
42. Zeidman SM, Ducker TB (1994) Rheumatoid arthritis. Neuroanatomy, compression and grading of deficits. Spine 19:2259–2266

3 Surgical techniques in cervical spinal canal stenosis

ULRICH KUNZ and CHRIS SCHULZ

Introduction

Degenerative changes of the cervical spine are diagnosed in more than 75% of the population older than 65 years of age. Spondylotic myelopathy induced by cervical spinal canal stenosis is a leading cause of cervical cord affection in the elderly. Myelopathy can also be caused by congenital stenosis in younger patients. The congenital narrowed spinal canal is more sensitive to additional slight degenerative findings. The severity and complexity of cervical spondylotic myelopathy (CSM) depends on the degree of cord dysfunction, which is caused by several static and dynamic mechanical components such as direct pressure and intermitting trauma due to instability, by vascular factors (reduction of arterial perfusion and venous outflow) and by an intramedullary edema.

Identification of myelopathic symptoms in early stages is difficult because clinical findings usually develop over a long period before they are noticed and initial findings are often misdiagnosed. The combination of myelopathic and radicular symptoms is common (myelo-radiculopathy). Intermitting sensory dysfunctions due to disturbance of the ascending posterior tracts can be the first symptom. In advanced stages the patients normally suffer from radicular pain and sensory and motor deficits on the upper and sometimes lower extremities. Gait and balance abnormalities are reported as well as clumsiness and numbness of the hands and bladder dysfunction. Different clinical stages of CSM are today classified according to an evaluation score of the Japanese Orthopaedic Association (JOA).

In correlation to these symptoms the physical examination shows motor weakness, spasticity and different kinds of sensory dysfunction. Often exaggerated reflexes and cloni or pathologic reflexes on the upper and lower extremities as well as gait ataxia are seen. Severely affected patients show spastic hemi- or quadriparesis and incontinence.

The "gold standard" of radiological diagnostics for CSM is nowadays magnetic resonance imaging (MRI) including MR-myelographic images (Figs. 3.1 and 3.2). In some cases a conven-

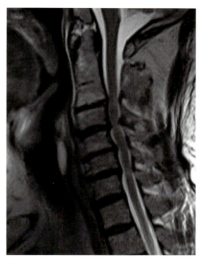

Fig. 3.1. Sagittal T2-weighted MRI-scan showing multilevel degenerative stenosis of the cervical spinal canal.

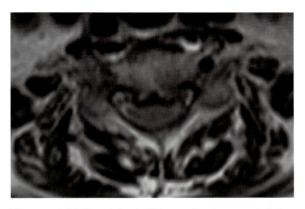

Fig. 3.2. Axial T2-weighted MRI-scan showing a typical dorsal spondylophyte with compression of the cervical cord.

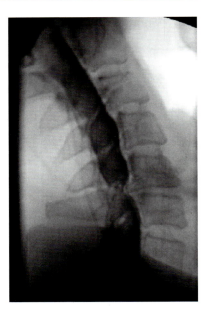

Fig. 3.3. Conventional cervical myelography showing a monosegmental degenerative spinal canal stenosis.

tional myelography is necessary (Fig. 3.3), but myelographic enhanced computed-tomography (CT)-scans should be added. In our opinion the native CT does not offer enough relevant information and is less important. Plain radiographs of the cervical spine and an electrophysiological examination of somato-sensory evoked potentials of the upper and lower limb should be performed in all patients with CSM.

Conservative treatment options

Mild clinical stages of CSM (JOA score >13–14) and a slow progression in very old persons should be treated with conservative methods. Treatment options include: analgetic and antiphlogistic medication, intermittent external immobilisation of the neck and physical therapy. Activities bearing the risk of advanced mobilisation or manipulation of the neck should be avoided.

Kadanka et al. [8] as well as Matsumoto et al. [10] did show that in patients with mild CSM conservative treatment leads to an improvement or a stabilization of clinical functions in more than 60%. The results of non-operative and operative therapy were similar in this subgroup of CSM, even in those patients, who were secondary operated on after progression of symptoms. This suggests that an initial trial of conservative treatment does not decrease the potential benefit of surgical procedures and should be performed in all patients with mild CSM. Close clinical, radiological and electrophysiological follow-up examinations are necessary [1].

Indications for surgical treatment

CSM is a progressive disease. The time course depends on several factors and varies, but spontaneous long-term reduction of clinical symptoms is extremely rare. An absolute indication for surgery is the rapid onset of sensory and motor deficits. Advanced stages or progressive symptoms of CSM (JOA score 8–13) after conservative treatment should be operated on electively, especially in the case of progressive radiological and electrophysiological findings. Whether patients with severe clinical symptoms (JOA score ≤7) and a long-term duration of CSM should be operated on or not is controversially discussed.

The aims of operative procedures are: decompression of the spinal cord, stabilization of pathological segmental instability and improvement of cord perfusion. This should result in the stabilization of or a recovery from clinical symptoms [2]. A wide variety of procedures are available to reach these aims. The surgical strategies are differentiated into anterior and posterior procedures or combined approaches. The definitive choice of the surgical procedure for CSM depends on several factors. The influence of the anatomic location of the pathology leading to CSM, the role of the dimension of the spinal canal, the alignment of the vertebral column and the extent of involved segments on the decision for each strategy are explained in the following chapters.

Anterior procedures

Anterior approaches are used in the treatment of CSM in patients with one to three involved segments, anterior location of the compressive pathology and straight or kyphotic alignment of the spinal column. Anterior procedures enable a direct access to disc herniations, osteophytes, thickened ligaments and ossifications of the posterior longitudinal ligament (OPLL) [11].

In some patients the identification of a single segment for the operative treatment is not possible because the extent of their CSM is across multiple levels. The tendency to operate on adjacent cervical levels showing mild radiographic findings is not generally accepted. On the one hand untreated segments can result in recurrent postoperative myelopathic changes, but on the other hand in extended surgical procedures the perioperative morbidity is increased and after multisegmental fusion the adjacent discs may become hyper-mobile and show a faster degeneration [4]. About 25% of ventrally fused patients develop a relevant discopathy in the adjacent segments. The potential benefit of multilevel approaches should therefore be carefully weighted against their potential risks [6].

After anterior decompression a stable fusion procedure is necessary. Otherwise instability persists, deformity increases and clinical symptoms will recur [13]. Different graft materials are available today. Mostly autogenous bone grafts harvested from the iliac crest or from the fibula are used. To avoid donor-site associated problems and to reduce operative time allogenic bone grafts can be inserted alternatively. They may show nearly the same fusion and failure rate compared to autogenous material but carry the (relatively low) risk of infectious disease transmission. Metallic or synthetic (polyether-ether-ketone (PEEK)) cages as well as polymethyl-methacrylate (PMMA) spacers show good postoperative results but long-term follow-up is needed to evaluate if they perform better than autogenous or allogenic bone grafts, which are still the "gold standard" for cervical interbody fusion procedures. The rate of graft failure (fracture, displacement, penetration, collapse, resorption or infection) increases with the number of levels involved. Therefore additional anterior plating is recommended in order to protect the position of the inserted grafts and to retain the spinal alignment.

For anterior procedures in cervical spine pathology mostly the antero-lateral approach is used. After induction of general anaesthesia the patient is placed in a supine position. In our opinion the administration of single-dose cortico-steroids and antibiotics as well as the insertion of a gastric tube for better palpation of the esophagus are reasonable. For exact radiological visualization during approaches to the lower cervical spine it may be useful to pull or tape both arms downwards; however there is a little risk of brachial plexus lesion in case of overstretching. Therefore we only pull the arms downwards for the phases of fluoroscopic control but not constantly. The location of the skin incision can be orientated according to anatomical landmarks: the hyoid bone corresponds to the level of C3/4, the thyroid cartilage to C4/5 and the cricoid cartilage to C5/6. The level of C6/7 is about two fingerbreadths above the jugulum. Since these marks may vary we sometimes prefer the fluoroscopical identification of the disc levels at the beginning of the operation.

A longitudinal skin incision is normally necessary for operations of more than three levels. Transverse skin incisions allow excellent cosmetic results and a sufficient exposure, even in three level approaches. The transverse incision usually is made in a skin fold on the right side from the midline to the anterior border of the sternocleidomastoid muscle. For approaches to the lower cervical spine a left sided approach is recommended by some authors to protect the recurrent laryngeal nerve, which is believed to be more at risk during right side approaches. After dissection of the subcutis, the platysma is transsected in the direction of its fibers. The subplatysmal soft tissue is divided into a lateral portion (sternocleidomastoid muscle and carotid sheath) and a medial portion (trachea, esophagus, larynx and thyroid gland) by blunt dissection beginning at the medial border of the sternocleidomastoid muscle. Crossing venous and arterial vessels should be carefully divided after ligation or coagulation. The lateral and medial portions are gently retracted to expose the prevertebral cervical fascia and the longus colli muscles. The correct disc level is controlled by fluoroscopy. After incision of the prevertebral fascia and dissection of the longus colli muscles from the underlying vertebral bone the branches of a self-retaining retractor are inserted under these muscles to displace the soft tissue portions. The anterior aspect of the cervical spine is now exposed and either a discectomy or a corporectomy can be performed.

■ Microsurgical cervical discectomy

After exposure of the spine the anterior longitudinal ligament (ALL) and the anulus fibrosus are incised. Ventrally located osteophytes, which

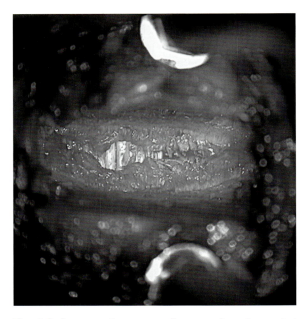

Fig. 3.4. Intraoperative aspect of an anterior microsurgical single-level discectomy: the disc is removed and the posterior longitudinal ligament is exposed.

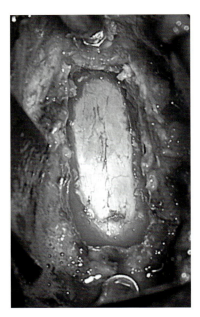

Fig. 3.5. Intraoperative aspect of a two-level cervical corporectomy: exposure of the dura after removal of the vertebrae and the posterior longitudinal ligament.

might aggravate the removal of the disc, need to be resected. The disc is removed onto the level of the posterior longitudinal ligament (PLL) (Fig. 3.4). Usually at this point the insertion of a distraction device is necessary. A high-speed drill is used for the resection of unarthrotic and spondylophytic bone but care must be taken to avoid relevant drilling of the osseous endplates since this might lead to an increased rate of graft complications. The PLL is opened and resected including the adjacent osteophytes. All structures, which might act compressively to the dura and spinal cord, need to be removed under fluoroscopic control. The clearance of the foramina of the segmental nerve roots and the epidural premedullar space should be controlled by palpation using a blunt hook. In cases of far lateral foraminotomy care must be taken to prevent lacerations of the vertebral artery.

After adequate decompression of the nerve roots and the spinal cord a disc spacer is inserted under radiographic control. The size of the graft should result in a spinal alignment as physiological as possible and should provide stable fixation after taking away the intervertebral distraction. In a single-level discectomy a stand-alone graft is normally sufficient to reach solid fusion. In multiple-level discectomy additional anterior plate support is recommended.

Finally the distraction device and the retractors are removed. We recommend the insertion of a vacuum drainage into the prevertebral space to prevent epidural or prevertebral hematoma. The platysma should be sutured as well as the subcutis and the skin.

Cervical corporectomy

In contrast to discectomy cervical corporectomy provides the possibility to remove cord-compressing structures not only at the disc levels but also behind the adjacent vertebral bodies. Comparing the effects of multiple-level discectomy and corporectomy one has to keep in mind that the increasing number of fusion sites results in a decreased fusion rate. Therefore corporectomy is the preferred treatment method of multi-level CSM.

After typical anterior exposure and removal of the involved discs (as described above) the vertebral body is resected to the level of the PLL using a high-speed drill and differently sized punches. The PLL is opened and gradually

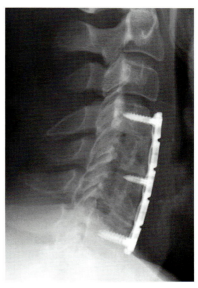

Fig. 3.6. Lateral radiograph after two-level corporectomy and insertion of a bone graft and application of a cervical ABC-plate.

Posterior procedures

Posterior approaches for the treatment of CSM are chosen in cases of dorsally located cord compression factors (thickened ligamentum flavum, hypertrophied laminae and facet joints) and hyperlordotic alignment. In straight or kyphotic deformity a posterior approach is normally contraindicated, because decompression will not lead to a sufficient translation of the cord away from the anterior border of the spinal canal. In contrast to anterior procedures the dorsal approach is recommended for the treatment of acquired CSM of more than three levels or severe developmental spinal canal stenosis [5]. The necessity of a supplemental instrumentation after decompression depends on the chosen manoeuvre and the presence of a pre-existing segmental instability. If a relevant number of posterior stabilizing elements is removed, further instrumentation results in a higher fusion rate, a better prevention of postlaminectomy kyphosis (especially if the laminectomy includes C2 and T1) and an improved capability of deformity correction [6]. The most effective instrumentation procedures are lateral mass screws and pedicle-based screw fixation as described in chapter 1.

For dorsal procedures a midline approach is used. The patient is placed in a prone position after induction of general anaesthesia. The head may be placed on a horseshoe-like holder but sharp fixation in a three-point fixation clamp is recommended. Fluoroscopy is used for correct identification of the involved cervical levels. After midline skin incision the subcutaneous tissue is dissected onto the dorsal cervical fascia, which is incised uni- or bilaterally. The paraspinal muscles are separated from the spinous processes and hemilaminae in a subperiosteal manner and retracted laterally using self-retaining retractors.

resected (Fig. 3.5). All bony and ligamentous material compressing the dura and the nerve roots has to be removed as far lateral as the entry of the foramina can be visualized. Otherwise a local compression can persist and the recovery from clinical symptoms may be incomplete. Care has to be taken to achieve adequate decompression especially on the side where the surgeon is standing during operation, since this is technically more demanding than at the contra-lateral side. The extent of the decompression should be controlled fluoroscopically using a blunt hook.

Adequate decompression is followed by graft interposition. We use autogenous bone in one- and two-level corporectomy and in-situ distractable metallic vertebral body replacement devices after corporectomy of two or more vertebral bodies. Anterior plating after corporectomy and bone graft interposition reduces the graft failure rate and takes only little additional operating time. A distance of about 5 mm from the end of the plate to the next intact disc level is necessary (Fig. 3.6) in order to avoid ossification of this disc resulting in further immobilisation. Whether semi-constrained, dynamic plate-screw systems increase the fusion rate is matter of a controversial debate because the believed lack of longitudinal rigidity may lead also to drifting of the plate and graft migration into the adjacent endplates.

Interlaminar approach (Fryckholm's procedure) and cervical hemilaminectomy

The interlaminar approach exposes the dorso-lateral aspect of the cervical spinal canal. It is normally used for the extraction of a herniated lateral soft disc fragment or for a decompression of a narrowed nerve root canal, which typically leads to radiculopathy but not myelopathy. However the combination of a large disc fragment and lateral canal stenosis or hypertrophic yellow ligament may produce cord compression, which can be released via such an interlaminar procedure. The Fryckholm approach traditionally focuses on removing the medial part of the facet joint and a lateral disc herniation to decompress the nerve root. Undercutting of the hemilamina, the facet joint and the spinous process can extend this procedure. If the interlaminar approach is too small for lateral spinal canal decompression a hemilaminectomy should be performed.

For an interlaminar approach the medial third of the facet joint as well as parts of the neighboured hemilamina are removed. In case of a hemilaminectomy the involved hemilamina is removed using the high-speed drill and punches. The ligamentum flavum is opened and resected, leading to a good exposure of the dura and the segmental nerve root. All bony material and ligaments with compressive effects on the dural structures are removed using an undercutting technique. The disc level is typically located in projection of the axilla of the nerve root. Protruded disc material is extracted and osteophytes are removed by drilling without displacement of the dura and only gentle retraction of the nerve root. Following decompression the retractors are removed, a suction drain is inserted and the fascia of the paraspinal muscles is sutured as well as the subcutis and skin.

Cervical laminectomy

For a cervical laminectomy a soft tissue approach as described above is performed bilaterally. After incision of the interspinous ligaments the spinous process can be removed. The spinal canal should be opened first in its lateral compartment at the junction of the lamina and the facet joint using a drill and small rongeurs. The yellow ligament is carefully resected beginning at the lateral side and then continued at the interlaminar space. This exposes the margins of the lamina. During removal of the lamina, care must be taken not to rupture the dura, which can be adherent. Therefore we recommend careful adhesiolysis using blunt hooks and microdissectors. If necessary, partial undercutting of the neighboured laminae and the facet joints can be added as well as foraminotomy.

The partial resection of the facet joints should not exceed 25% to 50% of the joint. Otherwise a supplemental instrumentation (lateral mass or pedicle screws) is advisable. Especially in younger patients or those with pathological segmental motion and pre-existing kyphosis stabilization is recommended because these patients carry an increased risk of postoperative instability (30% to 50% of treated patients) after laminectomy alone. They are also at a higher risk to develop a so-called swan-neck deformity.

Cervical laminoplasty

Laminoplasty is a dorsal decompressive procedure, which can sufficiently enlarge the spinal canal, but in comparison to laminectomy the dorsal elements, which cover the cord (laminae, interspinous and yellow ligaments) are not constantly removed. This anatomical restoration should result in a decreased postoperative instability rate [3, 9]. Single-door procedures can be distinguished from double-door procedures, however there is no difference in neurological long-term outcome between these techniques [12, 14]. The posterior exposure of the cervical spine is performed as mentioned above. A bilateral trough-hole onto the anterior laminar corticalis is drilled at the junction of the involved laminae and facet joints.

For single-door manoeuvres the bone is completely opened on one side. The ligamentum flavum is resected towards the adjacent segments. The posterior complex is then lifted dorsally using the contra-lateral trough as a hinge

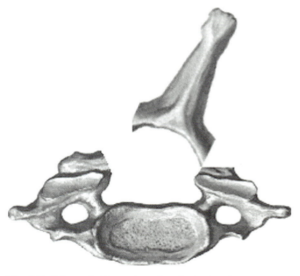

Fig. 3.7. Schematic illustration of a single-door laminoplasty.

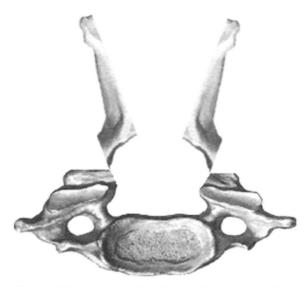

Fig. 3.8. Schematic illustration of a double-door laminoplasty.

(Fig. 3.7). The opening of the "single door" is secured by interposition of autogenous or allogenic bone or synthetic spacers and supplemental mini-plates and screws for fixation. Alternatively, the more traditional method of wiring of the "door" using a suture through the spinous process and the capsule of the facet joint is possible.

In double-door manoeuvres the bilateral troughs are not completely opened. The exposed spinous process is osteotomized in the midline and the resulting laminar halves are opened using the bilateral trough as hinges (Fig. 3.8). An interposition of suitable spacers into the "opened door" is necessary. This double-door technique does not require manipulation on the region of the lateral spinal canal, thus avoiding injury of the laterally located venous complex.

The wound closure includes adaptation of the paraspinal muscles after insertion of a suction drain followed by suturing of the fascia and multi-layer closure of the subcutis and skin.

References

1. Bednarik J, Kadanka Z, Dusek L, Novotny O, Surelova D, Urbanek I, Prokes B (2004) Presymptomatic spondylotic cervical cord compression. Spine 29:2260–2269
2. Ebersold MJ, Pare MC, Quast LM (1995) Surgical treatment for cervical spondylitic myelopathy. J Neurosurg 82:745–751
3. Edwards CC 2nd, Heller JG, Murakami H (2002) Corpectomy versus laminoplasty for multilevel cervical myelopathy: an independent matched-cohort analysis. Spine 27:1168–1175
4. Emery SE, Bohlman HH, Bolesta MJ, Jones PK (1998) Anterior cervical decompression and arthrodesis for the treatment of cervical spondylotic myelopathy. Two to seventeen-year follow-up. J Bone Joint Surg [Am] 80:941–951
5. Epstein N (2002) Posterior approaches in the management of cervical spondylosis and ossification of the posterior longitudinal ligament. Surg Neurol 58:194–207
6. Epstein N (2001) Anterior approaches to cervical spondylosis and ossification of the posterior longitudinal ligament: review of operative technique and assessment of 65 multilevel circumferential procedures. Surg Neurol 55:313–324
7. Houten JK, Cooper PR (2003) Laminectomy and posterior cervical plating for multilevel cervical spondylotic myelopathy and ossification of the posterior longitudinal ligament: effects on cervical alignment, spinal cord compression, and neurological outcome. Neurosurgery 52:1081–1087
8. Kadanka Z, Mares M, Bednanik J, Smrcka V, Krbec M, Stejskal L, Chaloupka R, Surelova D, Novotny O, Urbanek I, Dusek L (2002) Approaches to spondylotic cervical myelopathy: conservative versus surgical results in a 3-year follow-up study. Spine 27:2205–2211
9. Martin-Benlloch JA, Maruenda-Paulino JI, Barra-Pla A, Laguia-Garzaran M (2003) Expansive laminoplasty as a method for managing cervical multilevel spondylotic myelopathy. Spine 28:680–684
10. Matsumoto M, Chiba K, Ishikawa M, Maruiwa H, Fujimura Y, Toyama Y (2001) Relationship between outcomes of conservative treatment and magnetic resonance imaging findings in patients with mild cervical myelopathy caused by soft disc herniations. Spine 26:1592–1598
11. Mayr MT, Subach BR, Comey CH, Rodts GE, Haid RW Jr (2002) Cervical spinal stenosis: outcome after anterior corpectomy, allograft reconstruction, and instrumentation. J Neurosurg 96 (Suppl):10–16
12. Seichi A, Takeshita K, Ohishi I, Kawaguchi H, Akune T, Anamizu Y, Kitagawa T, Nakamura K (2001) Long-term results of double-door laminoplasty for cervical stenotic myelopathy. Spine 26:479–487
13. Sevki K, Mehmet T, Ufuk T, Azmi H, Mercan S, Erkal B (2004) Results of surgical treatment for degenerative cervical myelopathy: anterior cervical corpectomy and stabilization. Spine 29:2493–2500
14. Wang MY, Shah S, Green BA (2004) Clinical outcomes following cervical laminoplasty for 204 patients with cervical spondylotic myelopathy. Surg Neurol 62:487–492

4 Techniques of thoracic and lumbar pedicle screws, lumbosacral fixation, and costotransversectomy

BENJAMIN ULMAR

Historical development of pedicle screw instrumentation

As early as 1888, Wilkins treated a thoracolumbar vertebral fracture in a child, tying a silver wire around the spinal pedicles [26]. Hadra stabilised in 1891 a cervical fracture with wires placed around the spinous processes [6]. Lange used in 1910 metal rods fixed on the spinous processes, initially with silk and later with metal wires [13]. Henle reported in 1911 another procedure of spinal fixation without osteosynthesis using a transplanted bone bangle from the tibia to stabilize a C6 fracture [8]. This technique was enlarged in the following years for all spinal segments using anterior and posterior approaches. In 1907, Lambotte firstly reported the usage of transpedicularly placed screws combined with an external fixateur [12]. The same technique was described by Magerl in 1984, who inserted percutaneously or in an open approach "Schanz"-screws transpedicular into the vertebral bodies using an external fixateur [15]. This technique allowed a rigid screw anchorage in the vertebrae. The first use of the combination of transpedicular screws and an internal fixateur was described by Dick and Kluger in 1984 and in 1985, respectively [2, 3, 9]. After these publications, other authors described modified techniques of transpedicular screw placing also combined with an internal fixateur [7, 14, 21]. As an alternative method of fixation, Roy-Camille and co-workers [21] firstly reported the usage of transpedicularly placed screws combined with metal plates. The principles of the internal fixateur of Dick and Kluger [2, 3, 9] were followed by the development of various angle-stable rod-screw implant systems in the 1990's.

Anatomical background

Thoracic spine

The pedicles of the thoracic spine are smaller than at the lumbar spine. Therefore, the risk to injure the myelon and spinal nerves is higher. Tables 4.1 and 4.2 contain the morphometric parameters of the thoracic spine. The pedicle width determines the screw diameter. The transversal pedicle diameter ranges on average from 4.1 to 5.0 (at Th3 to Th8). Diameters of 4 mm and less are also possible. Krag and coworkers measured in computed tomography (CT)-analyses a transversal pedicle diameter of less than 3.9 mm between Th9 and L5 in two of eighteen cases [11]. In addition, the inner structure of the thoracic pedicles is different to that of the lumbar spine. The medial pedicle wall is two to three times stronger than the lateral wall. This explains why most pedicle fractures happen at the lateral wall.

When Roy-Camille et al. described the ideal pedicle entry point at the thoracic spine, they emphasized the usage of a point localised at the cross point of two lines between the midlines of the facet joints and the transverse processes [21]. Magerl reported at the lower thoracic spine the cross points of the lateral facet portions and the middle of the transverse processes as entry points [15]. Louis described various entry points for the different parts of the thoracic spine [14]. At Th1 to Th3 he emphasized an entry point 3 mm below the highest border of the joint of the adjacent upper vertebra and 3 mm medial to the lateral facet limitation. Between Th4 and Th10 the entry point should be localised medial to the lateral facet limitation and about 3 mm below the middle of the upper joint. This corresponds well with the horizontal line along the upper limitation of the transverse processes. In most cases a little deepening of

Table 4.1. Transversal and sagittal pedicle diameters of the thoracic spine according to Ebraheim et al. [5] and according to Panjabi et al. [20] in brackets.

Vertebra	Gender	Transversal pedicle diameter (mm)	Sagittal pedicle diameter (mm)	Pedicle length in axis (mm)
Th1	m	8.8 (8.5)	7.9 (9.6)	29
	f	10.4	8.5	27.3
Th2	m	6 (8.2)	9.8 (11.4)	29.4
	f	6.7	9.5	28.4
Th3	m	4.1 (6.8)	10.1 (11.9)	31.6
	f	5.3	9.9	29.6
Th4	m	3.9 (6.3)	10.9 (12.1)	31.7
	f	3.8	9.8	31.5
Th5	m	4.5 (6)	10.6 (11.3)	36.6
	f	4	10.1	32.5
Th6	m	3.6 (6)	9.5 (11.8)	37.9
	f	4	9.3	34.4
Th7	m	4.5 (5.9)	10.9 (12)	38.9
	f	4.6	9.8	37.3
Th8	m	5 (6.7)	11.8 (12.5)	41.9
	f	4.6	10.6	38.9
Th9	m	5.3 (7.7)	13.1 (13.9)	42.9
	f	5.5	12.4	38.9
Th10	m	5.6 (9)	14.5 (14.9)	44.2
	f	6	13.5	40.2
Th11	m	8.3 (9.8)	17.3 (17.4)	43.5
	f	8.8	14.8	39.5
Th12	m	8 (8.7)	16.6 (16.7)	44.1
	f	9.4	13.8	41.4

the bone (as a result of the pressure of the upper facet joint in hyperextension) is palpable. At Th11 and Th12 the entry point is similar. An additional orientation point can be determined lateral as a palpable little deepening, which is equivalent to the dorsal limitation of the articular processes. Ebraheim et al. gave a different description of the entry points with orientation to the lateral border of the lower facet [5]. The projection points are localised on average 7 to 8 mm medial to the lateral borders of the upper facet joint and 3 to 4 mm below the midlines of the transverse processes at the level of Th1 and Th2. At Th3 to Th12 these points are located 4 to 5 mm medial of the lateral facet borders and 5 to 8 mm above the midlines of the transverse processes.

The second parameter for the positioning of pedicle screws is the transversal (convergency) and the sagittal (inclination) angle. Roy-Camille et al. described an orientation of 90° to the facet plane [21]. Louis mentioned at the upper thoracic spine a medial angulation of 20° and caudal angulation of 10° [14]. At the medial and lower thoracic spine an orientation to the upper end plate (sagittal pedicle axis) of 90° was recommended. The differences in transversal and sagittal angles of different authors seem to result from different determinations of the pedicle entry points. According to Ebraheim and coworkers the transversal angle is about 30° to 40° and the inclination about 21° at the level of Th1/2 (Table 4.2) [5]. Between Th3 and Th11 the convergency ranges between 20° and 25° and the inclination between 20° and 17° [5]. At Th12 the average transversal angle is about 13° and the sagittal angle about 19° [5]. Panjabi et

Table 4.2. Transversal and inclination angles of the thoracic pedicle axis according to Ebraheim et al. [5] and according to Panjabi et al. [20] in brackets.

Vertebra	Gender	Transversal angle (°)	Inclination angle between pedicle axis and end plate (°)	Distance between the pedicle projection to the middle of transversal process (A) and to the lateral limit of the superior process (B) (mm)	
				A	B
Th1	m	39.4 (27.1)	23.3 (7.6)	2.1	9.1
	f	29.3	20.1	3.1	6.9
Th2	m	35.4 (28.6)	23.4 (17.9)	3.4	8.4
	f	27.6	20.1	4.5	5.4
Th3	m	27.1 (19.4)	22.1 (8.8)	5.5	5
	f	21.5	18.6	5.3	4.6
Th4	m	29.1 (19.5)	23.1 (8.5)	5	5.3
	f	18.8	17.4	6.3	4.3
Th5	m	24.3 (15.6)	24.6 (8.1)	6.2	6.5
	f	16.9	19	6.9	5.1
Th6	m	25.9 (16.4)	27.3 (8.6)	7.1	4.6
	f	15.4	24	7.4	4
Th7	m	24.8 (20.7)	23.6 (11.5)	7.3	5.4
	f	11.4	19	8	4.6
Th8	m	26.4 (19.6)	20.4 (11.6)	7.4	5
	f	9.4	18	8.1	3.4
Th9	m	21.1 (14.8)	17.9 (8.4)	8	5.5
	f	11.6	17.9	7.8	3.6
Th10	m	19.5 (12.4)	17.5 (7.1)	7.1	5.6
	f	16.5	17.1	6.3	4.5
Th11	m	21.5 (13.1)	19.9 (8.7)	6.3	5
	f	15.4	18.5	5.6	3.5
Th12	m	15.4 (9.8)	20.4 (5.1)	5	5.6
	f	10.8	17.5	5.1	4.4

al. described results, which are 10 to 15% lower on average [21]. The entry points for pedicle screws at the mid-thoracic spine as well as the screw trajectories are shown in Fig. 4.1.

Some criterions of the blood supply at the thoracic spine also are important with regard to the planning of a surgical procedure. The arteria radicularis magna is located anterior to the myelon. At the level of Th9 and Th10 it is the main vessel for the supply of the lumbosacral intumescentia. This artery develops mostly at the height of the costo-vertebral joints and in 80% at the left side. A vessel interruption by injury, fracture, tumor or spinal instrumentation may produce an ischemia of the myelon. Iatrogenic injury of vertebral arteries and the thyreo-cervical trunk is possible during an instrumentation of Th1/2 by mal-positioning of the pedicle screws.

Lumbar and sacral spine

The entry points for pedicle screws at the lumbar spine and at S1 as well as the screw trajectories are shown in Fig. 4.2 and Fig. 4.3. For a correct placing of pedicle screws the knowledge of anatomic landmarks as well as firm radiological image interpretation are essential. Tables 4.3 and 4.4 contain morphometric data of the

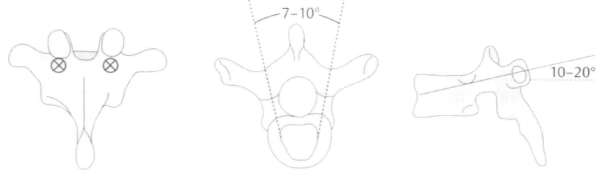

Fig. 4.1. Localisation of the entry point and screw trajectories at the mid-thoracic spine according to Matschke [16] (with permission of Thieme, Stuttgart, Germany).

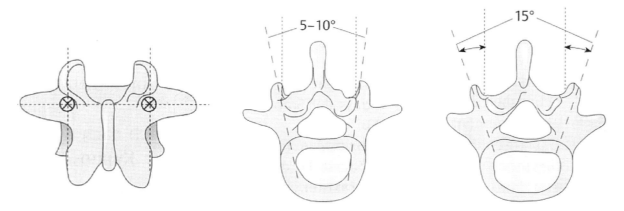

Fig. 4.2. Localisation of the entry point and screw trajectories at the lumbar spine according to Matschke [16] (with permission of Thieme, Stuttgart, Germany): Note the difference in convergency of the screw trajectories at the upper (middle) and lower lumbar spine (right side).

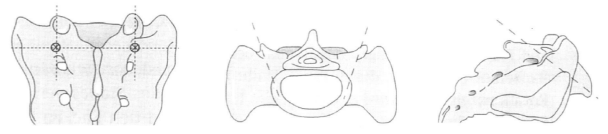

Fig. 4.3. Localisation of the entry point and screw trajectories at S1 according to Matschke [16] (with permission of Thieme, Stuttgart, Germany).

lumbar spine. The transversal diameters of the lumbar pedicles are important for the choice of the correct screw diameter. The anatomical diameter of the pedicle ranges at the lumbar spine from 7.4 mm (L1) to 18.3 mm (L5). The diameter for men is larger than for women. For preoperative planning the correct transversal diameter should be measured in CT-scans, reconstructed at the height of the isthmus. For attempting the screw size the endosteal diameter of the

Table 4.3. Transversal and sagittal pedicle diameters of the lumbar spine according to Ebraheim et al. [4] and according to Olsewski et al. [19] in brackets.

Vertebra	Gender	Transversal pedicle diameter (mm)	Sagittal pedicle diameter (mm)	Pedicle length in axis (mm)
L1	m	7.4 (9.5)	14.1 (17)	48.1 (45)
	f	7.5 (7.7)	14 (15.3)	47.1 (42.5)
L2	m	8.4 (9.6)	14.2 (16)	48.7 (46.8)
	f	7.9 (7.9)	13.8 (15.3)	48.5 (43.5)
L3	m	9.8 (11.7)	13.9 (16.1)	50.1 (49)
	f	9.7 (9.6)	13.8 (15)	49.6 (44.8)
L4	m	12.8 (14.7)	12.7 (16.4)	49.2 (50.4)
	f	12.5 (12.5)	12.8 (14.9)	49.3 (45.9)
L5	m	18.3 (21.1)	11.4 (17.4)	48.3 (46.2)
	f	17.6 (18.4)	11.4 (16.2)	48.3 (42.3)

Table 4.4. Transversal and inclination angles of the lumbar pedicle axis according to Ebraheim et al. [4] and according to Olsewski et al. [19] in brackets.

Vertebra	Gender	Transversal angle (°)	Inclination angle between pedicle axis and end plate (°)	Distance between the pedicle projection to the middle of transversal process (mm) += cranially; −= caudally
L1	m	25.8 (7)	6.7 (5)	+3.3
	f	24.9 (5)	6.1 (6)	+4
L2	m	27.3 (7)	5.1 (6)	+2.8
	f	27 (6)	4.6 (5)	+2.7
L3	m	29.4 (8)	3.9 (6)	+1.1
	f	33.6 (7)	3.6 (6)	+1.6
L4	m	33.6 (11)	3.6 (6)	−0.6
	f	33 (10)	3.2 (7)	−0.4
L5	m	40.6 (17)	2.7 (5)	−1.6
	f	39.6 (18)	2.6 (8)	−1.3

pedicle is used. According to Banta and co-workers, the effective transversal pedicle diameter is particularly smaller than the measure for the cortical boarder [1].

For the measurement of the intraoperative sagittal profile the different positions during the CT-scan and the intraoperative position (which has less lordosis) must be considered. According to Ebraheim and co-workers [4] and Olsewski et al. [19] the sagittal diameter of the lumbar vertebrae is the greatest. The distance between the frontal edge and the dorsal aspects of the vertebrae is maximal at L3 and L4 (50.1 and 50.4 mm). The pedicle screw should be inserted ideally enclosing the largest transversal diameter of the pedicle as well as the largest sagittal length of the vertebra. The entry points of the pedicle screws are determined by morphometric data: the convergency (transversal plane) and the inclination (sagittal plane) of the pedicle (Table 4.4). According to the studies cited above there is a large anatomical variability and difference of the transversal angles. Ebraheim et al. [4] reported an increasing transversal angle from 25.8° at the level of L1 to 40.6° at the level of L5, whereas Olsewski et al. [19] described that angle to be 7° in men at the level of L1 and 17° at the level of L5.

Generally, there are different possibilities to choose the entry point of the pedicle screw. Louis [15] described the direct entry-way ("tout droit") as the best for an optimal screw fixation.

Weinstein et al. [25] reported a more laterally and cranially placed screw entry point in order to avoid interferences between the pedicle screws and the facet joints. For a better orientation, the distance between the pedicle projection point and the midline of the transversal process is helpful. At the lumbar spine, the transverse process – anatomically correctly named as processus costarius – is a good landmark for the optimal definition of the pedicle screw entry point. Between L1 and L3 these points are located about 3.8 to 1.1 mm above the midlines of the transverse processes. At L4 and L5 these points are some millimeters (0.6 to 1.6 mm) below this orientation line.

The lumbar entry points are located at the cross point of two lines vertical to the superior articular processes and horizontal to the transverse processes. At the vertebrae L1 to L3, the pedicle screw entry points are located a little bit above and at the vertebrae L4 to L5 a little bit below the midline through the transverse processes. The sagittal orientation of the screw trajectories corresponds to the vertebral endplates. The sacral pedicle entry points at S1 are a little bit more below and lateral to the superior articular process. The insertion of the S1-pedicle screws can be done in convergency or divergency to the iliac-sacral joint and with a lateral and caudal direction of about 45°. Doing a divergent course of the screw, the length of the screws should not be longer than 45 mm to avoid an injury of the iliac-sacral joints. Generally an additional insertion of pedicle screws in S2 is possible. The pedicle diameter is clearly smaller than at S1.

After opening the pedicle channel a venous bleeding can be noted, because the pedicle is included in the posterior blood outflow. The bleeding usually stops after placing a screw through the pedicle. A potential injury of a committing vessel of the spinal nerves must be considered. The sagittal course of the pedicle screw should be controlled fluoroscopically during insertion. If a bicortical fixation of the screws is intended, it must be considered that the anterior vertebral cortex is convex and the sagittal radiographic image results from picture summation. An extensive anterior screw penetration must be avoided. In patients with poor bone quality due to osteoporosis a feeling of penetration of the anterior cortex of the vertebra during screw insertion is potentially not possible. Therefore, iatrogenic ventral vessel damage is more likely. The length of the pedicle screw and the final screw position should be controlled and documented using an image intensifier.

Implant components of the internal fixateur

One of the large number of multisegmental internal fixateurs is the krypton device (Ulrich medical, Ulm, Germany). This system is used in the same indications and pathologies as other implant systems and therefore is described with its components representatively for other transpedicular spinal internal fixateur systems. The system is modular and consists of the components pedicle screw, connector, locking screw, rod and a cross link system, which can be used optionally.

The pedicle screw

The screw is made of a titanium alloy. The conical head shows an angle of 45° to the axis of the screw. The pedicle screws are available in three different diameters: 5.0, 6.0 and 7.5 mm. The length is available in 5 mm increments: ⌀ 5.0 mm screws are available from 35 to 65 mm, ⌀ 6.0 mm and ⌀ 7.5 mm screws from 40 to 75 mm (Fig. 4.4).

The connector and the connecting screw

In an unconstrained position, the connector rotates 360° around the rod as well as around the conus. Therefore, a three dimensional adjustment is possible. The locking screw is equipped with a 3.5 mm hex. As a result, a rotation resistant connection is achieved between connector and screw. The assembly is easy because of the thread-less portion of the screw (Fig. 4.5).

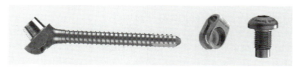

Fig. 4.4. Pedicle screw, connector and connecting screw of the krypton system (with permission of Ulrich medical, Ulm, Germany).

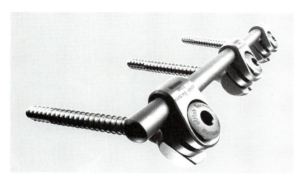

Fig. 4.5. Rod and assembled internal fixateur device of the krypton system (with permission of Ulrich medical, Ulm, Germany).

The rod, cross-link system and assembled krypton system

The rod is available in a length from 30 to 500 mm and with a diameter of 6.25 mm. It has a rough surface and can be cutted at the length needed for the assembled instrumentation. Like all other components of the krypton system it is made of a titanium alloy. To assemble the system, the locking screws are tightened in the conus using a 3.5 mm screw driver. Finally, a torque wrench is used to lock the screws by applying a force of 9 Nm. An additional cross-link system with an x-plate (length of 55 to 65 mm) hooks with break-off notches and nuts and locking plates is available for better control of rotational stability.

Indications for pedicle screws and transpedicular instrumentation

According to Matschke [16], Tscherne and Blauth [23], and Wagner and co-workers [24], indications for the usage of pedicle screws are spinal instability of different origins, fracture, degeneration, infection or inflammation like spondylitis and spondylodiscitis, tumor, spinal metastasis, kyphosis, scoliosis and spinal stenosis requiring decompression or laminectomy with the need for supplemental stabilization.

Surgical approach and handling of the transpedicular instrumentation

The goal of fusion surgery is to provide maximum stability, which can mostly be achieved by the insertion of transpedicular screws in combination with longitudinal rods via connectors and locking screws leading to an angle-stable anchorage [16, 23, 24]. To increase rotational stability the usage of a cross-link system (x-plate) is helpful.

The patient should be placed in a prone position. The shoulders, pelvis and lower limbs should be upholstered with cushions. The position must allow a free abdominal breathing and a hyperlordosis of the thoraco-lumbar spine. Fluoroscopy should be used right before skin incision in the operation theatre in order to identify the correct spinal level.

The classical approach to the thoracic and the lumbar spine is a midline incision. At the lumbar spine the paraspinal sacrospinalis-splitting approach according to Wiltse et al. can be used alternatively [27] as well as new minimally invasive approaches are possible.

After skin incision, the subcutaneous fat, the thoracolumbar and the paraspinous fascia must be incised. The supraspinous ligament should be preserved. The paraspinous muscles should be mobilised subperiosteal from the spinous processes and from the vertebral arches. Retractors can be used to keep the paraspinous muscles away. Optionally, parts of the intervertebral joints can be resected.

To verify the correct pedicle screw entry point, knowledge of the anatomical landmarks mentioned above is required. Additional lateral or biplanar fluoroscopy also might be helpful in order to identify the correct entry point and allows to control the correct inclination of the screw. The pedicle is opened and drilled. The route of the trephine should be controlled by insertion of a k-wire.

After positioning of the pedicle screws the montage of the fixateur interne can be done and the required lordosis or kyphosis can be fixed. If necessary, a repositioning of misaligned spinal segments or a correction of the sagittal spinal profile is possible, using a special repositor. This device connects the pedicle screws with external spindles, which transfer the correction forces of the spindle to the pedicle screws.

After sufficient and subtile blood coagulation, a stepwise wound closing needs to be done.

Costotransversectomy (postero-lateral approach to the thoracic spine)

History and indications

The lateral extracavitary approach to the thoracic spine was developed by Menard for the management of tuberculous spondylitis with neurological involvement [17]. Currently the costotransversectomy is also recommended for tumor resection and excision of vertebral fragments following vertebral fracture.

According to Torklus and Nicola [22] and Tscherne and Blauth [23] further indications for this approach are lesions with a lateral or anterior narrowing of the spinal canal and patients with contraindications for a thoracotomy. Using this approach with exposition of the antero-lateral part of most thoracic vertebrae removal of focal findings, revision of the disc, probe excision, abscess drainage, tumor debulking and tumor exstirpation are feasible. The costotransversectomy can be combined with a dorsal decompression and spinal instrumentation.

Surgical technique

According to Torklus and Nicola [22] the procedure starts with a curve-linear incision three to six centimeters lateral to the appropriate spinous process (Fig. 4.6, Incision A). The incision is placed over the rib involved in the pathologic process. For example, for a revision of the intervertebral disc space Th7/8 a preparation of the 7th rib is required. A second vertical skin incision is added. Alternatively an arched skin incision can be used (Fig. 4.6, Incision B). If it is necessary the incision can be enlarged by crosswise incision (Fig. 4.6, Incision extension). The incision of the subcutaneous fat and the fascia is in line with the skin incision. Depending on the level of the pathology and the approach, the rhomboid muscles and/or the trapezius need to be divided. After exposition of the rib and the transverse process the periosteum of the rib and the capsule of the costovertebral joint are divided and all muscle attachments are separated from the rib using subperiosteal dissection. The rib is incised about 6 to 8 centimeters from the midline and the posterior part is removed. If necessary, the posterior end of two or even three ribs can be resected. However, the intercostal vessels and nerves should be preserved. In case of difficult exposure, up to three nerves can be sacrificed. If extensive exposure is required, the transverse process should be resected. After this the lateral part of the disc, the aorta and the parietal pleura are visible. Generally, the left-sided postero-lateral approach should be preferred, since this allows for a better mobilization of the aorta. In addition, a costotransversectomy is technically less demanding at the upper levels of the thoracic spine because the paraspinous muscles are sparse compared to lower levels.

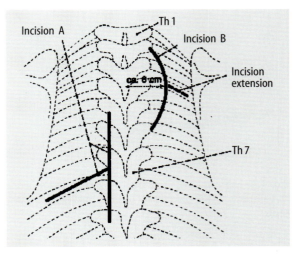

Fig. 4.6. Surgical approach of the costotransversectomy with variable incision lines according to Torklus and Nicola [22] (with permission of Urban & Schwarzenberg, München).

References

1. Banta CJ, King AG, Dabazies EJ, Liljeberg RL (1989) Measurement of effective pedicle diameter in human spine. Orthopedics 12:939–942
2. Dick W (1984) Internal fixation of the thoracic and lumbar vertebrae. Aktuelle Probl Chir Orthop 28:1–125
3. Dick W, Kluger P, Magerl F, Wörsdorfer O, Zäch G (1985) A new device for internal fixation of thoracolumbar and lumbar spine fractures, the fixateur interne. Paraplegia 23:225–232
4. Ebraheim NA, Rollins JR, Xu R, Yeasting R (1996) Projection of the lumbar pedicle and its morphometric analysis. Spine 21:1296–1300
5. Ebraheim NA, Xu R, Ahmad M, Yeasting RA (1997) Projection of the thoracic pedicle and its morphometric analysis. Spine 21:233–238

6. Hadra BE (1891) Wiring the spinous process in Potts disease. Trans Am Orthop Ass 4:206–211
7. Harms J, Stoltze D, Grass M (1985) Operative Behandlung der Spondylolisthesis durch dorsale Reposition und ventrale Fusion. Orthop Praxis 12:996–1002
8. Henle A (1911) Versteifung der Wirbelsäule durch Knochentransplantation. Verh Dtsch Ges Chir 40:118 ff
9. Kluger P (1985) Die Handhabung des Wirbelsäulenfixateurs nach Kluger. Endotec Produktinformation, Mühlheim/Ruhr, Germany
10. Kluger P, Gerner HJ (1988) Klinische Erfahrungen mit dem Fixateur interne und seine Weiterentwicklung. In: Schultiz KP, Winkelmann W (eds) Die instrumentierte Fusion von Wirbelsäulenfrakturen und -erkrankungen. Hippokrates, Stuttgart
11. Krag MH, van Hal ME, Beynnon BD (1989) Placement of transversal pedicular screws close to anterior vertebral cortex. Spine 14:879–883
12. Lambotte A (1907) Le traitment de fractures. Masson, Paris
13. Lange F (1910) Support of the spondylitic spine by means of buried steel bars to the vertebrae. Am J Orthop Surg 8:344
14. Louis R (1986) Fusion of the lumbar and sacral spine by internal fixation of screw plates. Clin Orthop 203:18–33
15. Magerl FP (1984) Stabilisation of the lower thoracic and lumbar spine with external skeletal fixation. Clin Orthop 189:125–141
16. Matschke S (2004) Verletzungen der Brust- und Lendenwirbelsäule. In: Everbeck V, Wentzensen A, Holz F, Krämer KL, Pfeil J, Sabo D (eds) Standardverfahren in der operativen Orthopädie und Unfallchirurgie. Thieme, Stuttgart
17. Menard V (1894) Causes de la paraplegie dans la mal de Pott. Rev Chir Orthop 5:47–64
18. Müller EJ, Muhr G (1997) Thorakale und lumbale Wirbelsäule. In: Müller EJ, Muhr G (eds) Wirbelsäulenverletzungen. Thieme, Stuttgart
19. Olsewski JM, Simmons EH, Kallen FC, Mendel FC, Severin C, Berens DL (1990) Morphometry of the lumbar spine: Anatomical perspectives related to the transpedicular fixation. J Bone Joint Surg Am 71:541–549
20. Panjabi MM, Takata K, Goel V, Federico D, Oxland T, Duranceau J, Krag M (1991) Thoracic human vertebrae. Quantitative three-dimensional anatomy. Spine 16:888–901
21. Roy-Camille R, Saillant G, Mazel C (1986) Internal fixation of the lumbar spine with pedicle screw plating. Clin Orthop 203:7–17
22. Torklus D, Nicola T (1985) Posterolateraler Zugang – Kostotransversektomie. In: Torklus D, Nicola T (eds) Atlas orthopädisch-chirurgischer Operationsschnitte und Zugangswege. Urban & Schwarzenberg, München
23. Tscherne H, Blauth M (1998) Wirbelsäule. In: Tscherne H (ed) Unfallchirurgie. Springer, Berlin
24. Wagner UA, Schmitt O, Schmidt HM, Wallny T (2000) Anatomische Grundlagen der thorakolumbalen Pedikelschraubenfixation und der dorsalen zervikalen Wirbelkörperverschraubung. In: Wagner UA (ed) Atlas der Pedikelschraubenimplantate. Thieme, Stuttgart
25. Weinstein JN, Rydevik BL, Rauschning WR (1992) Anatomic and technical considerations of pedicle screw fixation. Clin Orthop 284:34–46
26. Wilkins BF (1888) Separation of the vertebrae with protrusion of hernia between the same operation-cure. St. Louis Med Surg J 54:340
27. Wiltse LL, Bateman JG, Hutchinson RH, Nelson WE (1968) The paraspinal sacrospinalis-splitting approach to the lumbar spine. J Bone Joint Surg Am 50:919–926

5 Fusion procedures for degenerative disorders of the lumbar spine – indications, techniques, and results

Wolfram Käfer, Balkan Cakir, and Heiko Reichel

Introduction

For degenerative disorders of the lumbar spine, the rate of spine surgery increased by 55% from 1979 to 1990 in the United States (U.S.). With regard to the type of surgery, laminectomy or discectomy without fusion increased by 47% during this time, whereas surgery involving a lumbar fusion increased 100% during this decade [16]. Corresponding to this finding from the U.S., fusions for different degenerative disorders of the lumbar spine are among the most commonly performed spinal procedures worldwide. In addition, a dramatic increase of technology in lumbar fusion has been witnessed over the past two decades. Since then, different fusion methods, instrumentation types, and bone graft sources have been introduced and advocated to improve fusion rate and clinical outcome [7]. With the availability of such techniques, an increasing number of degenerative pathologies are considered to represent a reliable indication for a spinal fusion. For example, among patients with degenerative changes, 70% had a fusion procedure in 2001 in the U.S. For spinal canal stenosis, this proportion was 26%, and for patients with possible instability, 93% of operations included a lumbar fusion [16]. These numbers are impressive, however, one crucial question remains: What has been the impact of new technologies and innovations on the results of fusion procedures for degenerative disorders of the lumbar spine? At present, spine surgery is at a crossroad, where further technologic innovations need to be based on continuous and thorough investigation of the appropriateness of its indications and techniques as well as of its results.

Low back pain – definition and epidemiology

Low back pain (LBP) is defined as pain and discomfort, which is localized between the costal margin and the inferior gluteal folds, and which appears with or without referred leg pain. To fulfill the criterion of chronicity, duration of at least twelve weeks is required [2].

Based on a systematic review of the literature, point prevalence of LBP is estimated to range from 12% to 33%, 1-year prevalence from 22% to 65% and lifetime prevalence from 11% to 84% [56]. LBP tends to fluctuate over time and to show frequent recurrences and exacerbations [2].

With regard to its prognosis and its long-term course, one can assume that, after a first episode of LBP, the proportion of patients who still experience pain after twelve months is on average 62% (range 42% to 75%) and the percentage of patients sick-listed after six months is 16% (range 3% to 40%). The percentage of patients with relapses of pain is 60% (range 44% to 78%) and the percentage, which has relapses of work absence is 33% (range 26% to 37%) [31]. Referring to chronic LBP lasting longer than three months, its prevalence is about 23% [4].

A simple and practical classification to divide LBP into three categories is the so-called "diagnostic triage" according to Waddell: It differentiates non-specific low LBP from specific spinal pathology and nerve root pain/radicular pain [55]. Frequently, low back pain symptoms, pathology and radiological findings are poorly correlated, leading to a 85% rate of people, whose pain is not attributable to specific pathology or neurological encroachment [2].

Surgical techniques

To date, there are many surgical techniques with regard to lumbar fusion procedures. Many of them rely on the use of posterior instrumentation in order to improve stability in terms of biomechanics. However, fusion used to be frequently performed only by applying cancellous bone to the posterior elements of the lumbar spine. Nowadays, sophisticated interbody devices, which can be inserted from anterior, lateral or posterior, are available. Despite these advancements and the resulting diversity of implants, there is no clear evidence whether these innovations lead to a better outcome or not [7, 24]. Owing to the multitude of studies, dealing with the topic of lumbar fusion, but often just reviewing single cohorts of patients, treated with a specific implant, we will not try to give a comprehensive overview of the pertinent literature with regard to lumbar fusion procedures. Instead of this, this article's "Outcome" section provides relevant evidence-based information from two meta-analyses [7, 24] about the relative effectiveness of lumbar fusions.

Pedicle screws

The technique of posterior pedicle screw implantation is extensively described in this book's chapter "Techniques of thoracic and lumbar pedicle screws, lumbosacral fixation, and costotransversectomy".

Pedicle screws are very frequently used in lumbar fusions, since they enhance stability and enable deformity correction. Multiple designs are available, made out of titanium or stainless steel, with different shapes of the thread, cannulated or not, and with either a mono- or a polyaxial locking mechanism. However, there is no clinical evidence that a specific pedicle screw design might be clearly better than others.

Nevertheless, versatility of a pedicle screw system is important, since this allows the surgeon to address a variety of pathologies with

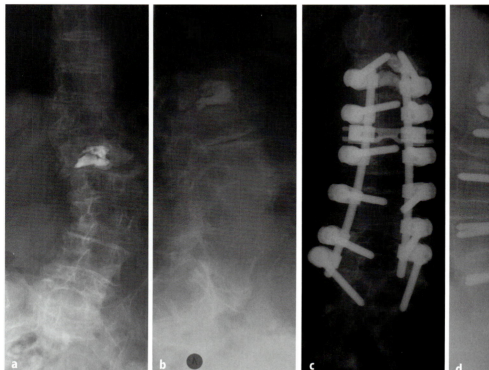
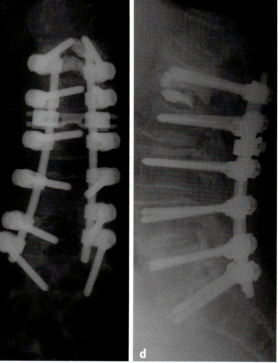

Fig. 5.1 a–d. Posterior-only correction of a degenerative lumbar scoliosis with posterior instrumentation and reduction L1–S1 (krypton, Ulrich medical) and postero-lateral fusion (PLF) with donor bone (preoperative a.p. (**a**) and lateral (**b**) and postoperative a.p. (**c**) and lateral (**d**) X-rays).

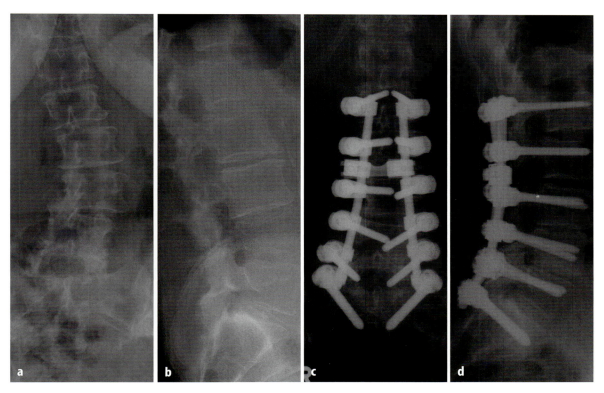

Fig. 5.2 a–d. Two stage correction of a de-novo scoliosis with initial posterior instrumentation and reduction L1–S1 (krypton, Ulrich medical) and secondary 5-segmental anterior lumbar interbody fusion (ALIF) with autologous iliac crest bone graft (preoperative a.p. (**a**) and lateral (**b**) and postoperative a.p. (**c**) and lateral (**d**) X-rays).

just one device, including for example multiple level reconstruction as well as percutaneous short-level stabilization.

Postero-lateral fusion

Postero-lateral fusion (PLF) was first introduced by Watkins in 1953 [57]. It uses the transverse processes, pars interarticularis, and facet joints after decortication as fusion site. It has become the most widely performed method of posterior lumbar fusion and can be performed for a variety of pathologic conditions. Application of supplemental posterior fixation is frequently performed nowadays, however, this technique can also be performed without any further stabilization. Interestingly, even recent publication could not demonstrate any better short-term clinical outcome of instrumented PLF compared to non-instrumented PLF [21]. However, supplemental instrumentation led to a higher fusion rate. Figure 5.1 a–d illustrates the example of PLF supplemental to the correction of a de-novo scoliosis.

Anterior lumbar interbody fusion

Anterior lumbar interbody fusion (ALIF) procedures can be divided by the choice of approach (open retro- and transperitoneal or laparoscopic) and the type of fusion graft (autologous bone or prefabricated allografts in contrast to synthetic cages). Since there is a wide variety of approaches and also numerous types of synthetic interbody devices (threaded cylinders or box type cages, solid or mesh, with or without additional screw fixation), we cannot give a comprehensive overview about that topic in this article.

Briefly, ALIF allows for a good reconstruction of the anterior spinal column, and maintained or increased spinal stability. Biomechanically, the anterior column is mainly responsible for load support. In addition, it provides a much bigger fusion site than the posterior elements. Autologous bone, machined allografts, and manufactured cages produce immediate structural support and adequate contact area. Synthetic cages mostly are filled with bone graft to enable a biologic fusion.

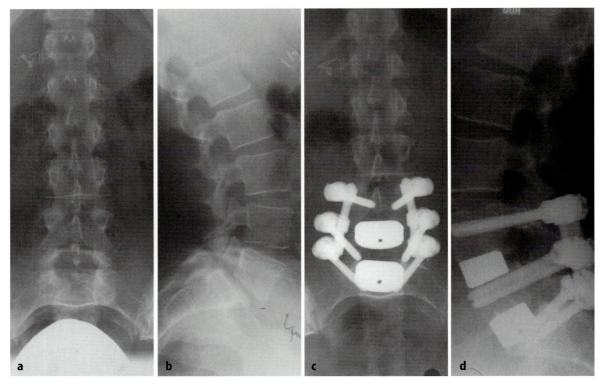

Fig. 5.3 a–d. Patient with symptomatic low-grade isthmic spondylolisthesis L5–S1 and symptomatic degenerative disc disease (DDD) L4–L5, operated on with posterior instrumentation L4–S1 (krypton, Ulrich medical), complete reposition L5–S1, and additional bi-segmental anterior lumbar interbody fusion (ALIF) L4–L5 and L5–S1 with trabecular metal cages (TM 400, Zimmer) in a two stage procedure (preoperative a.p. (**a**) and lateral (**b**) and postoperative a.p. (**c**) and lateral (**d**) X-rays).

With regard to the approach, the so-called mini-open retroperitoneal approach has become the standard procedure for anterior exposure of the lumbar spine. In contrast, exposure of the lumbar spine via an anterior transperitoneal approach may require extensive mobilization of the abdominal organs, which can be time consuming and technically demanding. A retroperitoneal approach maintains all abdominal viscera within their peritoneal envelope and thus decreases the operative trauma to the intestine. Regarding the procedure itself, lateral fluoroscopy is used to determine the level of incision. The incision itself can be performed horizontally, vertically or oblique depending on the level and the extension of the fusion site. Incision of the anterior, and if required, the posterior rectus sheath is followed by careful mobilization of the peritoneum to the medial. Depending on the spinal level to be accessed, the iliac vessels, ureter, sympathetic chain, and aorta need to be mobilized to gain satisfactory exposure. Disc space preparation strongly depends on the preferred interbody fusion device.

Especially in cases of multisegmental involvement (Fig. 5.2 a–d) and discogenic pain referring to degenerative disc disease (DDD) (Fig. 5.3 a–d), ALIF might have advantages compared to posterior-only fusion procedures. Nevertheless, anterior approaches are demanding and inhere the risk of damage to the great retroperitoneal vessels and visceral structures, i.e. the ureter. Especially in younger men, also the risk of retrograde ejaculation deserves attention.

Posterior lumbar interbody fusion

Cloward, in the 1930's, popularized the open bilateral posterior lumbar interbody fusion (PLIF) procedure [13]. At the beginning, iliac crest bone graft was packed into the intervertebral space after open discectomy without further stabilization. However, the complication rate was high, i.e. nerve root injury, dural laceration, and pseudarthrosis, and this procedure fell into disfavour. With the advent of spinal instrumentation techniques, PLIF became popular again as method of posterior-only lumbar fusion, since it enables posterior decompression, interbody fusion, correction of segmental deformity, and rigid internal fixation by means of supplemental pedicle screw instrumentation as one-stage procedure.

The technique of PLIF corresponds to that of TLIF, which is described further down. The essential difference is that a bilateral cage implantation is required through bilateral laminotomy and medial one-half facettectomy instead of a unilateral approach with complete facettectomy. In PLIF procedures, the size of bone graft or interbody fusion device substantially determines the amount of exposure and neural retraction. The latter is the key factor in this procedure with regard to neurologic complications. There are basic principles to be followed, such as adequate bleeding control, adequate amount of mobilization of the neural elements from the underlying disc and vertebral endplates, retraction only to the midline, and frequent intermittent release of retraction, which is limited to 30 minutes of duration at a time.

Preparation and dilatation of the disc space and insertion of the implant is comparable to the TLIF procedure, which is described further down.

PLIF can address a wide variety of pathologic conditions, such as DDD, degenerative spondylolisthesis (Fig. 5.4 a–d), and deformity, especially in combination with a spinal stenosis, since the procedure requires as constituting element the decompression of the spinal canal. It can also serve to create a solid base in a multisegmental fusion without need for interbody fusion of all levels (Fig. 5.5 a–d). PLIF is restricted to a lumbar level below L2 due to the conus medullaris. Complications include neuropraxia, dural lacerations, bone graft or spacer migration, and violation of retroperitoneal structures. In this context, a significantly increased complication rate for instru-

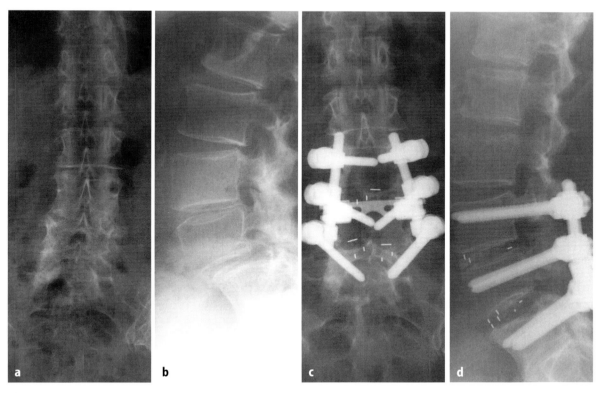

Fig. 5.4 a–d. Posterior-only fusion: posterior instrumentation L3–L5 (krypton, Ulrich medical), decompression L3–L5, and TLIF L3–L4 and PLIF L4–L5 with polyetheretherketone (PEEK) cages (Capstone, Medtronic) in a patient with degenerative spondylolisthesis L4–L5 and severe spinal canal stenosis L3–L5 (preoperative a.p. (**a**) and lateral (**b**) and postoperative a.p. (**c**) and lateral (**d**) X-rays).

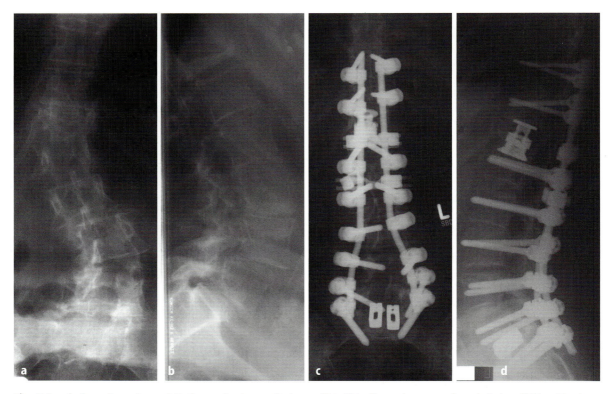

Fig. 5.5 a–d. Correction of an adult thoraco-lumbar scoliosis with sagittal instability L4–L5 and L5–S1 and concomitant osteoporotic T12 fracture with posterior instrumentation and reduction T10–S1 (krypton, Ulrich medical), posterior lumbar interbody fusion (PLIF) L5–S1 with trabecular metal cages (TM 500, Zimmer), postero-lateral fusion (PLF) with donor bone, and vertebral body replacement (VBR) of the fractured T12 with an in-situ distractible titanium spacer (obelisc, Ulrich medical) (preoperative a.p. (**a**) and lateral (**b**) and postoperative a.p. (**c**) and lateral (**d**) X-rays).

mented PLIF compared to instrumented and non-instrumented PLF was shown, clearly indicating the relation of complications with the grade of technicality of a procedure [21].

Transforaminal lumbar interbody fusion

Transforaminal lumbar interbody fusion (TLIF) was introduced in the 1980's in order to overcome the problem of neural retraction associated with use of PLIF procedures [29]. TLIF is a unilateral procedure, which requires supplemental instrumentation for stability reasons. The instrumentation can also serve to facilitate the TLIF procedure itself by means of temporary disc space distraction. Additional PLF is recommended, but not mandatory.

The TLIF approach usually utilizes complete resection of one facet joint in order to provide adequate exposure of the disc space. The working zone is limited by the thecal sac medially, the exiting nerve root supero-laterally, and the pedicle caudally. Due to the expanded exposure, TLIF provides radical decompression of the equilateral lateral recess and neuroforamen.

The procedure starts with a midline exposure and placement of pedicle screws. Afterwards, on one side the facet joint as well as parts of the lamina and the pars interarticularis region are removed using high-speed drills or osteotomes. The exiting nerve root should be identified, however, if possible the surrounding fat tissue sleeve should be retained. Starting from that point, protection of the thecal sac and the nerve root is accomplished with retractors. The discectomy starts with creating a window in the annulus, followed by sequential dilatation of the disc space and removal of the nucleus with aid of curettes and rongeurs. This can be supported by slight distraction of the disc space using the internal fixator. The cartilaginous endplates should be removed completely without violating the bony endplates, since destruction of their integrity might lead to subsidence of the cage. Referring to the avoidance of such an endplate violation, working parallel to the disc space trajectory is of utmost importance. Afterwards, the endplates need to be prepared for fusion by exposing the underlying cancellous bone at a limited area. An important step constitutes also the removal of the posterior and postero-lateral lips of the vertebral bodies, because this facilitates the cage implantation significantly. A trial implant is inserted with special regard to adequate reconstruction of the disc space height. Positioning of the template should be checked fluoroscopically in two planes. If the position is found to be correct, the template is removed and the definitive interbody cage gets packed with spongy bone and impacted in the disc space, which also should be filled with bone. However, care needs to be taken that the bonegraft is not placed adjacent to neural structures. The procedure is finished with mounting the rods to the pedicle screws and applying some compression to the construct.

TLIF provides anterior column support as ALIF and PLIF also do. However, analogously to PLIF it requires just a posterior-only approach, avoiding the risks of trans- and retroperitoneal approaches like major injury to the great vessels and visceral structures or retrograde ejaculation. Its advantages are those of all interbody fusion procedures compared to PLF like increased fusion site and improved ability for deformity correction. However, the latter might not be true in patients with severe osteoporosis and the risk of endplate violation with potential cage subsidence. Such initial or subsequent subsidence or dislocation is one of the major complications of TLIF. Another complication, which can become life threatening, is damage to the retroperitoneal vessels due to overly aggressive manipulation in the disc space. Intra-operative fluoroscopy can help in situations, when orientation in the disc space is difficult to obtain.

Good indications for TLIF procedures are mono- or bisegmental pathologies like instability, spinal stenosis, discogenic pain, and failed-

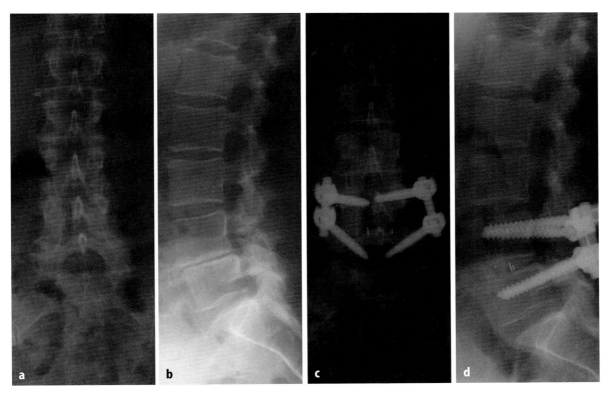

Fig. 5.6 a–d. Patient with failed-back-surgery syndrome (FBSS) L4–L5, operated on with monosegmental instrumentation and segmental distraction (Xia, Stryker) and transforaminal lumbar interbody fusion (TLIF) L4–L5 with a polyetheretherketone (PEEK) cage (AVS TL, Stryker) (preoperative a.p. (**a**) and lateral (**b**) and postoperative a.p. (**c**) and lateral (**d**) X-rays).

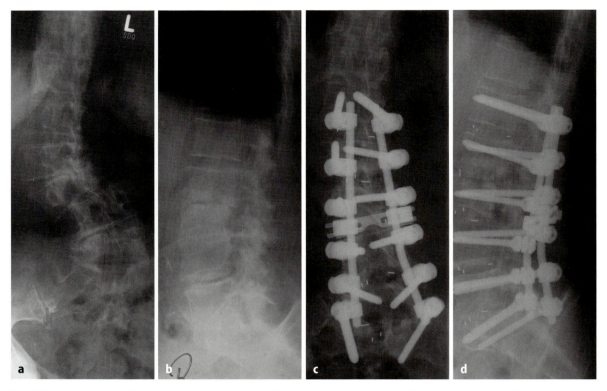

Fig. 5.7 a–d. Posterior-only correction of a de-novo scoliosis with severe translational instability L2–L3 in the frontal plane in a patient with mild osteoporosis; the procedure consisted of posterior instrumentation and reduction L1–S1 (krypton, Ulrich medical), 5-segmental transforaminal lumbar interbody fusion (TLIF) L1–S1 with polyetheretherketone (PEEK) cages (Capstone, Medtronic), and supplemental postero-lateral fusion (PLF) with donor bone (preoperative a.p. (**a**) and lateral (**b**) and postoperative a.p. (**c**) and lateral (**d**) X-rays).

back-surgery syndrome (FBSS) (Fig. 5.6 a–d). However, multiple level deformity can also treated successfully with instrumented TLIF, since this may allow for an even better control of correction compared to posterior instrumentation only (Fig. 5.7 a–d).

Indications for lumbar fusion procedures

The usefulness of surgical procedures for different disorders of the lumbar spine like fractures or tumor associated neural compressions is clear and undisputable. However, there is a controversial debate on the benefit of surgical procedures, particularly with regard to lumbar fusions in case of chronic LBP due to a variety of degenerative disorders. Considering the pathogenetic concept of segmental degeneration according to Kirkaldy-Willis, one can assume that instability, which is one step in the cascade of degeneration, leads to mechanical pain [32]. However, mechanical pain due to instability should be responsive to surgical stabilization of an unstable spinal segment. Therefore, orthopaedic surgeons strive for a clear and reliable attribution of the clinical symptoms LBP and posture-dependent sciatica to the alteration of a morphological structure in terms of degeneration and, in particular, segmental instability. Consequently, there has to be a differentiation of patients with chronic LBP due to a specific origin from those with a non-specific origin.

Generally, the surgical goals in lumbar fusion procedures include pain reduction, improvement of neurologic symptoms, and probably most important improvement in quality of life. If attainment of these goals is unlikely, surgery should be canceled and conservative treatment continued. On top of this, one should keep in mind that the primary focus in treating LBP should be placed on the prevention of disability, which is especially true when considering epidemiological data of this common entity.

Spinal stenosis

Spinal stenosis, which is a narrowing of the spinal canal or the intervertebral foramen at a single or at multiple levels, is classified as either primary or secondary [49]. Primary stenosis is a very uncommon condition and is caused by a congenital abnormality or a disorder in postnatal development leading to an altered intrinsic shape of the canal. In contrast, secondary stenosis is the most frequent form and usually results from degenerative changes. Consequently, it is most common in adults in their fifth and sixth decade of life. Secondary stenosis also may occur as a result of infection or trauma (e.g., fracture) and after surgery (due to inadequate decompression, or due to iatrogenic instability leading to pathological segmental movement, or from excessive scar tissue) [5].

Degenerative spinal stenosis is based on several distinct degenerative processes involving the facet joints, intervertebral discs, and intraspinal soft tissues. Especially hypertrophy of the ligamentum flavum and the facet joints narrows the lateral recess or the nerve root foramen, thus creating the trefoil-shaped narrowing of the canal. Aging also is associated with loss of disc height, which leads to narrowing of the foramen vertically. If disc height loss occurs pronouncedly, it can even allow buckling of the yellow ligament into the spinal canal. Facet degeneration can also be associated with degenerative instability, i.e. anterior spondylolisthesis, usually at the level L4–L5, contributing to further narrowing of the foramina [35].

Spinal stenosis frequently leads both to LBP and neurogenic claudication. The latter is the most specific symptom of spinal stenosis, although not all patients report it. It is defined as pain, paraesthesia, and cramping of the lower extremities due to neurologic compromise brought on by standing or walking and relieved by sitting. Neurogenic claudication may result from a mechanical irritation of the cauda equina or from ischemia caused by narrowing of small intraneural arterial branches and venous congestion, which is induced during exercise [50]. Posture-dependency of neurogenic claudication can be explained by the fact that extension of the lumbar spine leads to a marked decrease in the sagittal diameter of the spinal canal whereas flexion widens it with relief of nerve root involvement [47].

Imaging technologies like computed tomography (CT) and magnetic resonance imaging (MRI) have led to a marked increase in the diagnosis of spinal stenosis. To date, spinal stenosis is the most common diagnosis leading to lumbar spine surgery [16]. However, there is little evidence to guide clinical practice. For example, systematic reviews of treatment of spinal stenosis are faced with the problems of few randomized trials, heterogeneous patient populations, and outcome measures that frequently are not validated [5].

When it comes to treatment of spinal stenosis, the widely varying amount of back, groin, or leg pain and numbness among individuals, that means patients' clinical symptoms, but not their morphological changes, must be considered as a key factor in decision-making which treatment to have and when to have it.

Depending on the severity of symptoms, for most individuals, initial treatment should be non-surgical. However, such conservative treatment recommendations are based on expert opinion rather than evidence from controlled trials. Evidence from non-surgical treatment of non-specific LBP suggests efficacy for a variety of interventions. Therefore, for patients with spinal stenosis, non-surgical treatment should also focus on patient education, medication to control pain, and exercise and physical treatments to regain or maintain activities of daily living. Those treatment modalities may be used sequentially or in combination depending on the severity of symptoms and their change with time [5]. For some people, non-surgical interventions treat symptoms well.

For others, however, pain is not responsive to conservative treatment. For such individuals, surgical treatment is reasonable to consider.

Indications for surgical interventions include intolerable pain, which cannot be controlled by medications, and persistent or progressive neurogenic leg symptoms unresponsive to eight to twelve weeks of non-surgical treatment. Surgery for spinal stenosis should be approached cautiously in patients with other major co-morbid medical problems, predominantly lower-back pain as opposed to radicular pain, and advanced imaging findings that are inconsistent with symptoms or the examination findings.

Authors of some more recent studies suggest that surgical treatment provides better short- to mid-term outcomes than non-surgical treatment [3, 38, 58]. Comparisons between decompression alone and decompressions combined with a fusion procedure are rare. However, there is some moderate evidence that performing a fusion might improve the clinical outcome compared to decompression alone [30] and that patients perform better on the long run with a successful arthrodesis than with a pseudarthrosis regarding their back and lower limb symptoms [35].

To our understanding, in all cases of spinal stenosis with concomitant symptomatic degenerative instability, instrumented fusion should be added to decompression. The same is true in patients without previous degenerative instability, when decompressive surgery leads to iatrogenic spinal instability [33]. The choice of approach to the intervertebral space and the fusion site usually is determined by anatomical features like the extent of stenosis and instability. For example, PLIF or TLIF procedures are appropriate in mono- (Fig. 5.6 a–d) or bisegmental decompressions and stabilizations (Fig. 5.4 a–d), whereas multisegmental spinal stenosis normally should be operated on with multisegmental ALIF (Fig. 5.2 a–d) or just with instrumented PLF (Fig. 5.1 a–d), the latter possibly including optional interbody support of the most caudally located segment with a PLIF (Fig. 5.5 a–d).

Degenerative spondylolisthesis

Degenerative instability of the lumbar spine mostly is represented by degenerative spondylolisthesis [54] and to a lesser extent by the so-called de-novo scoliosis [36]. Especially spondylolisthesis is a common cause for chronic LBP, radicular pain, and neurogenic claudication among the adult population [54].

Recognizing the variety of spondylolisthesis types, Wiltse and co-workers established a comprehensive classification system in 1976, which divides spondylolisthesis in congenital, isthmic, degenerative, pathologic, iatrogenic, and traumatic etiologies [59]. Isthmic and degenerative causes, which are both acquired, are by far the most common in the adult population.

The most commonly affected level of the spine in degenerative spondylolisthesis is L4–L5. This entity is five to six times more likely to occur in women than men, which has been attributed to an increased ligamentous laxity compared with that seen in men [54]. Regarding to its pathogenesis, patients with sagittal development of their L4–L5 facets are believed to be at a higher risk for spondylolisthesis because they lack normal resistance to shear forces [26]. Such sagittal orientation of the L4–L5 facets combined with the more coronally situated L5–S1 facets results in hypermobility of the L4–L5 segment, particularly in the sagittal plane. If this hypermobility occurs in combination with other risk factors such as disc degeneration, facet joint arthritis, and ligamentous laxity, subluxation of the superior vertebra will take place [54]. This pathological mobility then leads to a narrowed canal and narrowed lateral recesses at the level of the slip.

The natural history of degenerative sagittal instability of the lumbar spine generally is favourable. Only 10% to 15% of patients seeking medical treatment eventually will have surgery. This might be due to hypertrophy and ossification of the intervertebral ligaments as well as development of osteoarthritic spurs and facet joint arthrosis, which may act as secondary stabilization with regard to a further slippage progression [41]. It can be assumed that a progressive slip appears in about one third of all cases. However, there seems to be no correlation between slip progression and clinical symptoms [41].

Referring to the amount of slippage, this rarely exceeds 25% in degenerative spondylolisthesis. Lateral X-rays in flexion/extension may serve to exclude dynamic instability in cases with a slip, but established secondary stabilization effect.

Since non-operative treatment is the mainstay of therapy for LBP, it also should be at the beginning of each course of action in patients with spondylolisthesis. There are, however, no controlled clinical trials establishing an optimal non-operative treatment protocol. Mostly, treatment is initiated with a short period of bed rest, followed by a course of anti-inflammatory medication. Physical therapy, i.e. aerobic conditioning, is another constituting element of conservative therapy. For example, stationary bicycling promotes spine flexion and consequently deconstriction of the thecal sac, and allows for more exercise before neurogenic claudication, which is a common clinical finding in degenerative spondylolisthesis, begins [54].

If this initial treatment fails, epidural steroid injections as well as facet joint blocks of the affected level might be administered. Nevertheless, there is lacking evidence of the efficacy of those treatment modalities.

When non-operative treatment finally fails, surgical options need to be considered. Relative indications for surgery include persistent radiculopathy, progressive neurologic deficit, and persistent and unremitting neurogenic claudication and LBP, all leading to a significant loss of quality of life. In those indications, it was shown that patients operated on for degenerative spondylolisthesis with concomitant stenosis do better than their conservatively treated controls with regard to pain relief and function [43, 58]. Absolute indications for surgical interventions include progressive neurologic deficit or cauda equina syndrome [54].

With regard to the type of surgery, pure decompressions can be distinguished from decompressions supplemented by fusion procedures, with or without instrumentation, and either purely posterior or as a circumferential 270° or 360° fusion.

Before the fusion era started, laminectomy was the mainstay for many years in the treatment of degenerative spondylolisthesis [17]. However, pure laminectomy soon was supplemented with postero-lateral fusion in order to address also the problem of LBP [30]. Since it was assumed at that time that instrumented fusion produces better fusion rates than non-instrumented spondylodesis, supplemental instrumentation in treating patients with symptomatic degenerative spondylolisthesis was also introduced. In 1997, Fischgrund and co-workers demonstrated that instrumented fusion leads to a higher fusion rate (82%) compared to non-instrumented fusion (45%); however, patient outcome was the same regardless of solid fusion or pseudarthrosis [19]. Interestingly, this patient sample was analyzed again a few years later, revealing a significantly better outcome in patients having a solid fusion compared to those with pseudarthrosis [35].

This finding is also reflected in a meta-analysis from 1994, which reviewed the literature pertaining to degenerative lumbar spondylolisthesis from 1970 to 1993 and which showed improved outcome when solid arthrodesis was achieved [39].

The most recent 2007 Cochrane meta-analysis of 13 randomized studies supports the results from the 1994 meta-analysis with regard to treatment modalities of degenerative spondylolisthesis [40]. A satisfactory clinical result was significantly more likely with fusion than with decompression alone as well as the use of supplemental instrumentation significantly increased the probability of attaining solid fusion. However, the authors stated that no conclusions about the real clinical benefit of applying supplemental instrumentation to a spinal fusion are possible beside the evidence that the use of instrumentation improves the chance of achieving solid fusion [40].

Since we believe that mechanical pain caused by instability is one major contributing factor to LBP, we try to achieve bony fusion in degenerative disorders of the lumbar spine. This is especially true in spondylolisthesis, which should be treated therefore with decompression in combination with instrumented fusion (ALIF (Fig. 5.3 a–d), PLIF, or TLIF (Fig. 5.4 a–d)). In addition, we strive for reduction of the slippage in order to enable a rebalancing of the lumbar spine (Figs. 5.3 a–d and 5.4 a–d). However, this personal opinion is just partially justified by the results from evidence-based medicine.

▌ Degenerative lumbar scoliosis

De-novo scoliosis, which is less frequent in an adult population than a pure sagittal translational instability like spondylolisthesis, is formed by a variety of degenerative changes including disc bulging, facet joint arthrosis, and ligamentum flavum hypertrophy, leading to mechanical insufficiency of the spine. These alterations contribute to the appearance of clinical symptoms like chronic LBP and neurogenic claudication, the latter due to central and/or lateral recess stenosis [48]. Nevertheless, neurological deficits are rare, and patients almost never complain about cosmesis, which is a typical finding in idiopathic adolescent scoliosis [36].

The asymmetric affection of anatomical structures, i.e. the disc and the facets, is of primary importance for the formation of the deformity and also for its progression, since asymmetric degeneration leads to increased asymmetric load and further asymmetric decompensation [1]. Deformity progression might be also supported by low bone density, as seen in many postmenopausal women with osteoporosis.

Decision-making with regard to therapy, which generally should be started with conservative treatment, needs to take into account symptomatology and in case of scheduled surgery radiologic measurements of deformity (scoliosis and kyphosis) and stenosis. Surgery for de-novo scoliosis is demanding and needs to take into account the co-morbidities, bone quality and more than anything else the required fusion site and length and the anticipated amount of correction. The main goal is beside decompression of the neural elements to achieve a stable and balanced spine. Therefore, it seems to be of crucial importance to tailor the treatment to the specific symptomatology of the patient. Consequently, surgical management can consist of pure decompressive surgery, correction and fusion, or a combination of all [1]. Despite the potential technical problems of such complex surgical procedures, satisfactory clinical results of operative therapy have been reported in retrospective studies in about 83% to 96% [48].

To our understanding, when it comes to surgery, adequate patient selection is of crucial importance in dealing with patients with degenerative lumbar scoliosis. The localization, amount, and the rigidity of the deformity are key factors in determining the surgical procedure. Also, curve progression pattern need to be taken into account. Prerequisite of any correction of such deformity is the technical feasibility based on the design of the applied internal fixator. Anterior release and structural support can be indicated in cases with flat back or kyphotic deformity (Fig. 5.2 a–d). Synthetic cages can facilitate deformity correction, either in PLIF or TLIF technique (Fig. 5.7 a–d). If it is reasonable, fusing the lumbo-sacral junction should be avoided, since this might lead to inferior functional outcome. On the other hand, one should not hesitate to expand the fusion to the thoracic spine if this is required in order to achieve a better fixation, especially in patients with osteoporosis (Fig. 5.5 a–d). Nonetheless, treatment should target in general a minimum rate of interventions.

▪ Non-specific low back pain

LBP has been considered to be a 20th century epidemic. Accordingly, the World Health Organization (WHO) has prioritized this entity, for example by prescinding it in the agenda of the Bone and Joint Decade. Many evidence-based systematic literature reviews have been published on LBP in different countries [34]. Their common finding was that dividing LBP into two categories referring to a specific and a non-specific origin plays a key role in determining therapy and outcome [45].

Non-specific LBP, which is characterized by pain, mainly localized at the back and radiating to the lower extremities, usually not below the knees, includes common diagnoses, such as lumbago, back sprain, back strain, myofascial syndromes, and muscle spasms. The term "non-specific" indicates that no precise structure can be identified causing LBP. Hence, LBP can be considered to be rather a symptom since direct causality cannot be determined.

The biopsychosocial model for non-specific LBP provides useful information in order to identify factors associated with delayed recovery. Such factors might be cultural beliefs, a high perception of disability, kinesiophobia, depression, stress from work or family, job dissatisfaction, anxiety, somatization, and lack of control [46]. This model serves to recognize the non-specific nature of LBP, and to identify and treat those underlying psychosocial factors, for example by means of behavioral treatment or ergonomic intervention [45].

The initial treatment of patients with acute LBP consists of over-the-counter medication and maintaining activity as tolerated. Also treatment with a limited number of sessions of manipulative therapy may be effective for pain relief. If pain persists over four weeks, a graded activity program including exercises and cognitive behavioral treatment should be administered.

However, some patients will experience further deterioration of their symptoms under conservative treatment. In those patients, LBP without sciatica might be attributable to degenerative disc disease (DDD) [15]. Even although DDD is a common finding also in asymptomatic subjects [6], one must consider surgery in those patients after careful assessment of potential pain generators, including facet blocks and provocative discography.

A systematic literature review in 1999 summarized that there is lacking evidence for using lumbar spine fusion in patients with lumbar spondylosis and LBP [23].

Nevertheless, there is now some evidence from a randomized controlled trial that surgery might lead to superior results in patients with

LBP due to DDD compared to a standard conservative treatment [20]. With regard to cognitive intervention and exercises, however, it seems that fusion surgery for DDD performs just equally, when comparing its results with such elaborated conservative treatment [8].

As a rule of decision-making, we try to continue conservative treatment in symptomatic patients with DDD if they can tolerate their LBP. However, after six to twelve months of unsuccessful conservative treatment, patients are scheduled for surgery. Since we believe that both the disc and the facet joints might play an important role as pain generators, in cases of scheduled fusion surgery, we always perform it with supplemental instrumentation and with removal of the disc and interbody fusion, either in ALIF (Fig. 5.3 a–d), PLIF, or TLIF technique. This recommendation is based on one hand on experimental analysis of the role of the disc [18] and on the other hand on our own empirical evidence as well as empirical evidence from other authors about the role of instrumentation and circumferential fusion in treating patients with LBP due to DDD [10]. However, pure disc degeneration, which becomes symptomatic, might also be a good indication for lumbar total disc replacement (TDR) [51].

Outcome

Outcome assessment

The two disease-specific questionnaires most commonly used and recommended in patients with LBP are the Oswestry Disability Scale and the Roland-Morris Disability Scale. These two self-reported measures link the functional impairment experienced by the patient to its back problem. Both instruments have very acceptable reliability and validity. Another crucial issue in outcome evaluation is health-related quality of life, which is related to patient functioning and which can be assessed through different generic questionnaires such as the commonly used Short Form series (SF-36 and SF-12) or the Euroqol. Both the SF-36 and Euroqol have shown good correlation with back-specific questionnaires, including the Oswestry Disability Scale and the Roland-Morris Disability Scale. Pain questionnaires are the third important outcome measure following lumbar fusion. Mostly, pain is assessed using a numerical verbal or visual rating scale [9]. Nevertheless, especially in randomized controlled trials of treatment for chronic LBP, patient global assessment also is a valid and responsive descriptor of the overall effect [27].

Global outcome

With regard to the global outcome of fusion procedures for degenerative disorders of the lumbar spine, the 2005 updated Cochrane Review "Surgery for degenerative lumbar spondylosis" from Gibson and Waddell [24] and the 2004 meta-analysis from Bono and Lee [7] serve as fundamental sources of information.

Gibson and Waddell identified a total of 31 randomized controlled trials, some of them dealing with different techniques of decompression or novel technologies like intradiscal electrotherapy (IDET) or total disc arthroplasty [24]. Just two studies reported on the outcome of lumbar fusion procedures compared to conservative treatment. One trial showed that fusion gave better clinical outcomes than conventional physiotherapy [20], and the other showed that fusion was no better than a modern exercise and rehabilitation program [8]. Gibson and Waddell summarized that no conclusions are possible about the relative effectiveness of anterior, posterior, or circumferential fusion, that there is conflicting evidence on the clinical effectiveness of fusion, and that instrumentation produces a higher fusion rate, whereas any improvement in clinical outcome is probably marginal [24].

Bono and Lee reviewed a much wider range of randomized and non-randomized, prospective and retrospective studies of lumbar fusion in degenerative disorders of the spine and found 84 articles published between the years 1979 and 2000, which fulfilled the inclusion criteria and which represented 7043 patients. The authors postulated in their comprehensive review that numerous deficiencies are present in the published results of fusion for lumbar degenerative disc disorders from the past 20 years. In addition they stated that despite a trend toward the increased use of internal fixation, an improvement in overall fusion rate or clinical outcome could not be demonstrated, and that a uniform system of outcome reporting which contains a core of critical demographic, perioperative, and post-surgical information is necessary to help improve the quality and usefulness of published results [7].

Complications

Complication rates also work as important variables of outcome assessment in patients following a spinal fusion procedure. Although such complication rates might be underestimated in administrative databases [16], they can provide meaningful contrasts in relative complication rates among different diagnoses, procedures, and demographic groups. For example, in patients operated on for spinal stenosis, complication rates increase steadily corresponding to an increasing burden of co-morbid medical illnesses. Equally, surgical mortality during hospitalization and within the first six weeks after discharge rises from about 0.5% among patients aged 65 to 69 years, to more than 2% among those 80 years or older [12]. Patients with re-operations do have complication rates, which are higher as in patients with first-time surgeries [14]. Referring to the type of lumbar spine surgery, one can assume that patients having lumbar spine fusion have approximately twice the risk of complications as those having just laminectomy or discectomy, which is true even after adjusting for co-variables such as age, sex, co-morbidity, race, previous back surgery, and diagnoses [12].

Predictors of outcome

Despite distinct advances in spinal surgery technology, there is still a considerable number of patients without marked improvement after spinal surgery for chronic LBP. Therefore it seems to be of crucial importance to determine potential outcome predictors. A special regard should be given to socio-demographic and psychological variables beside the technically orientated classical outcomes measures.

Hägg and co-workers in their study of patients with chronic LBP, randomized either to conservative treatment or lumbar spine surgery, found out that a personality characterized by low neuroticism as well as a low disc height predict functional improvement after surgical treatment, whereas depressive symptoms act as significant predictors after non-surgical treatment [28].

In another recent study, preoperative emotional status was also identified to be a significant predictor of pain and functional outcome two years after lumbar fusion. Other significant predictors included workers compensation status, smoking status, and preoperative pain and function [53].

Hopefully, such assessment of outcome prediction can facilitate the process of decision-making regarding surgical or non-surgical treatment in the future.

Trends

In the U.S., the rate of fusion procedures for degenerative disorders of the lumbar spine tripled during the 1990's, after already doubling during the 1980's, which made spinal fusion one of the most rapidly increasing forms of surgery. Fusion rates rose especially after 1996, when intervertebral fusion cages were approved by the Food and Drug Administration (FDA). Referring to all types of spinal fusion procedures, they increased by 77% between 1996 and 2001. In contrast, other major orthopaedic procedures, such as total hip and total knee arthroplasty, increased by only 13% to 15% during this time [16]. In addition to an increasing number of operations that involve fusion, an increasing proportion of all fusions involve posterior instrumentation. The reported rates of internal fixation nearly doubled from the 1980's to the 1990's [7]. These literature-based estimates are supported by population-based rates. During the last five years of the 1990's, a 40% increase in spine surgery rates took place, whereas a 70% increase in spine fusion rates and more than doubling of the rates of instrumented fusions was seen [37].

Future trends – beside the extensive use of instrumentation – in spine surgery for degenerative disorders of the lumbar spine might be the increased use of less or minimally invasive techniques [22], the application of bone substitutes in order to improve fusion rates [25, 52], and the implementation of an entire spectrum of non-fusion technology, which consists of pedicle screw-based posterior devices for dynamic stabilization [44], interspinous process technology [11], and different TDR designs [42].

Because new technology for spinal surgery is introduced at an ever-increasing pace, substantial changes in the surgical patterns in the future can be anticipated. The scenario of introduction of synthetic cages for lumbar spine surgery in 1996 in the U.S. [16] may serve as an example of how new technology relates to surgical rates and patterns. Most likely, the introduction of new implants, bone graft products, and surgical techniques will also have such an impact in the future.

Summary

LBP has been considered to be a 20th century epidemic and a nemesis to modern medicine. The key factor in dealing with this entity is to distinguish between the specific and the non-specific form. The latter is much more frequent and is characterized by a missing correlation between the clinical picture and structural morphological changes. The main problem of LBP is its tendency to chronicity. Therefore, both in specific forms due to degenerative disorders and in non-specific forms the main efforts should be placed on the prevention of disability. Conservative therapy consists of pain medication, physical therapy, and behavioral treatment. If these modalities fail, surgery should be considered. In case of spinal stenosis, decompressive surgery alone or in combination with fusion can be performed. In degenerative instability, which includes spondylolisthesis as well as de-novo scoliosis, deformity correction and stabilization with or without decompression might be required. Non-specific LBP due to DDD also can be addressed surgically by means of instrumented fusion or with dynamic devices. Single series have demonstrated good results for all these indications and surgical techniques. However, with regard to evidence-based outcome assessment, there is a considerable lack of high quality investigations of lumbar fusion for degenerative disorders.

References

1. Aebi M (2005) The adult scoliosis. Eur Spine J 14:925–948
2. Airaksinen O, Brox JI, Cedraschi C, Hildebrandt J, Klaber-Moffett J, Kovacs F, Mannion AF, Reis S, Staal JB, Ursin H, Zanoli G (2006) Chapter 4. European guidelines for the management of chronic nonspecific low back pain. Eur Spine J 15 (Suppl 2):192–300
3. Amundsen T, Weber H, Nordal HJ, Magnaes B, Abdelnoor M, Lilleas F (2000) Lumbar spinal stenosis: conservative or surgical management? A prospective 10-year study. Spine 25:1424–1435
4. Andersson HI, Ejlertsson G, Leden I, Rosenberg C (1993) Chronic pain in a geographically defined general population: studies of differences in age, gender, social class, and pain localization. Clin J Pain 9:174–182
5. Atlas SJ, Delitto A (2006) Spinal stenosis: surgical versus nonsurgical treatment. Clin Orthop 443:198–207
6. Boden SD, Davis DO, Dina TS, Patronas NJ, Wiesel SW (1990) Abnormal magnetic-resonance scans of the lumbar spine in asymptomatic subjects. A prospective investigation. J Bone Joint Surg Am 72:403–408
7. Bono CM, Lee CK (2004) Critical analysis of trends in fusion for degenerative disc disease over the past 20 years. Influence of technique on fusion rate and clinical outcome. Spine 29:455–463
8. Brox JI, Sorensen R, Friis A, Nygaard O, Indahl A, Keller A, Ingebrigtsen T, Eriksen HR, Holm I, Koller AK, Rise R, Reikeras O (2003) Randomized clinical trial of lumbar instrumented fusion and cognitive intervention and exercises in patients with chronic low back pain and disc degeneration. Spine 28:1913–1921
9. Carey TS, Mielenz TJ (2007) Measuring outcomes in back care. Spine 32:9–14
10. Christensen FB (2004) Lumbar spinal fusion. Outcome in relation to surgical methods, choice of implant and postoperative rehabilitation. Acta Orthop Scand (Suppl) 75:2–43
11. Christie SD, Song JK, Fessler RG (2005) Dynamic interspinous process technology. Spine 30:73–78
12. Ciol MA, Deyo RA, Howell E, Kreif S (1996) An assessment of surgery for spinal stenosis. Time trends, geographic variations, complications, and reoperations. J Am Geriatr Soc 44:285–290
13. Cloward RB (1985) Posterior lumbar interbody fusion updated. Clin Orthop 193:16–19
14. Deyo RA, Ciol MA, Cherkin DC, Loeser JD, Bigos SJ (1993) Lumbar spinal fusion. A cohort study of complications, reoperations, and resource use in the Medicare population. Spine 18:1463–1470
15. Deyo RA, Nachemson A, Mirza SK (2004) Spinal-fusion surgery – the case for restraint. N Engl J Med 350:722–726
16. Deyo RA, Mirza SK (2006) Trends and variations in the use of spine surgery. Clin Orthop 443:139–146
17. Epstein NE (1998) Decompression in the surgical management of degenerative spondylolisthesis: advantages of a conservative approach in 290 patients. J Spinal Disord 11:116–122

18. Fagan A, Moore R, Vernon Roberts B, Blumbergs P, Fraser R (2003) ISSLS prize winner. The innervation of the intervertebral disc. A quantitative analysis. Spine 28:2570–2576
19. Fischgrund JS, Mackay M, Herkowitz HN, Brower R, Montgomery DM, Kurz LT (1997) 1997 Volvo Award winner in clinical studies. Degenerative lumbar spondylolisthesis with spinal stenosis. A prospective, randomized study comparing decompressive laminectomy and arthrodesis with and without spinal instrumentation. Spine 22:2807–2812
20. Fritzell P, Hagg O, Wessberg P, Nordwall A (2001) 2001 Volvo Award winner in clinical studies. Lumbar fusion versus nonsurgical treatment for chronic low back pain. A multicenter randomized controlled trial from the Swedish Lumbar Spine Study Group. Spine 26:2521–2532
21. Fritzell P, Hagg O, Wessberg P, Nordwall A (2002) Chronic low back pain and fusion. A comparison of three surgical techniques. A prospective multicenter randomized study from the Swedish lumbar spine study group. Spine 27:1131–1141
22. German JW, Foley KT (2005) Minimal access surgical techniques in the management of the painful lumbar motion segment. Spine 30:52–59
23. Gibson JN, Grant IC, Waddell G (1999) The Cochrane review of surgery for lumbar disc prolapse and degenerative lumbar spondylosis. Spine 24:1820–1832
24. Gibson JN, Waddell G (2005) Surgery for degenerative lumbar spondylosis. Updated Cochrane Review. Spine 30:2312–2320
25. Glassman SD, Carreon L, Djurasovic M, Campbell MJ, Puno RM, Johnson JR, Dimar JR (2007) Posterolateral lumbar spine fusion with INFUSE bone graft. Spine J 7:44–49
26. Grobler LJ, Robertson PA, Novotny JE, Pope MH (1993) Etiology of spondylolisthesis. Assessment of the role played by lumbar facet joint morphology. Spine 18:80–91
27. Hagg O, Fritzell P, Oden A, Nordwall A (2002) Simplifying outcome measurement. Evaluation of instruments for measuring outcome after fusion surgery for chronic low back pain. Spine 27:1213–1222
28. Hagg O, Fritzell P, Ekselius L, Nordwall A (2003) Predictors of outcome in fusion surgery for chronic low back pain. A report from the Swedish Lumbar Spine Study. Eur Spine J 12:22–33
29. Harms JG, Jeszenszky D (1998) Die posteriore, lumbale, interkorporelle Fusion in unilateraler transforaminaler Technik. Operat Orthop Traumatol 10:90–102
30. Herkowitz HN, Kurz LT (1991) Degenerative lumbar spondylolisthesis with spinal stenosis. A prospective study comparing decompression with decompression and intertransverse process arthrodesis. J Bone Joint Surg Am 73:802–808
31. Hestbaek L, Leboeuf-Yde C, Manniche C (2003) Low back pain: what is the long-term course? A review of studies of general patient populations. Eur Spine J 12:149–165
32. Kirkaldy-Willis WH, Farfan HF (1982) Instability of the lumbar spine. Clin Orthop 165:110–123
33. Knaub MA, Won DS, McGuire R, Herkowitz HN (2005) Lumbar spinal stenosis: indications for arthrodesis and spinal instrumentation. Instr Course Lect 54:313–319
34. Koes BW, van Tulder MW, Ostelo R, Kim Burton A, Waddell G (2001) Clinical guidelines for the management of low back pain in primary care. An international comparison. Spine 26:2504–2513
35. Kornblum MB, Fischgrund JS, Herkowitz HN, Abraham DA, Berkower DL, Ditkoff JS (2004) Degenerative lumbar spondylolisthesis with spinal stenosis. A prospective long-term study comparing fusion and pseudarthrosis. Spine 29:726–733
36. Lonstein JE (2006) Scoliosis: surgical versus nonsurgical treatment. Clin Orthop 443:248–259
37. Lurie JD, Weinstein JN (2001) Shared decision-making and the orthopaedic workforce. Clin Orthop 385:68–75
38. Malmivaara A, Slatis P, Heliovaara M, Sainio P, Kinnunen H, Kankare J, Dalin-Hirvonen N, Seitsalo S, Herno A, Kortekangas P, Niinimaki T, Ronty H, Tallroth K, Turunen V, Knekt P, Harkanen T, Hurri H (2007) Surgical or nonoperative treatment for lumbar spinal stenosis? A randomized controlled trial. Spine 32:1–8
39. Mardjetko SM, Connolly PJ, Shott S (1994) Degenerative lumbar spondylolisthesis. A meta-analysis of literature 1970–1993. Spine 19:2256–2265
40. Martin CR, Gruszczynski AT, Braunsfurth HA, Fallatah SM, O'Neil J, Wai EK (2007) The surgical management of degenerative lumbar spondylolisthesis. A systematic review. Spine 32:1791–1798
41. Matsunaga S, Ijiri K, Hayashi K (2000) Nonsurgically managed patients with degenerative spondylolisthesis. A 10- to 18-year follow-up study. J Neurosurg 93:194–198
42. Mayer HM (2005) Total lumbar disc replacement. J Bone Joint Surg Br 87:1029–1037
43. Moller H, Hedlund R (2000) Surgery versus conservative management in adult isthmic spondylolisthesis – a prospective randomized study. Part 1. Spine 25:1711–1715
44. Nockels RP (2005) Dynamic stabilization in the surgical management of painful lumbar spinal disorders. Spine 30:68–72
45. Nordin M, Balague F, Cedraschi C (2006) Non-specific lower-back pain. Surgical versus nonsurgical treatment. Clin Orthop 443:156–167
46. Ostelo RW, van Tulder MW, Vlaeyen JW, Linton SJ, Morley SJ, Assendelft WJ (2005) Behavioural treatment for chronic low-back pain. Cochrane Database Syst Rev CD002014

47. Penning L, Wilmink JT (1987) Posture-dependent bilateral compression of L4 or L5 nerve roots in facet hypertrophy. A dynamic CT-myelographic study. Spine 12:488–500
48. Ploumis A, Transfledt EE, Denis F (2007) Degenerative lumbar scoliosis associated with spinal stenosis. Spine J 7:428–436
49. Porter RW (1996) Spinal stenosis and neurogenic claudication. Spine 21:2046–2052
50. Rydevik B, Brown MD, Lundborg G (1984) Pathoanatomy and pathophysiology of nerve root compression. Spine 9:7–15
51. Siepe CJ, Mayer HM, Wiechert K, Korge A (2006) Clinical results of total lumbar disc replacement with ProDisc II. Three-year results for different indications. Spine 31:1923–1932
52. Singh K, Smucker JD, Gill S, Boden SD (2006) Use of recombinant human bone morphogenetic protein-2 as an adjunct in posterolateral lumbar spine fusion. A prospective CT-scan analysis at one and two years. J Spinal Disord Tech 19:416–423
53. Trief PM, Ploutz-Snyder R, Fredrickson BE (2006) Emotional health predicts pain and function after fusion. A prospective multicenter study. Spine 31:823–830
54. Vibert BT, Sliva CD, Herkowitz HN (2006) Treatment of instability and spondylolisthesis. Surgical versus nonsurgical treatment. Clin Orthop 443:222–227
55. Waddell G (1987) 1987 Volvo award in clinical sciences. A new clinical model for the treatment of low-back pain. Spine 12:632–644
56. Walker BF (2000) The prevalence of low back pain. A systematic review of the literature from 1966 to 1998. J Spinal Disord 13:205–217
57. Watkins MB (1953) Posterolateral fusion of the lumbar and lumbosacral spine. J Bone Joint Surg Am 35:1014–1018
58. Weinstein JN, Lurie JD, Tosteson TD, Hanscom B, Tosteson AN, Blood EA, Birkmeyer NJ, Hilibrand AS, Herkowitz H, Cammisa FP, Albert TJ, Emery SE, Lenke LG, Abdu WA, Longley M, Errico TJ, Hu SS (2007) Surgical versus nonsurgical treatment for lumbar degenerative spondylolisthesis. N Engl J Med 356:2257–2270
59. Wiltse LL, Newman PH, Macnab I (1976) Classification of spondylolisis and spondylolisthesis. Clin Orthop 117:23–29

6 Herniation of the lumbar intervertebral disc – when is surgery required?

BALKAN CAKIR, HEIKO REICHEL, and WOLFRAM KÄFER

Background

Lumbar disc herniation (LDH) is the pathologic condition most commonly responsible for lumboradicular pain, and the condition for which lumbar surgery is carried out most frequently. The first description of a disc herniation was given by the anatomist Luschka [48]. In 1909 Krause was the first physician who performed a discectomy unwittingly as he thought that the removed material was a chondrom [56]. Therefore the first surgeons who performed and described a surgical excision of a ruptured intervertebral disc with knowledge of the pathophysiological interaction of radicular pain and LDH were Mixter and Barr in 1934 [52]. Since this time, many consider LDH to be a surgical issue.

But after the the landmark paper of Weber in 1983 [68] the pendulum regarding the best treatment has shifted from surgery towards nonsurgical treatment options. In this prospective study 126 patients were radomized from a series of 280 cases with herniated disc shown by myelographic assessment. These 126 patients with uncertain indications for sugery were allocated randomly to operative (60 patients) or conservative (66 patients) treatment. The 1-year follow-up showed better results in the operated group. However, the 4-year follow-up showed the same trend, but the difference between the two groups was no longer statistically significant. There was no difference between the two groups after ten years [68]. This study thus indicates that there is no significant difference at medium and long-term follow-up between the results of the operative and the non-operative treatment group.

In contrast to those findings, the long-term outcome of the Maine Lumbar Spine Study, a prospective cohort study, revelaed that surgically treated patients with a herniated lumbar disc had more complete relief of leg pain and improved function and satisfaction compared with non-surgically treated patients over ten years [4]. Nevertheless, improvement in patients predominant symptoms as well as in work and disability outcomes were similar regardless of treatment received.

These two scientific papers are symptomatic for the current therapeutical approach in LDH as they vary widely and as there is no general agreement on what is the preferred method of treatment, or at what stage of the illness various invasive treatments should be initiated. Probably this is the main reason why marked differences in the rates of surgery for LDH exist among western countries [17], which might reflect in part differences in attitudes of both physicians and patients. For instance the rate of back surgery in the United States was at least 40% higher than in any other country and it was more than five times higher than those in England and Scotland [17]. Moreover countries with high back surgery rates also had high rates of other discretionary procedures such as tonsillectomy and hysterectomy.

When comparing operative and non-operative treatment options the obvious and undisputable advantage of non-operative treatment is the absence of complications related to surgery. Any surgical procedure, no matter how carefully it is performed, has risks. Common complicatons in discectomy include wrong level surgery, missed pathology and/or retained disc, cerebrospinal fluid (CSF) leakage, epidural venous bleeding with epidural hematoma, iatrogenic instability with residual back pain, infection/discitis, thromb-embolism and postoperative epidural fibrosis [6]. The reported intra- and postoperative complication rate varies between 3% and 24.8% for standard nucleotomy and between 2.3% and 10.8% in microsurgical discectomy [8, 12, 43, 57, 65]. An argument for non-operative treatment is also the rate of re-operations after discectomy. With regard to the published data with sufficient follow-up period and sufficient number of patients, the revision rate after disc-

Table 6.1. Long term outcome and revision rate of lumbar discectomy.

Autor	Year	Patients (number)	Follow-up (years)	Success rate (%)	Revision rate (%)
Williams [71]	1990	989	~15	85.2	14.8
Pappas et al. [57]	1992	654	~4.5	76.3	9.3
Davis [18]	1994	984	⌀ 10.8	89	6
Jerosch and Castro [36]	1996	846	19–42	–	7.9

ectomy varies between 6% and 14.8% [18, 36, 57, 71] (Table 6.1).

With these figures in mind there is no doubt that surgery has to be reserved for patients who will not benefit from non-operative treatment. But nowadays there is still no consensus which criteria support or even justify the indication for surgery.

The purpose of this paper is to analyze some diagnostic findings, which are often considered as reliable criteria for decision-making in patients with LDH.

Paresis

Cauda equina syndrome (CES), which occurs in approximately 2% of all herniated lumbar discs [42], is thought to be the primary absolute indication for an acute surgical treatment of LDH [21, 42, 62–64]. The clinical features can include low-back pain, uni- or bilateral sciatica, saddle anaesthesia, motor weakness in the lower extremities that may progress to paraplegia with bowel and bladder dysfunction [2, 46, 50, 59].

Although there is common agreement that CES due to LDH should be treated with surgical decompression by means of lumbar laminectomy and discectomy, there is still controversial debate on the timing of surgical decompression, as some reports showed that delayed surgery may also provide satisfactory results [13, 14, 27, 42, 55, 64]. But the common problem of these studies is the limited number of patients included due to the rarity of this disorder. Therefore most of the published data inheres limited power and inability to achieve statistical significance. Ahn et al. were the first who conducted a meta-analysis of surgical outcome in CES secondary to LDH [1]. Forty-two articles met the criteria for inclusion in the study. In all studies included, CES was caused by LDH. Articles with CES caused by spinal stenosis, tumor, hematoma, fracture, infection, or ankylosing spondylitis were excluded. All patients were treated with surgical decompression and patients who refused surgery were also excluded. There was no difference in outcome between patients treated less than 24 hours after onset of CES and those treated within 24 to 48 hours. However, there was a significant advantage in treating patients within 48 hours, with improved outcome in resolution of sensory deficit, motor deficit, urinary function, and rectal function. The presence of preoperative chronic low back pain (LBP) was associated with poorer outcomes in urinary and rectal function. Preoperative rectal dysfunction was associated with a worsened outcome in urinary continence. Older patients were less likely to fully regain sexual function after surgery [1].

But even nowadays, the topic of an adequate time frame until surgery in CES is still controversial. In the recently published study by McCarty and co-workers the authors report about the results of 42 patients with evidence of a sphincteric disturbance who underwent urgent surgery [51]. 26 patients were operated on within 48 hours of onset of sphincteric symptoms, five of these within 24 hours. However, acute onset of sphincteric symptoms and the time to operation did not influence the outcomes two years after surgery [51].

Beside CES, paresis is also regarded as serious sign in patients with disc herniation. But does paresis justify surgery? Some authors regard surgery as the therapy of choice if the pressure on the root can be relieved immediately after its appearance [69]. Although the existence of paresis is a sign of seriousness, published data nonetheless indicate that paresis does require immediate surgery. The choice of treatment (operative versus non-operative) is not a prognostic factor for the recovery from or an improvement of paresis. Some authors reported about superior results by means of better motoric recovery or improvement after surgery in their retrospective studies, but they missed to include any statistical analysis. Bloch-Michel et al. reported about a recorvery/improvement rate of the paresis after surgery in 64% [9]. In contrast, the recovery/improvement rate was only 56% after non-operative treatment [9]. The same tendency was reported by Weigert and co-workers with recovery/improvement in 77% of the surgical treated patients versus 53% in the non-operatively treated patients [69]. On the other hand, there are also retrospective studies with contradictory findings. De Seze et al. reported about a lower recovery rate in patients treated operatively (54%) versus conservatively (63%) [19]. In the fundamental study of Weber, which had a prospective and randomized study design, the recovery rate was 70% in both groups (surgical and non-surgical) [68]. Therefore just the clinical presentation of paresis in LDH does not justify a surgical procedure.

But some authors still criticize the landmark paper of Weber [68] since neither criteria for recovery or improvement were defined nor the magnitude of paresis was considered. If the paresis itself would not justify an operative treatment, does the grading of paresis represent a good predictor for further treatment? Dubourg et al. addressed this problem in an open prospective multi-center study [22]. They enrolled patients with discogenic sciatica and concomitant paresis that had been present for less than one month and was rated ≤3 on a 5-point scale. Bilateral muscular testing of eleven lower limb muscles or groups of muscles was performed. Recovery and improvement were defined by pain not exceeding 20 mm on a visual analog scale (VAS) or pain ≤50% of the initial pain score and a score of either 5 (recovery) or 4 (improvement) for the weakest muscle at inclusion. At six month follow-up 14 of 25 patients (56%) of the non-operatively treated group had an improvement of the paresis and ten out of these 25 patients even a recovery (40%). 17 of 32 (53%) patients treated with discectomy had an improvement and eight out of these 32 patients (25%) had a recovery [22]. One of the major shortcomings of this study is the short follow-up period of six months. Therefore the recovery rate might have been underestimated. But on the other hand, Jonsson and co-workers reported about a recovery of the neurologic deficit in half of their patients two years after surgery, with the major part of this improvement occurring within four months after operation [37].

Although numerous bias might have affected the results of the study of Duborg et al. [22], like the lack of randomization, the missing evaluation of the intra- and inter-observer reproducibility of the muscle testing and the fact that patients undergoing surgery had sciatica for a longer time than the conservatively treated controls, it forms the basis for randomized studies in the future. Considering that no other conflictive data have been published in the literature until now, it seems that surgical treatment of sciatica with discogenic paresis is not more beneficial than non-operative treatment.

Although published data support the finding that paresis and paresis magnitude are not of relevant importance with regard to the therapeutical approach, the duration of paresis until surgery might be of crucial importance for neurological recovery? Therefore the question stated in the paper of Eysel and co-workers: "Should a patient with an acute paresis be treated surgically in an emergency procedure or is there any time left for a conservative attempt?" [25] is of substantial interest for the clinical setting. With regard to the published results in CES one might argue that it is obvious that the time frame between neurologic impairment and subsequent surgery should have a considerable effect on motoric recovery. But this impression is not supported by published data. There is no statistical proof for the influence of the duration of the paresis on its prognosis. Knutson et al. reported on 110 patients with paresis of the extensor of the great toe [40]. After operation paresis persisted in 26 patients, but the time from the first occurrence of the paresis did not have any influence on the motoric recovery. In a retrospective study, Eysel et al. analyzed the neurological recovery of 240 patients with radicular paralytic symptoms with regard to the grading of the paresis and the time elapsed since the occurrence of the paresis [25]. The distribution of the intensity of the paresis was as follows using a 5-grade scale: 111 patients grade 4, 99 patients grade 3, 66 patients grade 2, 13 patients grade 1 and six patients with grade 0 (paralysis). The distribution of patients with regard to the time delay until surgery was as follows: 77 patients less than one day, 73 patients less than three days, 55 patients less than one week, 55 patients less than four weeks and 35 patients more than four weeks. The grading of the paresis was a good prognostic criterion for the assessment of the postoperative course. Paresis grade 3 or 4 receded in more than 70% of the cases within six months, whereas the recovery rate in paresis grade 2 was 40% and in case of paralysis no complete neurological recovery was registered. However the period of time, which had elapsed since the occurrence of the paresis did not show any significant influence on motoric recovery.

An influence of duration between onset of the paresis and surgical treatment was reported by Weigert et al. [69]. In 344 patients treated surgically for L5 or S1 root compression, 58 patients had preoperatively a paresis. In 77% a complete recovery was assessed after operation. Referring to the duration of paresis there was no influence within the first year (recovery rate 80%) whether the paresis had existed for one month or one year. Only in patients with a paresis lasting longer than one year the recovery rate worsened (65%).

When analyzing the prognostic value of paresis one possible objective could be that especially in patients with paralysis, not with paresis, the time prior to surgery might be of crucial importance. Interestingly, in the afore mentioned study of Duborg et al. only patients with sciatic discogenic paresis, but not paralysis were involved [22]. Also when looking at the study of Eysel et al. only six out of 240 patients had a paralysis and the time frame until surgery was not reported in detail for these six patients [25]. Therefore these studies are not able to give strong evidence if the time frame until surgery is of predictive value in case of paralysis. The prognosis in case of complete paralysis has been evaluated by Andersson et al. [3]. However, they did not find any correlation between the time since onset of the symptoms until operation and the restitution of muscular function in patients operated on with complete paralysis of the dorsal flexors of the foot [3].

Although the duration of paralytic symptoms did not have any proven influence on motoric recovery after surgery, Woertgen et al. reported that it has a value as general predictive factor with regard to the clinical outcome after lumbar disc surgery [72]. In a prospective study with 121 patients they assessed the results after lumbar disc surgery with four different outcome measures (Prolo Scale, Low Back Outcome Score, Pain Grading Scale and Quality of Life) and concluded that predictive factors are different for different outcome scales. Nonetheless, the preoperative duration of paresis seemed to be a predictive factor of general relevance [72].

Pain

When conservative treatment for symptomatic disc herniation is considered, a question which needs to be addressed is: "What is a reasonable period of time for conservative treatement and how long should the treating physician council perseverance to a patient with severe sciatica? Is there a time limit when the results of subsequent surgery will deteriorate?"

It has been suggested that the probability of symptoms resolving with conservative treatment decreases progressively with time. Moreover in many studies prolonged pain has been regarded as a negative predictor for subsequent surgical therapy [36, 45, 53, 54, 58, 61, 72]. In his landmark paper, Weber proposed a period of three months to be sufficient to decide against surgery in four-fifths of the 60% conservatively treated patients with good and fair results [68]. But he also pointed out that if all patients with doubtful surgical indications had to wait for three months before a decision was made, 40% would spend this time in a more or less painful condition with possible psychosocial consequences. Therefore he advised to inform the patient so that he/she may be able to participate in the decision at an earlier stage. In conclusion the time limit of three months in the paper of Weber [68] is mainly based on the personal opinion of the author and is not proven by his data. The same is true for the period of two to three months proposed by Postacchini since he did not analyzed the outcome of the patients with regard to the time frame until surgery [58]. In contrast, Nygaard et al. analyzed in a prospective study of 132 consecutive patients the prognostic value of preoperative leg pain [54]. The authors came to the conclusion that leg pain lasting more than eight months correlates with an unfavorable postoperative outcome and with a high risk of not returning to work. Ng and Sell even proposed a threshold for the duration of sciatica of twelve months [53]. Some of the reported thresholds of the duration of sciatica, which is associated with poor outcome, are listed in Table 6.2.

The different boundary values reported in the literature for the duration of sciatica until the results of surgical intervention are expected to deteriorate may be partially explained by the results of the study of Woertgen and co-workers [72]. They analyzed the clinical results after discectomy with four different outcome measurements

Table 6.2. Reported thresholds of the duration of sciatica, which is associated with poor outcome.

Author	Year	Duration
Hurme et al. [34]	1987	> 2 months
Postacchini [58]	1996	> 2–3 months
Dvorak et al. [23]	1988	> 6 months
Jerosch et al. [36]	1996	> 6 months
Carragee [16]	1997	> 6 months
Nygaard et al. [54]	1994	> 8 months
Ng and Sell [53]	1996	> 12 months

and found that beside preoperative duration of paresis only the duration of preoperative pain was a predictive factor of the assessed outcome scales. They divided the clinical results in a dichotomic manner into good or poor results. With regard to the used scoring system the average duration of pain in patients with poor results differed markedly. When looking at the clinical results obtained with the "Quality of life score", patients with poor outcome had an average duration of pain of 209 days. In contrast, patients with poor results with regard to the "Low back out come score" had an average pain duration of 159 days prior to surgery. These numbers highlight that the main problem is still in assessing the clinical outcome of patients with LDH. Korres et al. already addressed this problem when they evaluated the results of lumbar discectomy using 15 different evaluation methods in 92 patients who had undergone a primary excision of a lumbar disc [41]. The satisfactory results ranged from 62% to 84% with regard to the evaluation method used. Therefore most of the studies analyzing the threshold of the duration of sciatica, which is associated with poor outcome, are not really comparable. In view of the favourable course of non-operative treatment in LDH, most authors recommend at least a period of conservative management of two months (Table 6.2). But with regard to the published data this threshold should not exceed twelve months since the risk of poor functional outcome then increases.

Beside a multitude of possible pre- and postoperative somatic causes of persistent pain, many studies have also addressed the importance of psychologic and social predictors of therapy outcome in lumbar disc prolapse [11, 23, 24, 29, 30, 32, 38]. Wilkinson, who focused attention on the problem of chronic pain after surgical and conservative treatment, introduced the term "failed back syndrome" (FBS), which is not a diagnosis but a collective term for patients with chronic pain after an acute LDH [70]. Between 10% and 60% of patients undergoing surgery or conservative treatment show signs of FBS during the months and years after treatment [23, 31]. In a systematic review Boer et al. analyzed eleven studies which addressed the predictive value of bio-psychosocial risk factors with regard to outcome after lumbar disc surgery [20]. The results indicated that socio-demographic, clinical, work-related as well as psychological factors predict lumbar disc surgery outcome. The findings showed relatively consistently that a lower level of education, a higher level of preoperative pain, less work satisfaction, a longer duration of sick leave, higher levels of psychological complaints and a more passive avoidance coping act as predictors of an unfavourable outcome in terms of pain, disability, work capacity, or a combination of these outcome measures. Junge and co-workers assessed 381 patients in six different spine centers after indication for discectomy was established [38]. The objective of the study was, beside others, to determine socio-demographic and psychological factors that might influence the outcome of lumbar disc surgery, as well as to develop a screening checklist and a score of reliable predictors to distinguish bad and good responders of surgery. At six months 89% and at twelve months, 86% of all operated patients were available for follow-up study. There was no significant difference in the outcome between the six and the twelve months follow-ups. At twelve months, 51.5% of the patients had a good, 28.4% a moderate, and 20.1% a bad outcome. The calculation of a predictor score gave an appropriate overall prediction of 80% as well as 76% for good outcome and for 79% for bad outcome, respectively. As final conclusion the authors proposed to include the Hannover mobility questionnaire, the Back depression inventory, and structured interviews in the process of preoperative assessment for disc surgery in addition to clinical and radiological examinations [38].

Type of disc herniation

Nowadays the definition of type of herniation is mainly based on magnetic resonance imaging (MRI) findings. Several definitions of disc herniation have already been introduced, understood and reported. These classifications compromise protrusion versus prolapse or contained versus non-contained herniation. Contained discs, which are wholly within an intact outer anulus or a capsule composed of the outer anulus and the posterior longitudinal ligament (PLL), are not in direct contact with epidural tissue, whereas non-contained discs are in direct contact. The discrimination of different types of disc herniation with MRI seems to be possible with acceptable sensitivity, specificity and accuracy. Kim et al. analyzed 211 patients with lumbar disc herniation at 242 levels and classified the type of herniations into five groups by their appearance on MRI [39]. The comparison with the findings at operation revealed 92% sensitivity, 91% specificity, and 92% accuracy of the MRI classification in distinguishing between protruded discs from other forms of LDH. For sequestrated discs these values were as follows: 92% sensitivity, 99% specificity, and 97% accuracy. In the extruded subligamentous type the values were 71% for sensitivity, 82% for specificity, and 79% for accuracy. Finally, in the extruded trans-ligamentous type the values were as follows: 52% sensitivity, 92% specificity, and 81% accuracy [39].

Although the classification of different types of disc herniation is possible on MRI with sufficient accuracy, the clinical meaningfulness, however, is uncertain. Gaetani et al. analyzed the records of 403 patients treated for LDH in a retrospective observational study in order to verify how three outcome measures, i.e. satisfaction with the outcome of surgery, the degree of return to activities of daily living including work (ADL), and duration of interruption of ADL, might be influenced by clinical variables [26]. The results of their study suggested that age and type of disc herniation were among the most important factors to consider when deciding whether or not to operate on patients with LDH [26].

However, the results of Gaetani and co-workers [26] are in contrast to the observations of Beattie et al., who compared in a MRI cross-sectional study of 408 symptomatic subjects the relationship of symptoms with anatomic impairment [7]. The presence of disc extrusion and/or equilateral severe nerve compression at one or at multiple sites was strongly associated with distal leg pain. In contrast, mild to moderate nerve compression, disc degeneration or bulging, and central spinal canal stenosis were not significantly associated with specific pain patterns [7]. Boos et al. confirmed these results in their prospective study of patients with symptomatic disc herniations and asymptomatic volunteers [10]. They came to the conclusion, that individuals with minor disc herniations (e.g., protrusion or contained disc) are at a very high risk that their MRI findings are not a causal explanation of pain because a high rate of asymptomatic subjects had comparable morphological findings [10].

The observations of Beattie et al. and Boos et al. [7, 10] are also supported when looking at the reported results after surgery with regard to the type of herniation. Carragee and co-workers analyzed the influence of anulus integrity and the type of herniation on the postoperative clinical outcome following lumbar discectomy [15]. On the basis of intraoperative findings disc herniations were classified into four categories:
1) fragment-fissure herniations,
2) fragment-defect herniations,
3) fragment-contained herniations, and
4) no fragment-contained herniations.

Patients in the fragment-fissure group, who had disc fragments and a small anular defect, had the best overall outcome and the lowest rate of re-herniations (1%) as well as re-operations (1%). Patients in the no fragment-contained group did poorly: 38% had recurrent or persistent sciatica [15]. Furthermore, Hirabayashi et al. reported about a higher incidence of second operations after lumbar micro-discectomy in patients with protrusion-type herniations than in those with extrusion-type or sequestration-type herniations [33].

But even a non-contained disc herniation with corresponding radicular pain or paresis is not an absolute indication for surgical intervention. Referring to Krämer, spontaneous resolution of symptoms and retraction of free fragments in LDH are possible, especially if the fragment is well hydrated (→ shrinkage), the whole volume of the fragment is less than 1/3 of spinal canal diameter and the fragment has a contact to the epidural membrane, which has a good blood supply (→ possible resorption) [44]. Ito et al. described an interesting phenomenon in their study population [35], which would support the hypotheses of Krämer [44]. Over seven years, they noted that surgeries for disc herniation most frequently encountered free fragments when done within two months after the onset of severe leg pain [35].

In a subsequent, prospective series, they found that free extruded fragments seldom were found at surgery, if the patient had been treated at least for two months conservatively. The authors' interpretation of these results is that disc resorption selectively targets these extruded fragments and that patients with non-contained lumbar disc herniations can be treated without surgery, if they can tolerate the symptoms for the first two months. The spontaneous disappearance or diminution of herniated discs in the lumbar spinal canal has also been described by others [28, 49, 60, 66, 67]. Autio et al. analyzed rim enhancement in herniated nucleus pulposus (HNP) in gadolinium diethylenetriamine pentaacetic acid MRI as neovascularization in the outermost areas of HNP, since such presentation of an enhancing rim is thought to be a major determinant of spontaneous resorption of HNP [5]. Thickness of rim enhancement was a stronger determinant of spontaneous resorption than extent of rim enhancement. In their study, higher baseline scores of rim enhancement thickness, higher degree of HNP displacement in the Komori classification, and age category 41 to 50 years were associated with a higher resorption rate. Moreover, clinical symptom alleviation occurred concordantly with a faster resorption rate. The final conclusion of their study was that MRI is a useful prognostic tool for identifying patients with HNP-induced sciatica and a benign natural course [5].

Conclusion

With regard to the literature the only clear indication for surgery in case of LDH is the CES. Even in this severe complication of LDH there is no strong evidence that emergency surgery is necessary. Nevertheless surgery should be performed as soon as possible and a delay should only be considered if the perioperative risk for the patient could be decreased markedly. Although paresis is regarded as serious sign in patients with disc herniation, neither the magnitude nor the duration of paresis constitute an indication for early surgery. Although there is no strong evidence in the literature, progression of paralytic symptoms should also be considered as indication for surgery.

Non-operative treatment methods should be applied at least over a time period of two months but should not be extended beyond one year if the patient shows only minimal improvement, since the results of surgery are diminished after this time.

With regard to published data the type of herniation on MRI seems not to be one of the most important factors to consider when deciding whether or not to operate on a patient with LDH.

The statement of Dr. John D. Lurie: "It can be far more difficult to rigorously evaluate commonly used interventions than novel approaches. When interventions are more familiar, there is always the impression that we already know how they work and how well they work. Even when there are little data to support such impressions" [47] should always be kept in mind when treating patients with LDH, especially when it comes to decision-making with regard to surgery.

References

1. Ahn UM, Ahn NU, Buchowski JM, Garrett ES, Sieber AN, Kostuik JP (2000) Cauda equina syndrome secondary to lumbar disc herniation: a meta-analysis of surgical outcomes. Spine 25:1515–1522
2. Andersen JT, Bradley WE (1976) Neurogenic bladder dysfunction in protruded lumbar disk and after laminectomy. Urology 8:94–96
3. Andersson H, Carlsson CA (1966) Prognosis of operatively treated lumbar disc herniations causing foot extensor paralysis. Acta Chir Scand 132:501–506
4. Atlas SJ, Keller RB, Wu YA, Deyo RA, Singer DE (2005) Long-term outcomes of surgical and nonsurgical management of sciatica secondary to a lumbar disc herniation: 10 year results from the maine lumbar spine study. Spine 30:927–935
5. Autio RA, Karppinen J, Niinimaki J, Ojala R, Kurunlahti M, Haapea M, Vanharanta H, Tervonen O (2006) Determinants of spontaneous resorption of intervertebral disc herniations. Spine 31:1247–1252
6. Awad JN, Moskovich R (2006) Lumbar disc herniations: surgical versus nonsurgical treatment. Clin Orthop 443:183–197
7. Beattie PF, Meyers SP, Stratford P, Millard RW, Hollenberg GM (2000) Associations between patient report of symptoms and anatomic impairment visible on lumbar magnetic resonance imaging. Spine 25:819–828
8. Best NM, Sasso RC (2006) Success and safety in outpatient microlumbar discectomy. J Spinal Disord Tech 19:334–337

9. Bloch Michel H, Cauchoix J, Benoist M (1967) A propos de 60 observations de sciatique paralysante. Sem Hop 43:2640–2646
10. Boos N, Rieder R, Schade V, Spratt KF, Semmer N, Aebi M (1995) 1995 Volvo Award in clinical sciences. The diagnostic accuracy of magnetic resonance imaging, work perception, and psychosocial factors in identifying symptomatic disc herniations. Spine 20:2613–2625
11. Boos N, Semmer N, Elfering A, Schade V, Gal I, Zanetti M, Kissling R, Buchegger N, Hodler J, Main CJ (2000) Natural history of individuals with asymptomatic disc abnormalities in magnetic resonance imaging: predictors of low back pain-related medical consultation and work incapacity. Spine 25:1484–1492
12. Bouillet R (1990) Treatment of sciatica. A comparative survey of complications of surgical treatment and nucleolysis with chymopapain. Clin Orthop 251:144–152
13. Buchner M, Schiltenwolf M (2002) Cauda equina syndrome caused by intervertebral lumbar disk prolapse: mid-term results of 22 patients and literature review. Orthopedics 25:727–731
14. Bues E, Markakis E (1969) Über die postoperative Rückbildung neurologischer Ausfälle und zur Frage des Operationstermines beim medialen lumbalen Bandscheibenvorfall. Dtsch Z Nervenheilkd 195:6–18
15. Carragee EJ, Han MY, Suen PW, Kim D (2003) Clinical outcomes after lumbar discectomy for sciatica: the effects of fragment type and anular competence. J Bone Joint Surg Am 85:102–108
16. Carragee EJ, Kim DH (1997) A prospective analysis of magnetic resonance imaging findings in patients with sciatica and lumbar disc herniation. Correlation of outcomes with disc fragment and canal morphology. Spine 22:1650–1660
17. Cherkin DC, Deyo RA, Loeser JD, Bush T, Waddell G (1994) An international comparison of back surgery rates. Spine 19:1201–1206
18. Davis RA (1994) A long-term outcome analysis of 984 surgically treated herniated lumbar discs. J Neurosurg 80:415–421
19. De Seze S, Guillaume J, Desproges Gotteron R, Jurmand SH (1957) Sciatique paralysante; etude clinique, pathogenique, therapeutique d'apres 100 observations. Sem Hop 33:1773–1796
20. den Boer JJ, Oostendorp RA, Beems T, Munneke M, Oerlemans M, Evers AW (2006) A systematic review of bio-psychosocial risk factors for an unfavourable outcome after lumbar disc surgery. Eur Spine J 15:527–536
21. Dinning TA, Schaeffer HR (1993) Discogenic compression of the cauda equina: a surgical emergency. Aust N Z J Surg 63:927–934
22. Dubourg G, Rozenberg S, Fautrel B, Valls Bellec I, Bissery A, Lang T, Faillot T, Duplan B, Briancon D, Levy Weil F, Morlock G, Crouzet J, Gatfosse M, Bonnet C, Houvenagel E, Hary S, Brocq O, Poiraudeau S, Beaudreuil J, de Sauvezac C, Durieux S, Levade MH, Esposito P, Maitrot D, Goupille P, Valat JP, Bourgeois P (2002) A pilot study on the recovery from paresis after lumbar disc herniation. Spine 27:1426–1431
23. Dvorak J, Gauchat MH, Valach L (1988) The outcome of surgery for lumbar disc herniation. I. A 4–17 years' follow-up with emphasis on somatic aspects. Spine 13:1418–1422
24. Dvorak J, Valach L, Fuhrimann P, Heim E (1988) The outcome of surgery for lumbar disc herniation. II. A 4–17 years' follow-up with emphasis on psychosocial aspects. Spine 13:1423–1427
25. Eysel P, Rompe JD, Hopf C (1994) Prognostic criteria of discogenic paresis. Eur Spine J 3:214–218
26. Gaetani P, Aimar E, Panella L, Debernardi A, Tancioni F, Rodriguez y Baena R (2004) Surgery for herniated lumbar disc disease: factors influencing outcome measures. An analysis of 403 cases. Funct Neurol 19:43–49
27. Gleave JR, Macfarlane R (2002) Cauda equina syndrome: what is the relationship between timing of surgery and outcome? Br J Neurosurg 16:325–328
28. Guinto FC Jr, Hashim H, Stumer M (1984) CT demonstration of disk regression after conservative therapy. Am J Neuroradiol 5:632–633
29. Hallner D, Hasenbring M (2004) Classification of psychosocial risk factors (yellow flags) for the development of chronic low back and leg pain using artificial neural network. Neurosci Lett 361:151–154
30. Hasenbring M, Hallner D, Klasen B (2001) Psychologische Mechanismen in Prozess der Schmerzchronifizierung – Unter- oder überbewertet? Schmerz 15:442–447
31. Hasenbring M, Marienfeld G, Kuhlendahl D, Soyka D (1994) Risk factors of chronicity in lumbar disc patients. A prospective investigation of biologic, psychologic, and social predictors of therapy outcome. Spine 19:2759–2765
32. Hasenbring MI, Plaas H, Fischbein B, Willburger R (2006) The relationship between activity and pain in patients 6 months after lumbar disc surgery: Do pain-related coping modes act as moderator variables? Eur J Pain 10:701–709
33. Hirabayashi S, Kumano K, Ogawa Y, Aota Y, Maehiro S (1993) Microdiscectomy and second operation for lumbar disc herniation. Spine 18:2206–2211
34. Hurme M, Alaranta H (1987) Factors predicting the result of surgery for lumbar intervertebral disc herniation. Spine 12:933–938
35. Ito T, Takano Y, Yuasa N (2001) Types of lumbar herniated disc and clinical course. Spine 26:648–651
36. Jerosch J, Castro WH (1996) Langzeitergebnisse von Reoperationen nach lumbalen Nukleotomien. Z Orthop 134:89–96

37. Jonsson B, Stromqvist B (1996) Neurologic signs in lumbar disc herniation. Preoperative affliction and postoperative recovery in 150 cases. Acta Orthop Scand 67:466–469
38. Junge A, Dvorak J, Ahrens S (1995) Predictors of bad and good outcomes of lumbar disc surgery. A prospective clinical study with recommendations for screening to avoid bad outcomes. Spine 20:460–468
39. Kim KY, Kim YT, Lee CS, Kang JS, Kim YJ (1993) Magnetic resonance imaging in the evaluation of the lumbar herniated intervertebral disc. Int Orthop 17:241–244
40. Knutsson B (1962) How often do the neurological signs disappear after the operation of a herniated disc? Acta Orthop Scand 32:352–356
41. Korres DS, Loupassis G, Stamos K (1992) Results of lumbar discectomy: a study using 15 different evaluation methods. Eur Spine J 1:20–24
42. Kostuik JP, Harrington I, Alexander D, Rand W, Evans D (1986) Cauda equina syndrome and lumbar disc herniation. J Bone Joint Surg Am 68:386–391
43. Kotilainen E, Valtonen S, Carlson CA (1993) Microsurgical treatment of lumbar disc herniation: follow-up of 237 patients. Acta Neurochir 120:143–149
44. Kraemer J (1995) Natural course and prognosis of intervertebral disc diseases. ISSLS Seattle, Washington, June 1994. Spine 20:635–639
45. Lewis PJ, Weir BK, Broad RW, Grace MG (1987) Long-term prospective study of lumbosacral discectomy. J Neurosurg 67:49–53
46. Love JG, Emmett JL (1967) "Asymptomatic" protruded lumbar disk as a cause of urinary retention: preliminary report. Mayo Clin Proc 42:249–257
47. Lurie JD (2006) Point of view. Spine 31:1380
48. Luschka H (1858) Die Halbgelenke des menschlichen Körpers. Reiner, Berlin
49. Maigne JY, Rime B, Deligne B (1992) Computed tomography follow-up study of forty-eight cases of nonoperatively treated lumbar intervertebral disc herniation. Spine 17:1071–1074
50. Malloch JD (1965) Acute retention due to intervertebral disc prolapse. Br J Urol 37:578
51. McCarthy MJ, Aylott CE, Grevitt MP, Hegarty J (2007) Cauda equina syndrome: factors affecting long-term functional and sphincteric outcome. Spine 32:207–216
52. Mixter WJ, Barr JS (1934) Rupture of the intervertebral disc with involvement of the spinal canal. N Eng J Med 211:210–215
53. Ng LC, Sell P (2004) Predictive value of the duration of sciatica for lumbar discectomy. A prospective cohort study. J Bone Joint Surg Br 86:546–549
54. Nygaard OP, Kloster R, Solberg T (2000) Duration of leg pain as a predictor of outcome after surgery for lumbar disc herniation: a prospective cohort study with 1-year follow up. J Neurosurg 92:131–134
55. O'Laoire SA, Crockard HA, Thomas DG (1981) Prognosis for sphincter recovery after operation for cauda equina compression owing to lumbar disc prolapse. Br Med J 282:1852–1854
56. Oppenheim H, Krause F (1909) Über Einklemmung bzw. Strangulation der Cauda equina. Dtsch Red Wochenschr 35:697
57. Pappas CT, Harrington T, Sonntag VK (1992) Outcome analysis in 654 surgically treated lumbar disc herniations. Neurosurgery 30:862–866
58. Postacchini F (1996) Results of surgery compared with conservative management for lumbar disc herniations. Spine 21:1383–1387
59. Ross JC, Jameson RM (1971) Vesical dysfunction due to prolapsed disc. Br Med J 3:752–754
60. Saal JA, Saal JS, Herzog RJ (1990) The natural history of lumbar intervertebral disc extrusions treated nonoperatively. Spine 15:683–686
61. Salenius P, Laurent LE (1977) Results of operative treatment of lumbar disc herniation. A survey of 886 patients. Acta Orthop Scand 48:630–634
62. Scott PJ (1965) Bladder paralysis in cauda equina lesions from disc prolapse. J Bone Joint Surg Br 47:224–235
63. Shapiro S (2000) Medical realities of cauda equina syndrome secondary to lumbar disc herniation. Spine 25:348–351
64. Shephard RH (1959) Diagnosis and prognosis of cauda equina syndrome produced by protrusion of lumbar disk. Br Med J 2:1434–1439
65. Silvers HR (1988) Microsurgical versus standard lumbar discectomy. Neurosurgery 22:837–841
66. Teplick JG, Haskin ME (1985) Spontaneous regression of herniated nucleus pulposus. Am J Roentgenol 145:371–375
67. Vucetic N, Maattanen H, Svensson O (1995) Pain and pathology in lumbar disc hernia. Clin Orthop 320:65–72
68. Weber H (1983) Lumbar disc herniation. A controlled, prospective study with ten years of observation. Spine 8:131–140
69. Weigert M (1967) Die Rückbildung der neurologischen Zeichen nach Bandscheibenoperation. Z Orthop 103:294–298
70. Wilkinson HA (1989) Failed-back syndrome. J Neurosurg 70:659–660
71. Williams RW (1990) Results of microsurgery. In: Williams RW, McCulloch JA, Young PH (eds) Microsurgery of the lumbar spine. Rockville, Aspen, 211–214
72. Woertgen C, Holzschuh M, Rothoerl RD, Brawanski A (1997) Does the choice of outcome scale influence prognostic factors for lumbar disc surgery? A prospective, consecutive study of 121 patients. Eur Spine J 6:173–180

7 Lumbar spinal canal stenosis – decompression with or without stabilization?

ULRICH KUNZ and CHRIS SCHULZ

Introduction

Lumbar spinal stenosis (LSS) implies spinal canal narrowing due to different conditions. The cause may be congenital, constitutional or developmental but most often it is a result of multifactorial degenerative changes in older patients. LSS is the leading diagnosis for adult persons older than 65 years undergoing spine surgery [2]. Throughout life, disc degeneration results in a loss of intervertebral height and bulging of the annulus, which causes segmental hypermobility and increased loads on facet joints leading to a hypertrophy of the facets and the capsular ligaments. The degenerative changes of the intervertebral discs, facet joints and surrounding soft tissues, especially the yellow ligament as well as pseudospondylolisthesis, lead to narrowing of the spinal canal, the nerve root canals and the intervertebral foramina with possible subsequent neural compression of different severity (Fig. 7.1). Proposed mechanisms for development of clinical symptoms include cauda equina microvascular ischemia, venous congestion, axonal injury and intraneural fibrosis [15].

Depending on the location of the compressive structures a central canal stenosis is distinguished from a lateral recess stenosis. The typical clinical end point of central LSS is the bilateral neurogenic claudication with a shortened walking distance due to diffuse pain and sensory and motor deficits on the legs [4]. Physical examination is usually unimpressive in those patients, especially if it is conducted without walking or standing stress. The recessal type of LSS frequently is associated with characteristic segmental radicular leg pain and sensory and motor deficits as well as positive straight leg raising test. In both types the examination of the distal pulses is necessary and in cases of doubt ultrasound control for vascular causes of claudication is recommended [11].

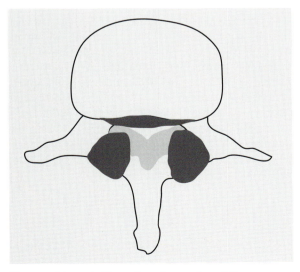

Fig. 7.1. Schematic illustration of narrowing of the lumbar spinal canal due to degeneration.

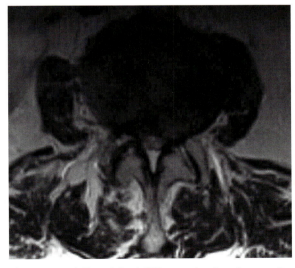

Fig. 7.2. Axial T2-weighted MRI-scan showing degenerative lumbar stenosis.

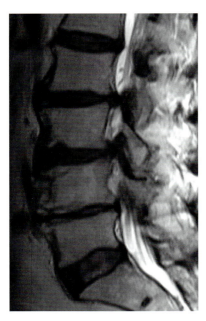

Fig. 7.3. Sagittal T2-weigthed MRI-scan of multi-level degenerative stenosis of the lumbar spinal canal.

Magnetic resonance imaging (MRI) is the mainstay of radiological diagnostics (Fig. 7.2–Fig. 7.4). Myelographic enhanced computed-tomography (CT) is performed in patients with contraindications for MRI. Beside this, the use of CT-scanning allows for a more accurate estimation of bony changes. The conventional myelography is replaced from primary diagnostics, whereas in difficult cases like multisegmental changes or recurrent disease it has proven useful, especially when a post-myelography CT-scan is applied. Electrophysiological examination is useful for discrimination of LSS from neuropathies and can help to identify the affected nerve roots in case of untypical clinical findings. Plain radiographs of the lumbar spine are unspecific but needed, especially those with flexion and extension manoeuvres in order to determine the extent of segmental instability.

Conservative treatment options

Since the symptoms of LSS often progress slowly, there is usually adequate time to pursue conservative treatment strategies. If the patients are not limited in their lifestyle by symptoms, reassurance and watchful waiting are appropriate [5]. There have been few reports of the results of conservative therapy including physiotherapy, anti-inflammatory medication and external immobilisation suggesting that many patients show symptomatic and functional improvement or remain unchanged over time. A study on the natural course of LSS reported unchanged symptoms in 70% of patients, improvement in 15%, and worsening in 15% after a 4-year observation period. Walking capacity improved in 37% of patients, remained unchanged in 33%, and worsened in 30% [1]. An additional course of epidural steroid injections and hyaluronidase application seems to offer a chance of temporary relief, but the stenosis itself cannot be structurally reduced and generally symptoms will recur with the risk of worsening.

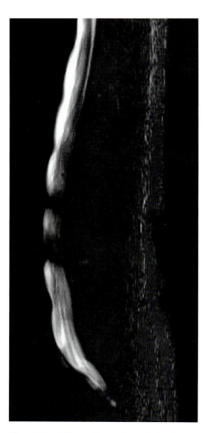

Fig. 7.4. MR-myelography of the lumbar spine as seen in Fig. 7.3.

Indications for surgical treatment

The goals of surgery are to decompress the thecal sac and the corresponding nerve roots while minimizing the risk of an iatrogenic spinal instability. A cauda equina syndrome or rapid deterioration of radicular deficits is a strict indication for immediate surgery. On the other hand, there is no widely accepted agreement upon indications for elective LSS surgery in patients with minimal complaint. Typically, patients undergo elective surgery to improve their pain free walking ability and to reduce disabling leg and back pain [13]. For patients who are persistently or increasingly symptomatic from LSS, the surgical decompression can be highly effective [3]. The greater the degree of osteoligamentous compression is prior to surgery, the better the chance of a satisfactory result will be, especially when the sensory and motor deficits are not very severe and long-standing.

The debate about the indications for conservative versus surgical treatment for LSS remains controversial. Generally, surgically treated patients tend to report greater improvement than those treated conservatively. However, surgical outcome literature is difficult to assess due to observer bias, inadequate outcome data categorization, vaguely defined outcome measures and inhomogenous study design. Consequently, reports show widely varying outcome due to such disparate research methodologies. Nonetheless, in extended stages of LSS with failure of conservative treatment the surgical therapy may result in good or excellent outcome in more than 75% of patients [16].

Surgical technique

The posterior decompression of LSS is not only the fastest but also the most effective approach. The compression due to hypertrophied bony and ligamentous material is mainly located dorsally and thus can easily be approached by dorsal procedures. Further anterior spinal canal compromise resulting from protruded discs and osteophytes also can be addressed via posterior approaches. There are two main concurring operative procedures: the laminectomy and the decompressive interlaminar fenestration. The definitive choice of the procedure depends on several factors: the extent of LSS (mono- or multisegmental), the main location of the compressive structures (central or recessal type), the distribution of symptoms (uni- or bilateral), and the co-existence and degree of spinal instability.

Whether a discectomy is required depends on the intraoperative aspect of the disc. In case of integrity of the annulus (a so called "hard" annulus) and the posterior longitudinal ligament without signs of sequestration no (potentially destabilizing) nucleotomy should be performed. If sufficient dorsal decompression can be achieved, the resection of small ventral lesions is not necessary.

In cases of relevant preoperative spinal instability and the need for a decompressive procedure due to LSS, additional intervertebral fusion should be performed (see also chapter 5, which describes fusion procedures in detail). Relevant postoperative instability also requires fusion. However, the necessity for such a procedure might be reduced if the facet joints are preserved. In addition, there is some moderate evidence that patients over the age of 40 years might develop relevant instability after laminectomy just in 15% of cases [6]. In our opinion, which means from a neurosurgical point of view, additional fusion or instrumentation is indicated only for a minority of patients. In cases of instability and subluxation spinal realignment is possible using distraction devices [9]. Such intervertebral spacers (bony, metallic or synthetic grafts) can be inserted either ventrally (ALIF – anterior lumbar interbody fusion) or – more often used – dorsally (PLIF – posterior lumbar interbody fusion). After fusion without additional posterior instrumentation an increased pseudarthrosis rate might occur [8]. Consequently, the fusion should be performed with use of additional posterior instrumentation (translaminar-transarticular screws or preferably transpedicular instrumentation) [7]. The adjacent lumbar levels might develop some faster degeneration and instability after fusion and instrumentation.

Interlaminar approach and hemilaminectomy

Keeping in mind that decompression of LSS can harbour the risk of symptomatic iatrogenic instability, is is from utmost importance to avoid any destabilization which is not required for an adequate clearance of the spinal canal. The bilateral interlaminar approach enables the sur-

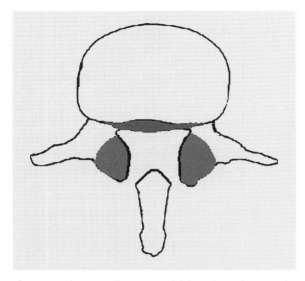

Fig. 7.5. Schematic illustration of bilateral interlaminar decompression: the facet joints are mainly preserved but compressive bony and ligamentous material can be removed.

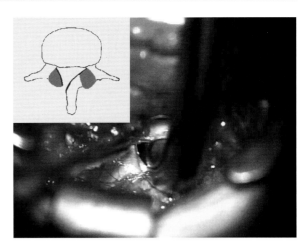

Fig. 7.6. Intraoperative aspect and schematic illustration (inset) of bilateral decompression via unilateral interlaminar approach: a curved punch is inserted for the resection of contralateral parts of the ligamentum flavum.

geon to adequately decompress the dural sac and the exiting nerve roots while preserving the dorsal coverage of the dura (protecting it from advanced epidural scaring). In addition it provides the reattachment of the paraspinal muscles (Fig. 7.5). This more difficult and more time-consuming but less destructive operative strategy is thought to assist in maintaining spinal stability – better than wide laminectomy can do. In our opinion the decompressive interlaminar approach shows the most favourable results for the treatment of LSS.

For dorsal procedures a midline approach is most commonly used. The patient is placed in a prone position with inclination of the spine and no pressure onto the abdomen. Fluoroscopy is used to confirm the proper lumbar levels and a midline skin incision is performed. The subcutaneous tissue is dissected onto the lumbodorsal fascia, which is incised uni- or bilaterally. The paraspinal muscles are separated from the spinous processes and hemilaminae in a subperiostal manner and reflected laterally using self-retaining retractors.

For an interlaminar approach the medial third of the facet joint as well as parts of the neighboured hemilaminae are removed. In cases of preplaned hemilaminectomy the involved hemilamina is removed using the high-speed drill and punches. The ligamentum flavum is carefully opened and resected. This presents the dural sac and the segmental nerve root(s). Care must be taken not to injure the dura because often adhesions between dural structures and ligamentum flavum exist, which need to be carefully separated. All bony and ligamentous material effecting compression on the dural structures is removed usually in an undercutting technique, which can be better performed using curved punches. The nerve root is decompressed in the lateral recess up to the foramen. An intraoperative control of the extent of the resection using blunt hooks is recommended. Extraction of protruded disc material and removal of osteophytes is rarely indicated.

For bilateral decompression via unilateral approaches the spinous process and the contralateral lamina(e) can be undercut (Fig. 7.6). However, such a procedure carries an increased risk of injury of the neural structures due to manipulation. The complete intraspinal decompression has to be confirmed by palpation using hooks of different length. The decompression procedure has to be continued until the contralateral recess can be visualized. The interspinous ligament as a stabilizing factor has to stay intact. If interlaminar decompression or hemilaminectomy provides inadequate decompression, a laminectomy should be performed.

Following decompression the retractors are removed, a suction drain is inserted and the fascia, subcutis and skin are sutured.

Laminectomy

This is the standard surgical approach for the relief of LSS, especially in older patients or those with severe developmental stenosis. It is highly effective in reducing clinical symptoms but in contrast to interlaminar decompression there is a significant risk to develop instability after laminectomy, even if the procedure is performed sparing the facet joints and intervertebral discs [10]. Especially in patients with significant preoperative pathological segmental motion the intervertebral stand alone-fusion or the combination with instrumentation is recommended because these patients carry the risk of a symptomatic postoperative instability after laminectomy alone [12].

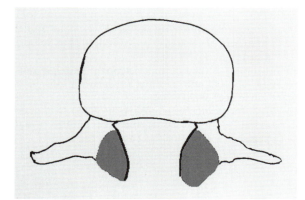

Fig. 7.7. Schematic illustration of lumbar laminectomy: the majority of the facet joints needs to be preserved.

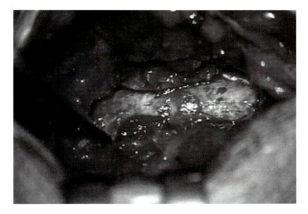

Fig. 7.8. Intraoperative aspect of lumbar laminectomy: all bony and ligamentous structures harbouring compression to the thecal sac is removed, which allows for expansion of the dura at the end of the operation; the hypertrophic facet joints are partially resected in an undercutting technique.

The soft tissue approach mentioned above is performed bilaterally in case of a planned laminectomy. After incision of the interspinous ligaments the spinous process is removed as well as the lamina is, usually with a micro-drill onto the niveau of the ligamentum flavum. The spinal canal should be opened first in its dorsal compartment. In the midline where the dural sac comes up, adhesions to the ligament frequently exist. Therefore the dural sac needs to be dissected carefully before the punch is used for the decompression. The ligamentum flavum is resected without producing pressure on the neural structures. Afterwards, the osteoligamentous resection is widened bilaterally to the facet joints (Fig. 7.7 and Fig. 7.8). The joints are usually hypertrophied and at least the medial parts of them have to be removed for adequate nerve root decompression. Using curved punches or by an angled use of the straight punch or a micro-drill, only the medial part of the facet, which builds the roof of the lateral recess, is removed. The partial resection of the facet joint should not exceed more than 50%, otherwise a relevant instability will persist, which requires fusion. Partial undercutting resection of the neighboured laminae and a foraminotomy should be added.

Summary

In summary, different types and degrees of LSS require different surgical procedures. Selective decompression – like the interlaminar approach – and non-selective procedures – like laminectomy – can be applied with mostly good results. However, one should keep in mind that LSS is part of the process of degeneration of a spinal segment, which has as one constituting element the phase of segmental instability. Therefore precise diagnostics are necessary in order to determine both the amount and localization of the stenosis and the degree of instability. In case of apparent pathological mobility, some fusion procedure should be added to the decompressive surgery. The same is true for non-selective decompressions, which might create significant iatrogenic instability even in the absence of degenerative instability and therefore might require additional stabilization. On the other hand, selective decompressions can lead to an adequate clearance of the spinal canal without the need for additional stabilization.

References

1. Atlas SJ, Delitto A (2006) Spinal stenosis. Surgical versus nonsurgical treatment. Clin Orthop 443: 198–207
2. Delank KS, Fürderer S, Eysel P (2004) Die lumbale Spinalkanalstenose (LSS). Z Orthop 142:19–30
3. Gibson JN, Waddell G (2005) Surgery for degenerative lumbar spondylosis. Updated Cochrane Review. Spine 30:2312–2320
4. Goh KJ, Khalifa W, Anslow P, Cadoux-Hudson T, Donaghy M (2004) The clinical syndrome associated with lumbar spinal stenosis. Eur Neurol 52:242–249
5. Gunzburg R, Szpalski M (2003) The conservative surgical treatment of lumbar spinal stenosis in the elderly. Eur Spine J 12(Suppl):176–180
6. Iguchi T, Kurihara A, Nakayama J, Sato K, Kurosaka M, Yamasaki K (2000) Minimum 10-year outcome of decompressive laminectomy for degenerative lumbar spinal stenosis. Spine 25:1754–1759
7. Knaub MA, Won DS, McGuire R, Herkowitz HN (2005) Lumbar spinal stenosis. Indications for arthrodesis and spinal instrumentation. Instr Course Lect 54:313–319
8. Kornblum MB, Fischgrund JS, Herkowitz HN, Abraham DA, Berkower DL, Ditkoff JS (2004) Degenerative lumbar spondylolisthesis with spinal stenosis. A prospective long-term study comparing fusion and pseudarthrosis. Spine 29:726–733
9. McCulloch JA (1998) Microdecompression and uninstrumented single-level fusion for spinal canal stenosis with degenerative spondylolisthesis. Spine 23:2243–2252
10. Niggemeyer O, Strauss JM, Schulitz KP (1997) Comparison of surgical procedures for degenerative lumbar spinal stenosis. A meta-analysis of the literature from 1975 to 1995. Eur Spine J 6: 423–429
11. Richter M, Kluger P, Puhl W (1999) Diagnostik und Therapie der Spinalstenose beim älteren Menschen. Z Orthop 137:474–481
12. Rompe JD, Eysel P, Zollner J, Nafe B, Heine J (1999) Degenerative lumbar spinal stenosis. Long-term results after undercutting decompression compared with decompressive laminectomy alone or with instrumented fusion. Neurosurg Rev 22:102–106
13. Sengupta DK, Herkowitz HN (2003) Lumbar spinal stenosis. Treatment strategies and indications for surgery. Orthop Clin North Am 34:281–295
14. Szpalski M, Gunzburg R (2003) Lumbar spinal stenosis in the elderly: an overview. Eur Spine J 12(Suppl):170–175
15. Truumees E (2005) Spinal stenosis: pathophysiology, clinical and radiologic classification. Instr Course Lect 54:287–302
16. Yuan PS, Booth RE Jr, Albert TJ (2005) Nonsurgical and surgical management of lumbar spinal stenosis. Instr Course Lect 54:303–312

8 Spondylolisthesis – diagnosis and therapy

Thomas Mattes and Heiko Reichel

Introduction

Herbiniaux, a Belgian obstetrician, reported in 1782 about a narrowed birth canal caused by a displacement of the fifth lumbar vertebra over the sacrum [8]. An acute slip was thought at that time as an explanation. In 1854 Kilian broke with that theory and first described the theory of a steadily subluxation of the lumbo-sacral joint [11]. He coined the concept and the term of spondylolisthesis. In 1858 Lambl described the defect in the intraarticular portion of the neural arch, the spondylolysis, as a main factor for occurrence of spondylolisthesis [13].

Classification and grading

A classification system of spondylolisthesis was given by Wiltse and co-workers in 1976 [26]:
- Dysplastic form,
- Isthmic form,
  - Lytic form,
  - Elongation without lysis,
  - Acute traumatic form,
- Degenerative form (pseudospondylolisthesis),
- Traumatic form (pedicle, lamina, facet joint),
- Pathological form.

Grading of spondylolisthesis according to Meyerding [18] is based on the amount of vertebral slippage: Grade 1 indicates that up to 25% of a vertebra has slipped forward over the vertebra below. Grade 2 represents a slip of 25% to 50%, grade 3 a slip of 50% to 75% and grade 4 a slip of 75% to 100%. Spondyloptosis is a condition, where the entire L5 vertebra translates past the anterior edge of the sacrum, thereby "falling of" the sacrum.

Etiology

Since the first reports about isthmic spondylolisthesis, different etiologies, either congenital or acquired, have been intensively discussed with regard to their causative relevance. However, there is not a proven single etiology for this form of spondylolisthesis. A real congenital defect in the intraarticular portion seems to be very rare and if existing, frequently connected with other malformations of the spine.

Dysplastic form

Dysplastic spondylolisthesis results from congenital hypoplasia or aplasia in the posterior part of the vertebral articulation. As described by Taillard [22], all parts of the neural arch can be affected. A hypoplastic spondylolysis zone in the intraarticular portion can lead to a slip of more than 50%. In those cases, spina bifida is a frequent radiological finding. A gap in the pedicular region is seldom and if it occurs, the amount of slippage is little. It also has to be mentioned for this condition, that the neurocentral synchondrosis persists up to the age of six years, which might contribute to that finding. Consequently, radiological abnormalities without relevant instability, especially seen in computed tomography (CT) and magnetic resonance imaging (MRI), are frequent.

Isthmic form

Isthmic form of spondylolisthesis, which is considered to be the true form of spondylolisthesis, is acquired and occurs in children after onset of their walking age. The most frequent localization is the lumbo-sacral junction, which is mostly represented by the L5–S1 segment. It is the most common form in patients younger than 50 years. Therefore causative factors are assumed which result from the upright gait, since this posture is associated with a lumbar lordosis and a horizontal position of the lumbar facet joint, which might lead to chronic notching or repetitive microfractures followed by elongation of the pars interarticularis and gradual slipping [14].

Degenerative spondylolisthesis

Degenerative spondylolisthesis is a special form of acquired spondylolisthesis, also called "pseudo"-spondylolisthesis. In contrast to the isthmic form it is localized mostly at the level L4–L5 or L3–L4 as well as multisegmental affection also is possible. The causative factors are degenerative changes in the spine with decrease of disc height and degeneration of the facet joints leading to symptomatic segmental instability. The amount of slippage is normally less than 25%. Usually patients are older than 50 years.

Traumatic and pathological spondylolisthesis

Traumatic spondylolisthesis normally requires a severe injury, which also serves as self-explaining causative factor. The pathological form of spondylolisthesis depends on structural changes of the bone, which take place in different diseases like rheumatoid arthritis, Paget's disease, primary and secondary bone tumors, osteogenesis imperfecta and others. Iatrogenic spondylolisthesis is a special condition of pathological spondylolisthesis and is caused by wide dorsal decompression with weakening of the articular region.

Prevalence and localization

The prevalence of spondylolisthesis in the general population is assumed to be around 4% to 7%, but in most cases, spondylolisthesis is asymptomatic. Higher prevalence is known in athletes reported over all disciplines with about 27% [10] up to 47% in athletes performing javelin [21]. A coexisting spondylolisthesis is furthermore found with a high prevalence in patients with Scheuermann's disease [20]. It has been estimated that 80% of people with a spondylolisthesis will never have symptoms, and if it becomes symptomatic, only 15% to 20% will ever need surgical repair.

Almost 90% of all cases of spondylolisthesis are located in the lower lumbar spine with about 90% in the segment L5–S1 and nearly 10% at the level L4–5. Occurrence at levels above L4–L5 is rare.

Diagnosis

Clinical findings

Like in all other disorders of the spine clinical findings are various and manifold. In addition, an estimated number of unreported cases must be considered to be without any symptoms [1, 15]. Especially in children, spondylolisthesis is often without any symptoms. In mild spondylolisthesis the clinical examination may be inconspicuous. Tenderness of the paravertebral muscles in the lower back could be an unspecific sign. A lumbo-sacral kyphosis, a pelvic tilt, an increased abdominal skin crease and a dorsal lumbo-sacral step are more intrinsic and make the diagnosis supposable.

Patients often suffer from unspecific low back pain. Secondary hamstring tightness is the result of tilting of L5, which leads to a compensatory tilt of the pelvis. This could also induce even in mild cases gait abnormalities without neurological disturbances. In severe cases with a grade 2 or higher slippage a fairly recognizable deformity of the low back, especially if the slip is accompanied by a very vertical angle, can be seen. The patient appears to have a short trunk and a large abdomen. They will also have an accompanying large lordosis, and a vertical pelvis. The typical Z-posture with inclination of the trunk over a tilted pelvis with flexion contracture of the hips and flexed knees can also be seen. If the hamstrings become very tight they may also have a waddling gait.

In severe cases neurological deficits caused by stress to the nerve roots during slipping or bulging are possible.

Radiological findings

X-rays in anterior-posterior (a-p) (Fig. 8.1a) and lateral views (Fig. 8.1b) are the standard radiological examination. The radiolucent defect

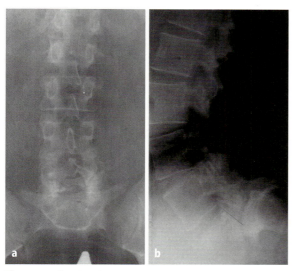

Fig. 8.1 a, b. Anterior-posterior (**a**) and lateral (**b**) X-ray showing a grade 4 isthmic spondylolisthesis L5/S1 with the typical radiographic finding of the a.-p. over-projection of L5 and S1, also referred to as the inverted Napoleon's hat sign.

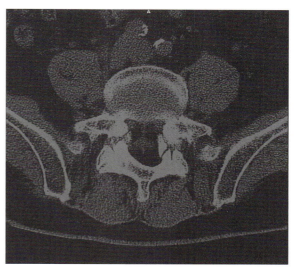

Fig. 8.3. Hypertrophic pseudarthrosis in the spondylolysis zone shown in the CT-scan.

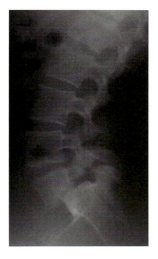

Fig. 8.2. Lateral X-ray of a grade 3 isthmic spondylolisthesis L5/S1 already showing the lysis in the isthmic region; sometimes oblique X-rays are required to fully ascertain the isthic defect (the so-called "Scotty dog" with the "collar" defect in the dog's neck).

in the zone of lysis often is visible in the lateral view (Fig. 8.2). Additional oblique planes can help detecting the lysis showing the "Scotty dog" with the defect (collar) in the dog's neck. Especially in children with a dysplastic type of spondylolisthesis a slip without lysis can be found.

CT and MRI give additional information about the lysis zone and its relation to the cauda equina and the respective nerve roots [7]. A hypertrophic pseudarthrosis (Fig. 8.3) frequently can be seen nearby the nerve roots. In patients without neurological symptoms, primary multiplanar imaging is not mandatory. Nevertheless, such reconstructions are necessary for preoperative assessment and decision-making.

Conservative treatment

Treatment of spondylolisthesis depends on symptoms, age of the patient and its grading and must be determined individually [24, 25]. A general consent does not exist in literature [4, 23]. However, in severe cases and relevant slippage progression a trend towards surgical treatment with good results can be seen. In all other cases non-surgical treatment is favoured after onset of symptoms.

Most slips are grade 1 or grade 2, and can be treated without surgery when they become symptomatic, provided that there is no relevant progression of the slip.

In some patients without any symptoms, diagnosis of spondylolisthesis will be a secondary finding due to diagnostics intended for other reasons. A clinical and radiological monitoring in regular intervals is sufficient and may detect progression.

In symptomatic cases without neurological disorder, non-surgical therapy is the treatment of choice and corresponds to treatment modalities in other chronic low back pain conditions.

Ambulant treatment with a combination of physical therapy, manipulation, and analgetics are adequate. Strengthening of the abdominal and back muscles and particular attention to stretching the hamstrings will alleviate stress on the low back.

In severe pain, in-patient treatment might be necessary. Facet joint injections, infiltration of the lysis zone and epidural steroid injections can help decrease inflammation in these areas.

In addition, patients should be given the advice to avoid overload. Choice of profession needs to be done careful in younger patients as well as an occupational retraining in adults may be adjuvant to reduce suffering. Avoidance of lifting heavy items, doing strenuous sports, and excessive bending and twisting seems to be important, which is also true with regard to attain and maintain a normal body weight.

In most cases non-surgical treatment is successful in relieving patient's pain. If not or in case of progression of slip under non-surgical treatment, surgery has to be considered. However, there remains significant variation in surgical strategies, and limited evidence to guide decision-making.

Surgical treatment

Isthmic spondylolisthesis during adolescence

For a very small minority of adolescents surgery is necessary in case of a progressive slip to grade 2 ore more that is symptomatic. Direct repair of the lysis zone is described [2], however spinal fusion is generally recommended to prevent further progression of the slippage [6]. This is the one situation where progression is felt to be likely and the morbidity (undesirable side effects and potential complications) of a spinal fusion surgery is outweighed by the risk of progression of the deformity.

Spondylolisthesis in adults

In adults spinal fusion surgery would be the choice likewise in higher grading and in symptomatic spondylolisthesis. Goal of surgery is the correction of the kyphosis and reduction of the slip with restoration of the sagittal spinal profile [9]. The role of complete reduction and restoration of lumbo-pelvic relationship remains to be established [17]. Nevertheless, surgical treatment and complete reduction of spondylolisthesis is technically difficult and needs high experience in spinal surgery and advanced instrumentation devices. In-situ fixation with posterolateral fusion, non-instrumented anterior interbody in-situ fusion, and treatment with or without decompression also has been described.

We recommend a posterior reduction with use of instrumentation with pedicle screws followed by anterior lumbar interbody fusion (ALIF) with a bone graft form the iliac crest (Fig. 8.4 a–g). Alternatively, a single posterior approach is possible with spinal instrumentation and interbody fusion in a posterior technique (posterior lumbar interbody fusion (PLIF) or transforaminal lumbar interbody fusion (TLIF)) using synthetic cages [3, 5, 12]. In severe slips (Meyerding grade 3 or 4) sometimes sacral doming impends reduction [16] and a ventral release with a partial resection of L5 or sacral dome resection might be necessary before reduction, which can also be assessed preoperatively with MRI. We suggest for this situation a one stage dorso-ventro-dorsal approach, doing the instrumentation with pedicel screws and if necessary posterior decompression first, followed by anterior release with partial resection of L5 (in spondyloptosis seldom complete resection of L5) and ALIF procedure. After this, reduction can be completed using the dorsal approach.

In all surgical procedures the hypertrophic lysis zone must be noticed and posterior decompression with removal of the lamina, facets and lysis zone is mandatory. A nerve root compression during reduction otherwise appears.

Special intraoperative complications and surgical failures must be considered and discussed with the patient prior to initiating surgical treatment. Non-union with or without hardware failure, continued pain, adjacent segment degeneration occur as well as operative complications e.g. infection, bleeding, cerebro-spinal-fluid (CSF) leak, nerve root damage and all possible general risks [19].

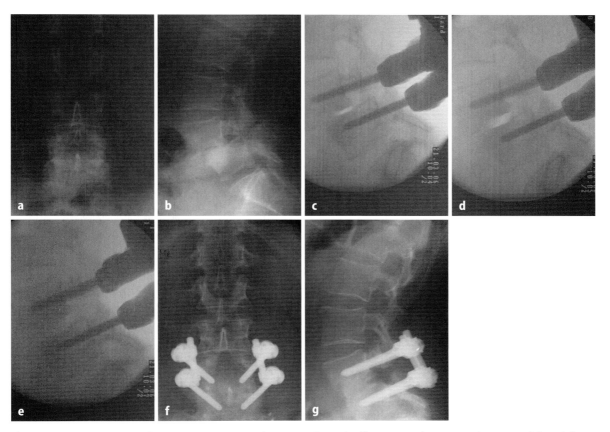

Fig. 8.4 a–g. Pre-, intra- and postoperative X-rays of a patient with grade 3 spondylolisthesis receiving one stage dorso-ventral spondylodesis using the krypton internal fixator (Ulrich medical, Ulm, Germany) and an autologous bone graft from the iliac crest; **a, b:** preoperative a-p and lateral X-rays; **c–e:** intraoperative fluoroscopy, showing the distraction (**c**) and sequential reposition (**d, e**); **f, g:** postoperative a-p and lateral X-rays showing the complete reduction.

Results in spinal fusion procedures for spondylolisthesis are generally good and superior to the outcome in other patient groups. Normal activity after surgery can be anticipated. In degenerative spondylolisthesis surgery also is quite successful even though degeneration of the adjacent segment still may cause suffering. Consequently, multisegmental fusion sometimes is necessary. Patients with degenerative spondylolisthesis with failure of non-surgical treatment frequently will gain improved function and a substantial decrease in their pain after surgery.

Summary

Like in all spinal disorders, spine surgery is seldom the initial treatment for spondylolisthesis. An estimated number of non-symptomatic cases, sometimes seen as incidental radiological findings, show that surgical stabilization and reconstruction of spinal profile is not always necessary.

In a considerable number of cases non-surgical treatment including advise about activity and application of load is successful in relieving the patient's pain. If non-surgical treatment fails to improve suffering from symptoms caused by spondylolisthesis spine surgery might be beneficial.

Nevertheless spinal surgery in spondylolisthesis is technically demanding and numerous risks and complications are possible. Especially patients with a severe slip over 75% make high demands on surgical skills and therefore should only be operated on in specialized spinal surgery departments.

References

1. Alyas F, Turner M, Connell D (2007) MRI findings in the lumbar spines of asymptomatic, adolescent, elite tennis players. Br J Sports Med 41:836–841
2. Bradford DS, Iza J (1985) Repair of the defect in spondylolysis or minimal degrees of spondylolisthesis by segmental wire fixation and bone grafting. Spine 10:673–679
3. Dantas FL, Prandini MN, Ferreira MA (2007) Comparison between posterior lumbar fusion with pedicle screws and posterior lumbar interbody fusion with pedicle screws in adult spondylolisthesis. Arq Neuropsiquiatr 65:764–770
4. Deyo RA (2007) Back surgery – who needs it? N Engl J Med 356:2239–2243
5. Ekman P, Möller H, Tullberg T, Neumann P, Hedlund R (2007) Posterior lumbar interbody fusion versus posterolateral fusion in adult isthmic spondylolisthesis. Spine 32:2178–2183
6. Farfan HF, Kirkaldy-Willis WH (1981) The present status of spinal fusion in the treatment of lumbar intervertebral joint disorders. Clin Orthop 158:198–214
7. Fatyga M, Majcher P, Krupski W, Gawda P (2002) Value of the CT and MRI evaluations in diagnosis of the patients with spondylolisthesis. Orthop Traumatol Rehabil 4:575–578
8. Herbiniaux G (1782) Trait sur divers accouchments laborieux, et sur les poypes de la matrice. JL De Boubers, Bruxelles
9. Hsieh PC, Koski TR, O'Shaughnessy BA, Sugrue P, Salehi S, Ondra S, Liu JC (2007) Anterior lumbar interbody fusion in comparison with transforaminal lumbar interbody fusion: implications for the restoration of foraminal height, local disc angle, lumbar lordosis, and sagittal balance. J Neurosurg Spine 7:379–388
10. Ichikawa N, Ohara Y, Morishita T, Taniguichi Y, Koshikawa A, Matsukura N (1982) An aetiological study on spondylolysis from a biomechanical aspect. Br J Sports Med 16:135–141
11. Kilian HF (1854) Schilderung neuer Beckenformen und ihres Verhaltens in Leven. Bassermann & Mathy, Mannheim
12. Kluger P, Weidt F, Puhl W (1997) Spondylolisthesen und Pseudospondylolisthesen. Behandlung durch segmentale Reposition und interkorporelle Fusion mittels Fixateur interne. Orthopäde 26:790–795
13. Lambl W (1858) Das Wesen und Entstehen der Spondylolisthesis. Beitr Geburtsh Gynäk 3:1–79
14. Letts M, Smallmann T, Afanasiev R, Gouw G (1986) Fracture of the pars interarticularis in adolescent athletes: A clinical biomechanical analysis. J Ped Orthop 6:40–46
15. Libson E, Bloom RA, Dinari G (1982) Symptomatic and asymptomatic spondylolysis and spondylolisthesis in young adults. Int Orthop 6:259–261
16. Mac-Thiong JM, Labelle H, Parent S, Poitras B, Jodoin A, Ouellet J, Duong L (2007) Assessment of sacral doming in lumbosacral spondylolisthesis. Spine 32:1888–1895
17. Martin CR, Gruszczynski AT, Braunsfurth HA, Fallatah SM, O'Neil J, Wai EK (2007) The surgical management of degenerative lumbar spondylolisthesis: a systematic review. Spine 32:1791–1798
18. Meyerding HW (1932) Spondylolisthesis. Surg Gynecol Obstet 54:371–377
19. Ogilvie JW (2005) Complications in spondylolisthesis surgery. Spine 30 (suppl):97–110
20. Ogilvie JW, Sherman J (1987) Spondylolysis in Scheuermann's disease. Spine 12:251–253
21. Steinbrück K, Krahl H, Rompe G (1980) Bedeutung mechanischer Faktoren bei der Entstehung der Spondylolyse (Untersuchungen an Leistungssportlern). Z Orthop 118:456–457
22. Taillard WF (1976) Etiology of spondylolisthesis. Clin Orthop 117:30–39
23. Transfeldt EE, Mehbod AA (2007) Evidence-based medicine analysis of isthmic spondylolisthesis treatment including reduction versus fusion in situ for high-grade slips. Spine 32 (suppl):126–129
24. Vialle R, Benoist M (2007) High-grade lumbosacral spondylolisthesis in children and adolescents: pathogenesis, morphological analysis, and therapeutic strategy. Joint Bone Spine 74:414–417
25. Weinstein JN, Lurie JD, Tosteson TD, Hanscom B, Tosteson AN, Blood EA, Birkmeyer NJ, Hilibrand AS, Herkowitz H, Cammisa FP, Albert TJ, Emery SE, Lenke LG, Abdu WA, Longley M, Errico TJ, Hu SS (2007) Surgical versus nonsurgical treatment for lumbar degenerative spondylolisthesis. N Engl J Med 356:2257–2270
26. Wiltse LL, Newman PH, Macnab I (1976) Classification of spondylolysis and spondylolisthesis. Clin Orthop 117:23–29
27. Ciullo JV, Jackson DW (1985) Pars interarticularis stress reaction, spondylolysis, and spondylolisthesis in gymnasts. Clin Sports Med 4:95–101

9 Current concepts in scoliosis surgery

JENS SEIFERT and PETER BERNSTEIN

Indications for surgery

Non-treated scoliotic spine deformities may result in life-threatening chronic pulmonary heart disease due to ventilation disorder [15].

Scoliotic deformity also accelerates the degeneration of intervertebral discs, leading to more severe morphological changes of the affected vertebral joints. This degeneration can lead to chronic local, pseudoradicular and radicular back pain [5].

In late adulthood, decompensation of the thoraco-lumbar scoliotic spine might occur in the same way as in degenerative scoliosis [6, 14]. Sufficient, pain-relieving treatment of such problems remains a demanding task and might not be accomplished in all cases. In respect to the just mentioned natural course of the scoliotic spine disease, stage-dependent recommendations for treatment had been established, which are based on the Cobb angle and its progression. Table 9.1 summarizes the stage-dependent recommendations for treatment of scoliotic deformity.

Onset of fast progression of the scoliotic deformity should not be missed. Therefore a quite frequent radiographic assessment of the Cobb angle is necessary in adolescents and pre-adolescent children. In case of more than 10° progression in the angle range of 40–50° one must assume further worsening and should indicate surgery early. Pain in post-adolescents with a slowly progressing 50° scoliosis might also be indicative for surgery.

Care must be taken when treating very young children. If high angle values are observed, initial brace therapy can be promising, but one always has to keep in mind that the risk of progression is higher than in adolescent scoliosis. If this is the case despite brace therapy, non-fusion deformity controlling surgery and/or early fusion surgery should be considered.

Surgical approaches

Anterior approach

The patient is placed on the side on the operating table with the convex curvature pointing upwards and overbending of the patient. Incision is made cephaled over the 10th rib and might be extended towards the abdominal wall [2].

After resection of the rib, opening of the thoracic cavity and splitting of the external oblique, internal oblique and transverse muscles, the plane between the retroperitoneal fat and the fascia that overlies the psoas muscle is developed. Following the psoas muscle in the retroperitoneum, the diaphragm should be exposed digitally. Incision of the diaphragm is started at the bone-cartilage transition and continued arche-shaped until reaching the crossing of the diaphragm, psoas muscle and the 12th vertebra. The pleura is incised laterally, followed by ligatures of the segmental vessels of the vertebrae that are to be instrumented later. Little psoas incisions can be helpful in lumbar vertebral exposure. Division of the ligated vessels can be done using an electrosurgical knife. We recommend the use of an ultrasound scalpel. A

Table 9.1. Stage-dependent recommendations for treatment of scoliotic deformity.

Cobb angle	0–10°	10–20°	20–40°	40–50°	Over 50°
Therapy	No scoliosis	Physiotherapy	Physiotherapy and brace	Borderline	Indication for surgery

good ventral release of the soft tissue layers can be achieved when using this technique.

After resection of the intervertebral discs and abrasion of the end plates of the vertebrae, segmental mobilization is done with a Luer. Using an AO-distractor might be helpful. Implants can now be positioned to correct the deformity.

Posterior approach

According to the length of the planned instrumentation, an enlargement of the commonly used posterior midline approach is necessary. Care should be taken for exact subperiosteal preparation and control of haemorrhage. To allow for implant positioning, correction and spondylodesis the following steps are mandatory: All joints to be corrected have to be opened. The surgeon should take care to remove interlaminar and interspinous soft tissue completely to be able to expose the transverse (lumbar spine) and costal (thoracic spine) processes. Every step should be followed by sufficient coagulation measures.

After reaching this point of surgery screw or hook fixation can be performed.

Implants and fixation techniques

Modern implants are composed of titanium or titanium alloy. There is a large pool of different implant systems available. One should be familiar with different implants to be able to use their different correction, extension and stabilization potential.

Antero-lateral instrumentation

Basically two techniques are commonly known: the single-rod (Zielke) and dual-rod (Halm-Zielke, HZI) ventral derotating spondylodesis (VDS) [12]. Correction is accomplished from anterolateral using different implant designs (HZI, Kaneda, etc.).

When resecting the intervertebral discs the posterior longitudinal ligament is left in place. This already determines the direction of the screws. Single screws should be positioned right into the vertebra parallel to its posterior border. When using a dual-rod system, convergent placement of the screws is advantageous. Bicortical anchorage should be achieved [3].

Also, radiographic control of the vertebrae and the intervertebral spaces can be helpful. Rods are flexible and are used for compression in conjunction with the screws and plates. The second rod is being used for augmentation and derotation. Figure 9.1 a, b illustrates the correction potential of HZI-VDS.

Posterior instrumentation

Screw fixation

The technique of pedicle screw fixation is commonly known and described in detail in chapter 4 of this book. There are some supportive measures that might be helpful: image amplifier,

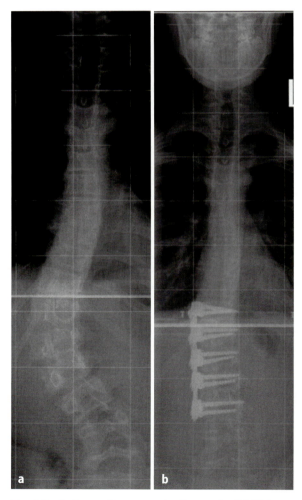

Fig. 9.1 a, b. Pre- and postoperative X-rays of a HZI-VDS.

intraoperative computed tomography (CT) or neuro-navigation. Vertebral rotation should be considered when placing the screws. In the convex part of the deformity screws can diverge while on the inside of the curvature screws should be placed with more convergence. Experience, sufficient imaging and sound palpation are the basis for success.

Thoracic pedicles might be smaller than 4 mm [11]. This requires different fixation methods, e.g. hooks or the so-called tricortical anchorage (double-perforation of the lateral process and re-entry in the vertebral body coming from lateral).

We recommend the following procedures in scoliosis surgery:

Lumbar spine: Opening of the accessory process on the crossing between articular and transverse process. Extension of the pedicle canal with a conical, blunt instrument. Sound palpation. Extension of the hole with an awl and hole preparation with a screw tap. Stepwise fluoroscopic control with lateral view, final control with frontal view.

Thoracic spine: Opening of the articular process with a chisel down to the pedicle. Palpation of the pedicle from caudal. The further steps correspond to the lumbar procedure.

▮ Hooks

Hooks are spine implants that can be inserted easily. Drawbacks are a lower corrective force transmission and a higher risk of outbreak. Nevertheless they are routinely used for three-dimensional corrections [10]. Many authors use some kind of hybrid technique without adverse effects in respect to safety and correction potential [9].

Different fixation techniques like laminar hooks, pedicle hooks, transverse process hooks, and articular hooks are available. Hooks have a higher risk of loosening and outbreak. Therefore it is necessary to "brace" the instrumentation ends by implanting the hooks against each other (in means of compression and distraction).

▮ Sublaminar wires

In the treatment of patients with severe scoliotic deformities or when using dynamic (growth following/growth conducting) implants, some centers still prefer the older technique of Luque [8]. In this procedure a preparation of the verte-

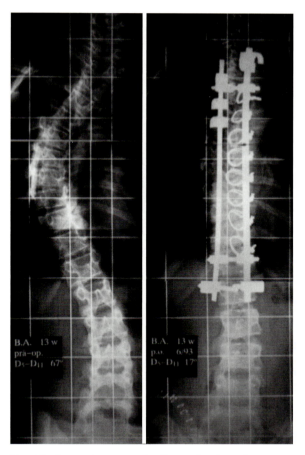

Fig. 9.2. Pre- and postoperative X-rays showing a Luque-procedure in combination with hooks and screws.

bral arches over a number of segments is necessary. The arches are undermined with wires, which are then attached to rods that are placed on both sides of the vertebral column.

Figure 9.2 illustrates such a Luque-procedure, which is performed in combination with hooks and screws.

Correction principles

▮ Posterior techniques

▮ Harrington-technique [7] (Fig. 9.3)
- Principle: Distraction of the concave part and compression of the convex part.
- Advantage: Effective correction.
- Disadvantage: Generation of a flat back with a reduced kyphosis in the thoracic and reduced lordosis in the lumbar spine.

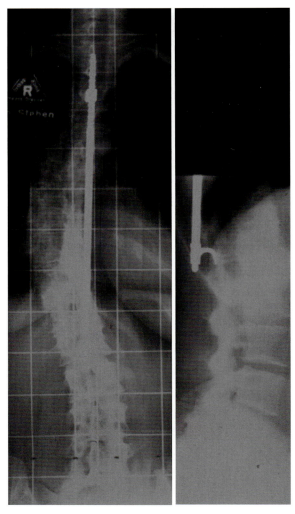

Fig. 9.3. X-rays showing the surgical result of a Harrington-procedure 22 years postoperatively.

■ **Cotrel-Dubousset-technique** (Fig. 9.4 a, b)
■ Principle: Preparation of the rod system following the scoliotic deformity with rotatable fixation of the rods at hooks and/or screws; 90° rotation from scoliosis into kyphosis or lordosis without great distraction.

■ **Luque-technique**
■ Principle: Sublaminar wires are used to hold the spine and corrective rod together.
■ Advantage: High corrective potential with predictable result.
■ Disadvantage: Distinct risk of neurological damage and demanding revision.

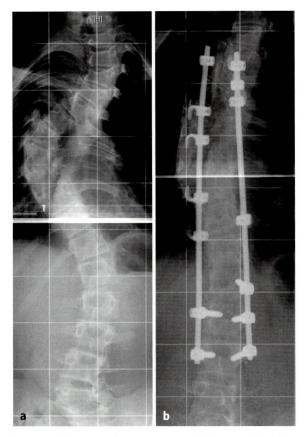

Fig. 9.4 a, b. X-rays of a posterior Cotrel-Dubousset-hybrid-instrumentation two years postoperatively.

Techniques:
– Convex-side-technique: A straight erected rod is brought towards the spine segment-wise from one end to the other.
– Concave-side-technique: the rod is fixed on both ends and is drawn towards the spine from the middle of the curvature.

Wires are twisted around themselves and shortened. The second rod is used as a fixation rod [8].

■ **Anterior techniques**

The principle of the ventral derotating spondylodesis (VDS) consists of compression of the outer curve and derotation from scoliosis into lordosis. At first the intervertebral discs are removed and segmental mobilization is performed. After that compression of the outer curve with flexible rods (Zielke) or translation of the outer curve with stiff rods into a less scoliotic deformed spine is achieved. The remaining deformity is rotated ventrally using a derotator in the single-rod technique or using the second rod in the dual-rod technique. Before performing this step it is necessary to place bone chips between the vertebrae. They provide anterior support and enable persistent lordosis of the lumbar region. The thoracic procedure is performed contrary in direction of the kyphosis.

Combination of different techniques

Modern implant systems allow for a broad combination of posterior fixation techniques and corrective principles. We recommend the combination of the compression-distraction forces of pedicle screw based techniques with the rotatory forces of the Cotrel-Dubousset-technique. By combining these principles the surgeon may be able to correct according to the sagittal profile and the curve architecture of the scoliosis.

Anterior release surgery in conjunction with VDS might facilitate mobilization of the vertebrae. This technique is applied in severe forms of scoliosis [1]. In addition, correction and stabilization problems of severe scoliosis and double curvatures can be solved by a combination of the anterior and posterior techniques (Fig. 9.5 a–c). In such a case, advantages of each system/technique can be used for the respective main curve [3]. Operations can be performed in a one- or two-stage procedure.

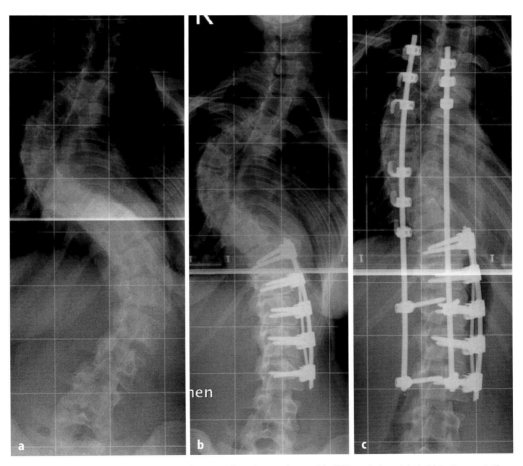

Fig. 9.5 a–c. Pre- and postoperative X-rays of a combined ventro-dorsal procedure with VDS and dorsal hybrid-instrumentation.

Spondylodesis

The above mentioned techniques are based upon a correction of the spine with different stabilization systems and the following bony stiffening of the spine, the so-called spondylodesis.

Spondylodesis is required for long-term spinal stability.

The "Gold-standard" is the autologous spondylodesis by using autologous spongiosa chips and blocks that are harvested from the iliac crest or from the rib. Recent studies could not prove that bone substitute materials and their mixture with autologous bone or osteoinductive substances may guarantee for long-term stability of spondylodesis [13].

Especially in case of the isolated dorsolateral, long-range instrumented spondylodesis oscillation and biological reorganization can lead to hardware breakage and pseudarthrosis. Those forms of pseudarthrosis can only be successfully avoided when using autologous bone for spondylodesis [10].

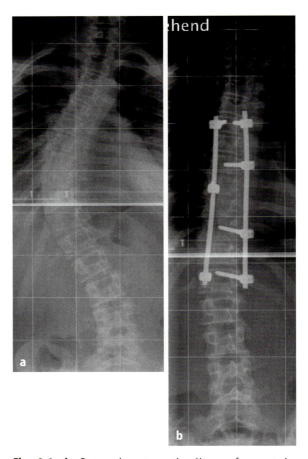

Fig. 9.6 a, b. Pre- and postoperative X-rays of a posterior correction spondylodesis only with pedicle screws.

New concepts in scoliosis surgery

Only pedicle-screw-guided correction

The principle of the posterior scoliosis correction depends upon tight fixation points for implants. Only if this is secured, the high corrective forces of the posterior instrumentation can be transmitted to the spine (Fig. 9.6 a, b). To accomplish this task, instrumentation of the thoracic and the lumbar spine is necessary. Thoracic pedicles are in some cases smaller than the available screws. To avoid neurological damage, certain supportive measures can be taken:
- Radiographic assessment in two planes;
- Neuronavigation;
- Broad exposure of pedicles;
- Tricortical anchorage of the screw.

If those measures are taken, all the above-mentioned correction procedures can be applied. If anchorage of the screws is sufficient, this method allows for brace-free rehabilitation.

Growth Conduction (VEPTR)

The application of growth conduction techniques is still a matter of debate. In the last few years, Campbell and co-workers developed the "vertical expandable prosthetic titanium rib" (VEPTR) for severe scoliosis in childhood [4].

In this technique, a distraction rod is being placed subcutaneously on the inner (concave) side of the curve, following the old Harrington-principle. The next – and new – step consists of the implantation of a so-called titanium rib on the concave side, which can be adjusted according to growth and correction needs.

References

1. Arlet V, Jiang L, Ouellet J (2004) Is there a need for anterior release for 70–90 degrees masculine thoracic curves in adolescent scoliosis? Spine 13:740–745
2. Bauer R, Kerschbaumer F, Poisel S (1991) Orthopädische Operationslehre – Band I: Wirbelsäule. Thieme, Stuttgart
3. Bullmann V, Halm HF, Schulte T, Lerner T, Weber TP, Liljenqvist UR (2006) Combined anterior and posterior instrumentation in severe and rigid idiopathic scoliosis. Eur Spine J 15:440–448
4. Campbell RM, Hell AK, Hefti F (2005) The vertical expandable prosthetic titanium rib implant for the treatment of thoracic insufficiency syndrome associated with congenital and neuromuscular scoliosis in young children. J Pediatr Orthop B 14:287–293
5. Danielsson AJ, Nachemson AL (2003) Backpain and function 22 years after brace treatment for adolescent idiopathic scoliosis. Spine 28:2078–2085
6. Goldberg CJ, Fogarty EE, Moore DP, Dowling FE (1997) Scoliosis and developmental theory: adolescent idiopathic scoliosis. Spine 22:2228–2237
7. Harrington PR (1962) Treatment of scoliosis. Correction and internal fixation by spine instrumentation. J Bone Joint Surg Am 44:591–610
8. Heini PF, Locher S, Schede CP, Anderson S, Slongo T (2004) Surgical treatment with the technique of Galveston-Luque of spine deformities associated with prune belly syndrome. J Pediatr Orthop 13:231–237
9. Kim YJ, Lenke LG, Kim J, Bridwell KH, Cho SK, Cheh G, Sides B (2006) Comparative analysis of pedicle screw versus hybrid instrumentation in posterior spinal fusion of adolescent idiopathic scoliosis. Spine 31:291–298
10. Lepsien U, Bullmann V, Hackenberg L, Liljenqvist U (2002) Langzeitergebnisse dorsaler Instrumentationsspondylodesen mit dem Cotrel-Dubousset-Instrumentarium bei idiopathischen Thorakalskoliosen. Z Orthop 140:77–82
11. Liljenqvist U, Hackenberg L (2002) Morphometric analysis of thoracic and lumbar vertebrae in idiopathic scoliosis. Studies Health Technol Inform 88:382–386
12. Liljenqvist U, Halm H (1998) Augmentation der VDS durch Doppelstabinstrumentation. Eine kritische Analyse der 2- bis 4-Jahresergebnisse. Z Orthop 136:50–56
13. Price CT, Connolly JF, Carantzas AC, Ilyas I (2003) Comparison of bone grafts for posterior spinal fusion in adolescent idiopathic scoliosis. Spine 28:793–798
14. Weinstein SL (1999) Natural history. Spine 24:2592–2600
15. Zhang JG, Wang W, Qiu GX, Wang YP, Weng XS, Xu HG (2005) The role of preoperative pulmonary function tests in the surgical treatment of scoliosis. Spine 30:218–221

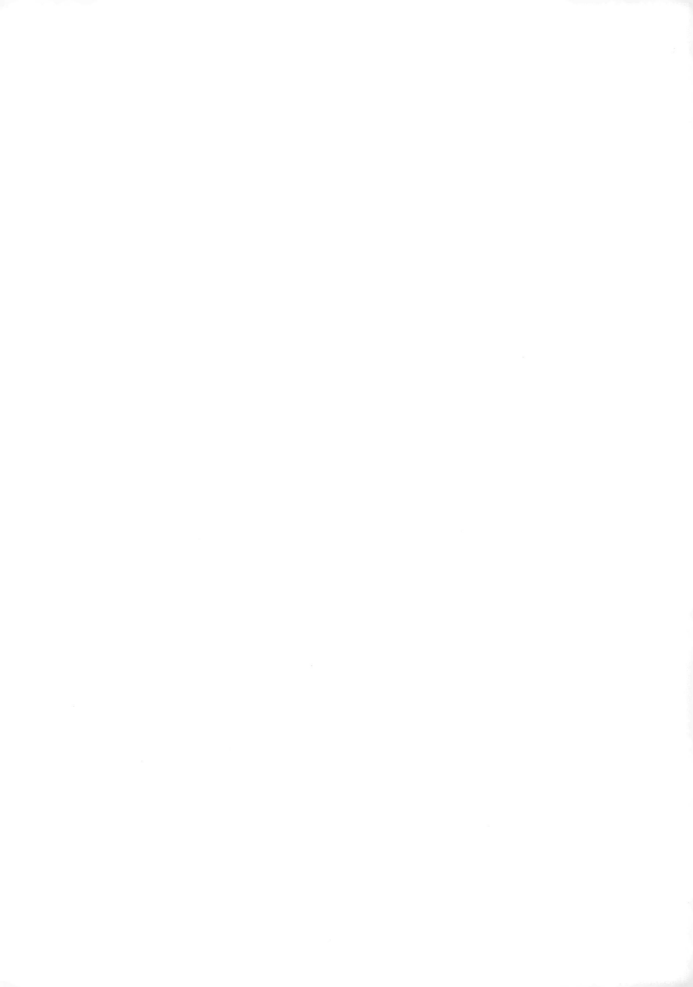

10 Syringomyelia – causes and treatment

Uwe Max Mauer

Definition

Syringomyelia is a cystic cavitation of the spinal cord, containing fluid similar to the cerebrospinal fluid (CSF). This cavity may be formed by dilatation of the central canal or may lie within the substance of the spinal cord. The typical clinical course of syringomyelia is progressive with a slow but progressive deterioration. The morphological feature is a slow increase of the cavity with clinical symptoms worsening with time. Usually, the spinal level of symptoms is ascending, which is the major difference to myelomalacia.

Pathophysiology

The history of syringomyelia is a history of numerous hypotheses. The pathophysiology is still not completely understood. However, idiopathic syringomyelia does not exist.

Generally accepted is that the underlying condition is an obstruction of the flow of the CSF. The most recent hypothesis of developing a syringomyelia is the following: During heart cycle blood enters the brain and the spinal column with a resulting volume increase. As a consequence, the subarachnoid space (SAS) is compressed and CSF is pushed from intracranial through the foramen magnum to the spinal space. Fluid is also pushed from the extracellular space to the SAS along the arterioles of the spine. At the end of the heart cycle blood returns, volume decreases and the CSF pulses back [2, 5, 8]. In syringomyelia this pulsation of the CSF from the cerebrum to the spine and from extracellular to the SAS is obstructed. Therefore the flow of the fluid has to find another way. The extracellular fluid is trapped in the spinal cord and cannot be pushed in the SAS outside the spinal cord.

We can summarize all reasons for a syringomyelia by this hypothesis (Table 10.1) as well as we are able to conclude the causal therapy of

Table 10.1. Diseases associated with syringomyelia (according to Klekamp J, Samii M (2002) Syringomyelia – Diagnosis and treatment. Berlin, Heidelberg).

Diseases of the craniocervical junction

■ Malformation
- Chiari malformation
- Basilar invagination
- Small volume of the posterior fossa
- Rhombencephalic malformations

■ Arachnopathy
- Post meningitic
- Post surgical
- Post hemorrhagic
- Post traumatic

■ Tumour
- Posterior fossa
- Supratentorial

Diseases of the spinal canal

■ Malformation
- Spina bifida
- Tethered cord syndrome
- Diastematomyelia

■ Tumour
- Intramedullary
- Extramedullary
- Extradural

■ Arachnopathy
- Post meningitic
- Post surgical
- Post hemorrhagic
- Post traumatic

■ Degeneration
- Disc disease
- Scoliosis
- Kyphosis

syringomyelia by this hypothesis. Therefore syringomyelia is not an independent disease but only a symptom of another disease, which also leads to the fact that the prognosis of the course of the disease is not only depending on the prognosis of syringomyelia but also on the prognosis of the underlying disease.

The typical reason for obstruction of the flow of CSF is a Chiari malformation. The entire concept of these malformations emerged toward the end of the 19th century from Chiari's initial description of alterations in the cerebellum resulting from cerebral hydrocephalus [1]. In the era of magnetic resonance imaging (MRI) it can be shown that in Chiari I malformation the tonsils extend 5 mm or more below the foramen magnum [2].

Another typical reason for disturbance of the flow of the CSF is arachnoidal scarring. Arachnoidal scarring may be caused by a variety of mechanisms. Such mechanisms might be inflammation due to bacterial, fungal or viral infections, chemical substances like contrast media, breakdown products of blood after subarachnoidal hemorrhage or due to mechanical irritation related to trauma, degenerative disease of the spine or indural surgery. Depending on the cause of the pathology, the scarring may be limited to a very circumscribed area of just a few millimeters or may extend over several spinal segments.

Clinical history of posttraumatic syringomyelia

Posttraumatic syringomyelia requires a traumatic lesion of the arachnoid. It does not necessitate spinal cord injury. If spinal cord tissue is damaged severely a defect inside the spinal cord – a myelomalacia – will result. As a general rule the extent of myelomalacia is restricted to the spinal levels of the cord injury and does not progress. A syringomyelia may progress from the level of injury in both directions. Progressive clinical symptoms start to develop after an interval, which typically lasts several years.

In most instances posttraumatic syringomyelia starts mainly with severe pain followed by progressive motor weakness. Sensory problems, sphincter disturbances, swallowing problems or cardio-pulmonary dysfunction are rarely part of the initial presentation.

Diagnostics

Main diagnostic tool in assessing patients with syringomyelia is the MRI (Figs. 10.1 and 10.2). MRI is the only method to detect syringomyelia directly in its whole extension and to monitor its progress at any time. In addition it allows for diagnosing most of the reasons for syringomyelia (Table 10.1) and to exclude a number of other lesions, which may be mistaken for syringomyelia (e.g. intramedullary tumors, cysts, hematomyelia etc.). Therefore in every case of suspected syringomyelia MRI with contrast medium (gadolinium) should be used.

If the diagnosis of syringomyelia has been made and tumor is excluded, the localisation of the CSF flow obstruction needs to be determined. In posttraumatic syringomyelia signs of a locally restricted focal area of arachnoidal scarring may be difficult to detect on standard MRI scans. T2-weighted MR images are the preferred method to show radiological signs of

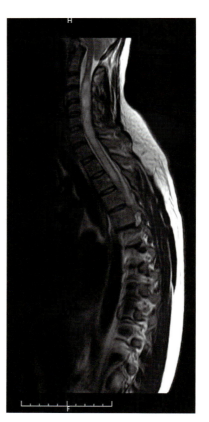

Fig. 10.1. Syringomyelia in Chiari I malformation.

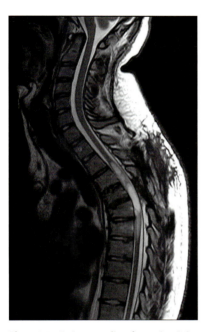

Fig. 10.2. Syringomyelia after spine injury.

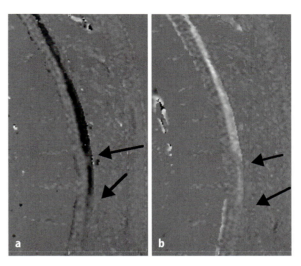

Fig. 10.3 a, b. Typical adhesion in cardiac gaited phase contrast MRI of the thoracic spine.

such a scarring, like adhesions of the spinal cord to the dura, abrupt changes in spinal cord caliber, and irregularities of the cord contour. Additionally, dynamic imaging with phase contrast MRI [3, 4] can be used to search for an area of CSF flow obstruction as an indirect indicator of a focal area of arachnoid pathology (Fig. 10.3 a, b). Such imaging will also demonstrate flow phenomena inside the syrinx itself. In doubt of the localization of the CSF flow disturbance conventional myelography and postmyelography computed tomography (CT) is to our opinion and experience not a reliable diagnostically tool.

Since 2003, we established in our hospital a standard investigation protocol for patients with suspected syringomyelia. We perform in those patients MRI of the head and the whole spine with gadolinium and in addition cardiac gaited phase contrast CSF flow studies of the cranio-cervical junction, the cervical, thoracic and lumbar spine in median sagittal view for the cranio-caudal flow direction. If there is aliasing in the flow studies we perform another study with a range of higher velocity. Usually we start with 3 cm/s, and increase the velocity in case of aliasing to 5 cm/s, 8 cm/s and 10 cm/s, respectively. If there is no flow visible at 3 cm/s we control both the cardiac gait and the position of the field of view and perform another study with 1 cm/s. In addition we investigate the CSF and serum state to exclude demyelination, vasculitis, and immune and infective disorders, respectively.

Surgical management

The goal of surgery is to establish a reliable pathway for the CSF flow to treat the underlying cause of syringomyelia.

If surgery of a Chiari malformation is performed there are three major points to consider: Firstly the reconstruction of a more capacious posterior fossa, secondly the normalization of CSF flow from the fourth ventricle into and out of the cranio-cervical subarachnoid space, and thirdly the identification and correction of any chronic pathological entity that could prevent the success. The operation consists of a sub-occipital craniectomy, which usually is a C-1 laminectomy followed by an intradural lyses of arachnoid adhesions between the cerebellar tonsils and the floor of the fourth ventricle (Fig. 10.4). In some cases shrinkage of the prolapsed cerebellar tonsils with bipolar electrocautery and duraplasty might be necessary [5, 6]. The bony decompression needs to create an sufficiently enlarged foramen magnum, but care must be taken to prevent a cerebellar slump, a rare but difficult to treat complication of an overly aggressive craniectomy [7]. Plugging of the obex still is a matter of controversial debate.

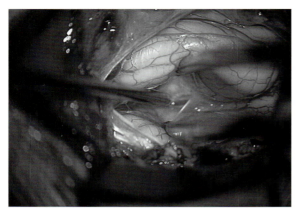

Fig. 10.4. Typical arachnoid adhesions between the cerebellar tonsils in Chiari I surgery.

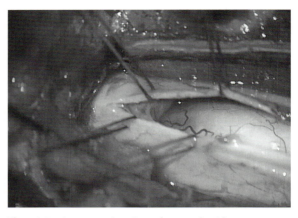

Fig. 10.5. Intraoperative view of an arachnoid cyst.

In arachnoid cysts or webs like in posttraumatic syringomyelia decompression of the SAS and arachnoid dissection are performed as the first surgical option (Fig. 10.5). The operation can be done in the prone position. Head may be fixed with a Mayfield clamp. In some hospitals cervical cases are performed in the semi-sitting position. Median- and tibial-SSEP are employed for neurophysiologic monitoring. Great care is taken to achieve a good haemostasis. Before opening the dura the intradural situation can be assessed with ultrasound. After opening the dura and opening the rostral and caudal SAS, CSF usually flushes into the surgical field and often the cord starts to pulsate and begins to collapse. To limit the risk of postoperative scarring and tethering of the spinal cord an extensive duraplasty is indicated.

If the underlying reason of a CSF flow disorder cannot be corrected, direct syrinx drainage is indicated. This requires a myelotomy, which may be performed in the midline or the dorsal root entry zone.

In a small number of cases the only option for treatment is to insert a tube for a subarachnoid or peritoneal shunt, which has the disadvantage that such a silicon catheter may cause additional arachnoidal scarring [8]. If a shunt is indicated it should be inserted at a spinal level, which is not affected by arachnoidal changes.

Aim of the surgery in syringomyelia is firstly to prevent deterioration, and secondly to ameliorate the neurological function. However, the latter cannot be achieved in all patients.

References

1. Chiari H (1891) Über die Veränderungen des Kleinhirns in Folge von Hydrocephalie des Grosshirns. Dtsch Med Wschr 17:1172–1175
2. Bejjani G (2001) Definition of adult Chiari malformation: A brief historical overview. Neurosurg Focus 11:1–12
3. Edelman R, Wedeen VJ, Davis K, Widder D, Hahn P, Shoukimas G et al (1986) Multiphasic MR Imaging: A new method for direct imaging of pulsatile CSF flow. Radiology 161:779–783
4. Schroth G, Klose U (1992) Cerebrospinal fluid flow – I. Physiology of cardiac-related pulsation. Neuroradiology 35:1–9
5. Klekamp J, Batzdorf U, Samii M, Bothe H (1996) The surgical treatment of Chiari I malformation. Acta Neurochir 138:788–801
6. Oakes W, Tubbs R (2004) Management of the Chiari malformation and spinal dysraphism. Clin Neurosurg 51:48–52
7. Holly L, Batzdorf U (2001) Management of cerebellar ptosis following craniovertebral decompression for Chiari I malformation. J Neurosurg 94:21–26
8. Sgouros S, Williams B (1995) A critical appraisal of drainage in syringomyelia. J Neurosurg 82:1–10

11 Computer navigation in spine surgery

Thomas Mattes

Introduction

Surgical failure with major and minor complications caused by misplaced implants is well known in spinal surgery. Especially in pedicle screw based spinal instrumentations violation of the spinal canal with neurological compromise is dreaded [5, 14, 23]. Poor placement of pedicle screws can also lead to early failure of the instrumentation or reduced stability with the risk of subsequent pseudarthrosis. In addition, intraoperative screw loosening might occur, especially if reduction is necessary. A rate of up to 30% of misplaced screws while performing a conventional technique is reported in the literature, depending on anatomical variations and individual experience [4, 13, 21]. The use of intraoperative fluoroscopy is useful but gives just a two-dimensional (2-D) image of a complex three-dimensional (3-D) structure. Consequently the surgeon needs to assemble both the radiological pictures and his anatomical knowledge in order to create an image of this third dimension. However, depending on the personal experience and the individual anatomy a certain inaccuracy is known. For example, a lumbar pedicle perforation rate of up to 30% has been described [24].

To improve surgeon's orientation in complex anatomical situations, computer-based surgical technologies have been developed. Due to continuous advancements these computer-assisted surgery (CAS) technologies became more and more common in the last decade. At present several hundreds of navigation systems are in routine use during spinal surgery and total knee and hip arthroplasty as well as in trauma surgery and neurosurgery.

In mid 90's, navigated pedicle screw implantation was one of the first clinical applications of this new technology; soon after integration in the clinical routine use a reduced screw misplacement rate compared to the conventional technique was shown [1, 11, 12, 15, 16]. Since then efforts have been made in order to improve also the ergonomics and the safety of these navigation systems.

In principle, there are two different methods of navigation available [1, 10, 12, 22]. One option is a computed tomography (CT)-based system with the necessity of a preoperative CT-scan and creation of 3-D CT-data, which is matched with the anatomy of the patient intraoperatively. Alternatively, fluoroscopy-based navigation systems do not require a preoperative CT-scan and allow the visualisation and navigation of instruments on the basis of intraoperatively acquired 2-D fluoroscopic images.

In both systems the perception of surgical tools and anatomical structures follows the principle of dynamic referencing (tracking). Most navigations systems work at present with a passive optical tracking technique. The interaction of an infrared emitting camera and reflector balls on instrument and patient side enables the detection of the 3-D position of the related objects. These systems are easy to use; in addition reflector balls are reusable and can be changed each by each. Hindrance of such reflector balls is their sensitivity to contamination with fluids. Consequently, the perceptibility of the reflector balls can be reduced during surgery and time-consuming cleaning sometimes extends the real surgery time. Newer passive reflector arrays, like the Navitrak-ER device (ORTHOsoft Inc., Montreal, Canada) compensate for the disadvantages of common reflectors with a special geometry and fluid insensible reflecting surface. Active optoelectronic tracking and electromagnetic tracking also is available for some systems.

Besides the afore-mentioned components, dedicated instruments are essential parts of the navigation system. In spinal navigation systems special pointers, drilling guides and awls are available. Some of them are pre-calibrated or easy to calibrate with automatic calibration tools.

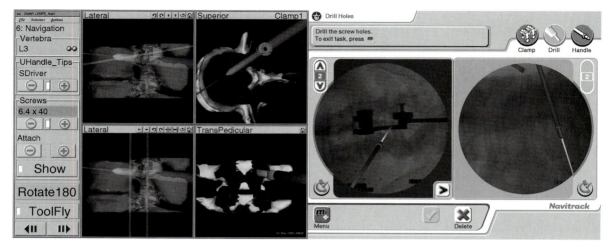

Fig. 11.1. Monitor screen shot with an intraoperative aspect of visualization of the targeted structure and surgical devices: CT-based navigation on the left side and fluoroscopy-based navigation on the right side.

Computed tomography (CT)-based navigation

CT-based navigation enables intraoperatively a real 3-D visualisation based on a 3-D reconstruction of a CT-data set with possibility of 3-D surface view and multiplanar viewing (Fig. 11.1). CT-data can be transferred into the navigation system using CD-Rom, USB-stick or direct network transfer. Preliminary an automated or semi-automated segmentation and control of the quality of CT-data is required. In our experience the quality of the virtual 3-D model as well as the time needed for segmentation and intraoperative referencing correlates with the quality of the CT-data. For CT-based navigation of the cervical and upper thoracic spine we recommend a 1 mm thin slice CT-scan, and for the lumbar spine a 2–3 mm scan. Based on the segmented data the navigation software calculates a 3-D model using an automatic rendering algorithm. Afterwards, preoperative planning with use of the virtual CT-data, e.g. the planning of the size and the position of a screw, is possible.

During surgery, a reference clamp (dynamic reference base (DRB)) is attached to the spinous process (Fig. 11.2). Afterwards a surface matching or a paired point matching is necessary to equalize the CT-model with the real anatomy. For that reason, a predefined number of surface points (matching points) on the bony surface of the vertebra to be instrumented must be probed with the pointer. Alternatively, some systems provide a contact free Fluoro-CT matching. After successful registration a clinical validation of the estimated accuracy is mandatory. Depending on the chosen surgical technique and the applied implant system the use of either navigated drill guides or pedicle awls is feasible. Figure 11.1 illustrates the overlay of instrument position in the virtual model, which enables a real-time 3-D view for safe instrumentation.

There are several studies pointing out that the use of CT-based navigation improves accuracy, precision, and reproducibility of pedicle screw positioning compared to a fluoroscopic controlled manual technique [1, 20, 21]. Some

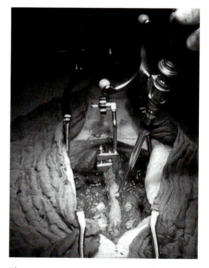

Fig. 11.2. Dynamic reference clamp attached to the spinous process L3 and navigated pointer during validation.

complications can be avoided at the cost of increased expense, additional X-ray exposure of the patient, and an extended duration of surgery due to time consuming intraoperative referencing; in addition, technical errors and screw mal-positioning are still possible despite use of navigation systems [8, 19].

Fluoroscopy-based navigation

Compared to CT-based navigation, a less elaborate application is available with fluoroscopy-based navigation [6, 17]. A preoperative CT-scan is not necessary. Contrary, fluoroscopic images in different planes are acquired intraoperatively with a calibrated C-arm after fixation of the DRB. Unlike normal intraoperative fluoroscopy, simultaneous displaying of different planes is possible without strenuous and repetitive repositioning of the C-arm. In addition, X-ray exposure is reduced.

Similar to other studies [7, 17] we were able to demonstrate a comparable accuracy of lumbar pedicle instrumentation using the Dynesys dynamic stabilization system (Zimmer, Warsaw, USA) using CT-based and fluoroscopy-based navigation (Navitrack navigation system (Orthosoft, Montreal, Canada)) and a manual technique. Screw position was assessed in postoperative CT-scans with multiplanar reconstruction. For evaluation of the screw position a special scoring system (Table 11.1) was designed with a maximum of six points per pedicle screw. An optimal result corresponds to a small number of points, whereas a bad result is denoted by a high number of points.

In the conventional surgery group (group 1), eleven segments received instrumentation (on average 1.6 per patient with a range of one to two segments). The CT-based navigation group (group 2) comprised seven segments (average: 1.4, range: 1–2) and the fluoroscopy-based navigation group (group 3) another twelve segments (average: 1.7, range: 1–3). Navigation was technically feasible in all cases, and technical break-off did not occur. Postoperative analysis revealed that the best results referring to the postoperative screw position were obtained with the CT-based navigation, followed by the fluoroscopy-based navigation. The worst results with regard to accuracy were achieved in the group

Table 11.1. Score for the postoperative identification of the screw position with CT measurement, maximum six points per pedicle screw.

	Points
Pedicle	
– no perforation	0
– perforation of 1 and 2 mm	1
– perforation of 3 and 4 mm	2
– perforation >4 mm	3
Entrance point of the screw	
– in the vertebral body	0
– perforation of vertebral body	1
Facet joint contact	
– ideal	0
– non-ideal	1
Inclination of the screw	
– no	0
– yes	1

operated on with the conventional technique. However, none of the patients suffered from neurological complications or postoperative wound infection.

Fluoroscopic 3-D navigation

Fluoroscopic 3-D navigation represents a new technology, which enables intraoperative 3-D imaging and further multiplanar reconstructions through acquisition of a set of 2-D fluoroscopic images by an isocentric 3-D C-arm.

The fusion of an existing navigation system and 3-D fluoroscopy, which has been realized with the VectorVision fluoro 3D spine system (BrainLAB AG, Feldkirchen, Germany), was proven to be efficient in trauma surgery. However, reports of its use in spinal surgery are rare [18]. The mean benefit compared to CT-based navigation is to obviate the highly susceptible process of intraoperative referencing, which is especially true in patients with poor bone quality. Further development in order to enable simultaneous registration of multiple vertebra, e.g. for navigated fracture repair or deformity correction, as well as to adapt the size of instruments to minimal-invasive surgical approaches still is necessary.

Restriction of this technology may be reduced image quality in obese patients and those with osteopenia and tumors. Movements during image acquisition might also influence the result. In such conditions, CT-based navigation still is the benchmark.

Furthermore, application of such a system requires the purchase of an isocentric C-arm, a computer-navigation system, the respective fusion technology interface and carbon OR-tables.

Summary

The main goal of the application of navigation systems in different surgical procedures is to achieve a higher precision of implant positioning and a reduction of technical complications. New tracking technologies, dedicated instruments and ergonomic software facilitate the application of these systems and might improve their results. Another beneficial aspect might be some support in performing traditional procedures (like total hip arthroplasty) via minimally invasive approaches. With regard to spine surgery, the use of navigation systems can lead to a decreased screw misplacement and complication rate. However, like in all new technologies, a learning curve must be considered. Possible errors need to be anticipated and corrected on the base of the surgeon's personal experience. It must be pointed out that navigation should be used as a tool, which might enable the experienced surgeon to improve his results, but not for a beginner, who would not be able to perform a surgical procedure at all without navigation.

Based on our experience, we recommend the routine use of CT-based navigation in cervical and upper thoracic spinal surgery with application of pedicle screws and in patients with complex anatomy, e.g. due to prior surgery. Intraoperative generation of a 3-D dataset using an isocentric 3-D C-arm is optional and deserves specific consideration of the generated expenses. Fluoroscopy-based navigation improves the surgical accuracy and holds the positive side effects of a reduced X-ray exposure, a minimized need for intraoperative handling of the C-arm and the synchronous provision of multiplanar images.

To justify the expense of this new technology against the background of reduced budgets in health care systems, prospective controlled and randomized studies are advocated.

References

1. Amiot LP, Lang K, Putzier M, Zippel H, Labelle H (2000) Comparative results between conventional and computer-assisted pedicle screw installation in the thoracic, lumbar and sacral spine. Spine 25:606–614
2. Arand M, Schempf M, Fleiter T, Kinzl L, Gebhard F (2006) Qualitative and quantitative accuracy of CAOS in a standardized in vitro spine model. Clin Orthop 450:118–128
3. Arand M, Schempf M, Hebold D, Teller S, Kinzl L, Gebhard F (2003) Präzision der navigationsgestützten Chirurgie an der Brust- und Lendenwirbelsäule. Unfallchirurg 106:899–906
4. Castro WH, Halm H, Jerosch J, Malurs J, Steinbeck J, Blasius S (1986) Accuracy of pedicle screw placement in lumbar vertebrae. Spine 21:1320–1324
5. Esses SI, Sachs BL, Dreyzin V (1993) Complications associated with the technique of pedicle screw fixation. Spine 18:2231–2239
6. Foley KT, Rampersaud YR, Simon DA (2001) Virtual fluoroscopy: computerassisted fluoroscopic navigation. Spine 26:341–351
7. Fritsch E, Duchow J, Seil R, Grunwald I, Reith W (2002) Genauigkeit der fluoroskopischen Navigation von Pedikelschrauben. Orthopäde 31:385–391
8. Gebhard F, Kinzl L, Arand M (2000) Grenzen der CT-basierten Computernavigation in der Wirbelsäulenchirurgie. Unfallchirurg 103:696–701
9. Gertzbein SD, Robins SE (1990) Accuracy of pedicle screw placement in vivo. Spine 15:11–14
10. Kosmopoulos V, Schizas C (2007) Pedicle screw placement accuracy: a meta-analysis. Spine 32: 111–120
11. Laine T, Schlenzka D, Mäkitalo K, Tallroth K, Nolte LP, Visarius H (1997) Improved accuracy of pedicle screw insertion with computer-assisted surgery. Spine 22:1254–1258
12. Laine T, Lund T, Ylikoski M, Lohikoski J, Schlenzka D (2000) Accuracy of pedicle screw insertion with and without computer assistance: a randomised controlled clinical study in 100 consecutive patients. Eur Spine J 9:235–240
13. Liljenqvist UR, Halm HFH, Link TM (1997) Pedicle screw instrumentation of the thoracic spine in idiopathic scoliosis. Spine 22:2239–2245
14. Lonstein JE, Denis F, Perra JH, Pinto MR, Smith MD, Winter RB (1999) Complications associated with pedicle screws. J Bone Joint Surg Am 81: 1519–1528
15. Merloz P, Tonetti J, Pittet L, Coulomb M, Lavallée S, Sautot P (1998) Pedicle screw placement using image guided techniques. Clin Orthop 354:39–48
16. Nolte LP, Zamorano LJ, Jiang Z, Wang Q, Langlotz F, Berlemann U (1995) Image-guided insertion of transpedicular screws. A laboratory set-up. Spine 20:497–500

17. Nolte LP, Slomczykowski MA, Berlemann U, Strauss MJ, Hofstetter R, Schlenzka D, Laine T, Lund T (2000) A new approach to computer-aided surgery: fluoroscopy-based surgical navigation. Eur Spine J 9:78–88
18. Rajasekaran S, Vidyadhara S, Shetty AP (2007) Intra-operative Iso-C3D navigation for pedicle screw instrumentation of hangman's fracture: a case report. J Orthop Surg 15:73–77
19. Richter M, Cakir B, Schmidt R (2005) Cervical pedicle screws: conventional versus computer-assisted placement of cannulated screws. Spine 30:2280–2287
20. Richter M, Mattes T, Cakir B (2004) Computer-assisted posterior instrumentation of the cervical and cervico-thoracic spine. Eur Spine J 13:50–59
21. Robins SE, Gertzbein SD (1987) Accuracy of pedicle screw placement in vivo. Proc Orthop Trauma Assoc 1:27–28
22. Sasso RC, Garrido BJ (2007) Computer-assisted spinal navigation versus serial radiography and operative time for posterior spinal fusion at L5-S1. J Spinal Disord Tech 20:118–122
23. Schizas C, Theumann N, Kosmopoulos V (2007) Inserting pedicle screws in the upper thoracic spine without the use of fluoroscopy or image guidance. Is it safe? Eur Spine J 16:625–629
24. Weinstein JN, Spratt KF, Spengler D, Brick C, Reid S (1988) Spinal pedicle fixation: reliability and validity of roentgenogram-based assessment and surgical factors on successful screw placement. Spine 13:1012–1018

Trauma

12 Treatment of cervical spine injuries

Christoph Ulrich

Introduction

As regards the thoraco-lumbar spine, a high incidence of injuries is associated with a low incidence of neurological complications. When we look at injuries of the cervical spine, however, we find that the ratio is precisely the opposite. About 15% of spinal injuries are located here, but in 70% of the cases, they are associated with concomitant neurological symptoms. This is for one thing due to the high number of disco-ligamentous injuries in this area, which will rather permit translatory dislocation than axial compression – and, of course, this is due to the presence of the spinal cord. As quasi-peripheral nerve (at L1), the cauda equina is much more likely to tolerate major compressions than the sensitive spinal ganglion cells.

A uniform classification of injuries of the entire cervical spine is prevented by its individual structure, especially in the head-neck transition area. Injuries of the upper cervical spine (C0–C2) must be differentiated from injuries of the lower cervical spine (C3–C7).

Only the lower cervical spine can be classified analogous to the thoraco-lumbar spine. As regards the upper cervical spine, knowledge of the layer as well as segment-dependent injury potentials is indispensible.

While conservative therapy with external fixation is more often indicated for the osseous injuries of the upper cervical spine, operative fixation of two adjacent segments will be indicated on the lower cervical spine and on the thoraco-lumbar spine, because disco-ligamentous healing will not result in reliable, long-term stability. Anterior stabilization with angular-stable plates is the standard procedure for monosegmental instabilities without posterior fragment compression.

Without doubt, posterior screw-based fixation methods provide more biomechanical stability than anterior implants; however, their placement is much more difficult. Especially as regards C1/2 fixation and transpedicular C3–C7 fixation, computer navigation is superior to the conventional procedure in terms of radiation exposure and precision.

Analogous to the thoraco-lumbar spine, instabilities as well as neurological deficiencies must be considered as emergency indications, since recovery of a damaged spinal cord can only be expected through restoration of the original width of the spinal canal and segmental stability. Small cages or tricortical corticospongious grafts may be used intervertebrally to replace a destroyed disc.

Especially patients with a high paraplegia require quick stabilization to prevent paralysis from ascending, and for early rehabilitation and mobilization of the patient to be initiated.

When cervical spine injury is suspected, stiff neck immobilization of the cervical spine at the scene of the accident is indicated as primary treatment. Closed reduction of dislocations must not be performed if no precise diagnosis is available, for the possibility must be ruled out that retrovertebrally dislocated disc material is pressed into the spinal canal during repositioning, which could cause additional paraplegia.

Diagnostics

Medical history, physical examination, and selective imaging methods are the three pillars of diagnostics; they provide the basis for the classification of injuries and the resulting therapeutical decisions.

Owing to the frequently combined occurrence of skull and cervical spine injuries, additional cervical spine injury must be ruled out for each skull injury.

The intense pain in the back of the neck, which may point to cervical instability of both the upper as well as the lower cervical spine, is another characteristic feature of a cervical-spine injury.

Neurological examination must be performed by a specialist prior to surgical measures and if the findings are not clear, especially also for forensic reasons.

Imaging methods

Radiographs

Conventional radiographs always constitute the basis of the diagnostics of spinal injuries, as a rule after clinical examination.

A lateral radiograph of the cervical spine, an anterior-posterior (ap)-radiograph of the lower cervical spine, and a transoral ap-radiograph of atlas and axis are part of the standard program for all patients with suspected spinal injury. Valuable first informations are provided by the extension lines and standardized measuring values from the standard radiographs (Fig. 12.1 a–d).

Lateral imaging of the cervical spine must always include the 7th cervical vertebral body, the intervertebral disc C7/T1 and the cranial endplate of T1. Because injuries near the cervicothoracic transition are common, this area is of extreme diagnostic relevance.

Computed tomography (CT)

CT-scanning, as spiral CT with multiplanar reconstruction, is an indispensable element of radiological cervical spine diagnostics. Especially the cervico-thoracic transition, which tends to evade diagnostic distinctness, can be fully imaged, both coronarily as well as in its lateral reconstruction. A high level of diagnostic certainty is realized, and injuries can be clearly classified both on the lower as well as the upper cervical spine.

Magnetic resonance imaging (MRI)

As for the thoraco-lumbar spine, the benefits of MRI lie in the imaging of the soft-tissue structures and the radiation-free imaging even of longer sections of the spinal column. MRI is therefore the preferred indication for neurological symptoms without morphologic correlate (e.g. SCIWORA or cervical spine whiplash), for ligamentous instabilities and intervertebral disc injuries, for tumors und metastases, as well as for the clarification of posterior components when an isolated anterior approach is planned for B and C injuries.

The sensitivity of the method is very high; the osseous specificity, however, is significantly lower. The traumatological "gold standard" is therefore reserved for CT.

Functional examinations

Since the cervical spine is particularly frequently the location of purely disco-ligamentous lesions, which after spontaneous reduction through contraction of the nuchal musculature

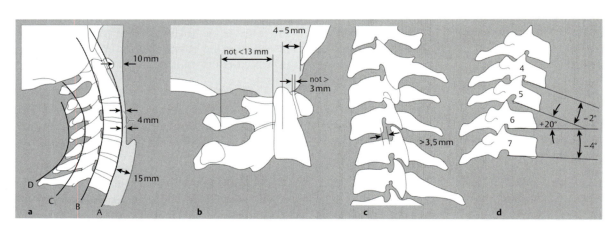

Fig. 12.1 a–d. Extension lines for assessment of the alignment of the cervical spine (**a**); extension lines for assessment of instability on the upper cervical spine (**b**); maximally tolerable translation on the lower cervical spine according to White and Panjabi (**c**); maximally tolerable kyphosis on the lower cervical spine according to White and Panjabi (**d**) (from: Ulrich C. Verletzungen der Halswirbelsäule. Orthopädie und Unfallchirurgie update 2006; with permission of Thieme, Germany).

in supine position escape detection on survey radiographs, standard radiographs are supplemented by functional examinations. Especially the passive functional examination, which must be performed on the conscious patient, is of great value.

Conservative treatment

Most injuries on the upper cervical spine are osseous injuries. The emphasis is therefore on conservative treatment since restoration of the original stability of the injured structure is most likely achieved by osseous healing.

External fixation, which is the basis of conservative treatment, can be performed with the Schanz collar (practically only for the prevention of extreme flexion), with the stiff neck, which supports also the chin (for the prevention of flexion, extension and rotation), and with the Halo vest. However, Halo vest treatment is associated with a considerable number of complications (loosening of pins (30%), infections (20%), pressure sores under the Halo vest, traumata to nerves, and cicatrization).

For children, there is also the Minerva plaster, which includes the head, shoulders and the thorax, and which for hygienic reasons is less indicated for adults.

It is important to know that with this type of external fixation only the upper cervical spine can be immobilzed. The lower cervical spine cannot be safely immobilized by means of external fixation until healing. The postoperative Schanz collar used after interventions on the lower cervical spine serves more as a means to immobilize soft tissue.

Surgical treatment

The indication for operative treatment is based on the assessment of the following three criteria:
- Neurology,
- Instability,
- Malposition.

Neurology is clinically assessed while abnormal position is radiographically evaluated. Instability is quantified by means of a valid classification system.

The diversity of injuries on the cervical spine is matched by the same diversity of individual posterior and anterior stabilization and spondylodesis methods. Based on biomechanical and clinical tests, the following general principles can be stated for the surgical procedure:
- The surgical technique is to bring about decompression and stability. Anterior as well as posterior approaches are possible. Reliable implant fixation is performed with screws.
- Stabilizations on the upper cervical spine are demanding and complicated. In contrast to the lower cervical spine, direct posterior or anterior screw fixations are possible in addition to specific spondylodesis techniques.
- On the lower cervical spine, the anterior access should be the first choice. In terms of surgery as well as fixation, this involves significantly fewer problems than the posterior approach. Additional decompression of the myelon is possible without restriction if needed. Implant fixation is technically simple, and the knowledge of instability and type of implant allows functional therapy to be performed – also and especially on the paraplegic.
- Posterior methods are indicated under trauma conditions only for special injury constellations. As single procedures they require an intact anterior spine. Wire cerclage techniques require intact osseous posterior elements and should only be applied as additional method.
- Combined stabilization methods are indicated for highly unstable or specific complex injuries. Especially on the cervicothoracic transition and when Bechterew's disease is involved, such procedures, which can be performed in one or two stages, are indicated.
- In view of the foreseeable necessities of repeat examinations required later, especially with regard to the modern imaging methods, the implants chosen should be made of titanium whenever possible.

Stabilization techniques

Anterior instrumentation

Anterior spondylodesis of C2–T2
The anterior access permits stabilization of C2–T2. After exposure of the injured motion segment, the disc is excised and a tricortical graft

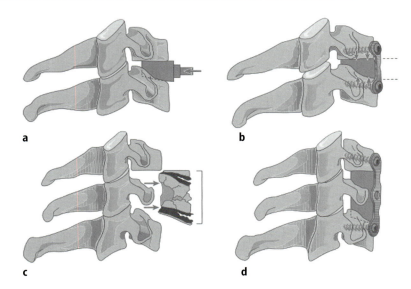

Fig. 12.2 a–d. Monosegmental (**a**, **b**) and bisegmental (**c**, **d**) cervical spondylodesis (from: Ulrich C. Verletzungen der Halswirbelsäule. Orthopädie und Unfallchirurgie update 2006; with permission of Thieme, Germany).

of a suitable size from the right or left iliac crest is inserted into the injured motion segment, with the spongy surfaces facing cranially and caudally (Fig. 12.2 a, b).

Angle-stable plates are to be preferred. The position of the plate is to be checked intraoperatively in both planes, since oblique position of the plate may result in incorrect drilling and injury to the A. vertebralis. Occasionally, removal of an entire vertebral body may be required (teardrop fracture). Replacement is possible by means of a cage or an autologous tricortical bone graft (Fig. 12.2 c, d).

Screw placement in C2 (odontoid fractures)

Direct screw fixation of an odontoid fracture type 2 or type 3 across the intervertebral space C2/3 is an elegant but also complicated method because the function of both the vertebral body and the motion segment is retained. Many single steps must be observed.

Whether one screw is used or two is not of any significance for primary stability or healing. Cannulated screws with self-tapping thread are recommended. Minimally invasive methods may only be applied if the trocars can be firmly anchored in the intervertebral disc space C2/3 and this ensures that no soft tissue is coiled up during drilling or screwing. The traction screw must be inserted via the baseplate of C2. This is achieved through removal of a small piece of the disc C2/3, which creates a corridor for the screw. This corridor may later result in spontaneous stiffening of segment C2/3 via an osseous bridge. If the dens screws are inserted too far anteriorly, i.e. through the anterior wall of C2, the heads will inevitably break through the thin cortical bone. Odontoid osteosynthesis is only possible if the fracture involved can be directly exposed to compression, i.e. if it is a transverse fracture without dislocation tendency under compression (Fig. 12.3 a–c).

With regard to both anterior procedures, the following mistakes and risks may be involved and therefore require clarification: hematomata, lesion of the N. recurrens (temporarily in almost 50% of cases), postoperative ventilation disturbances, persistent dysphagia (in over 20% of cases), a permanent Horner syndrome, injury of the A. vertebralis, and intraoperative injury to the esophagus.

Posterior instrumentation

The posterior access to the cervical spine is suited for all methods of fixation of the cervical spine from the occiput (C0) to the cervico-thoracic transition.

A screw-fixed implant with two longitudinally connecting paraspinal rods is to be preferred to all wire cerclage techniques because of the reliable stability provided. Screw application, however, is very demanding and is performed in the area of the upper cervical spine following to the individual anatomy of each vertebral body and on the lower cervical spine on the lateral mass or transpedicularly.

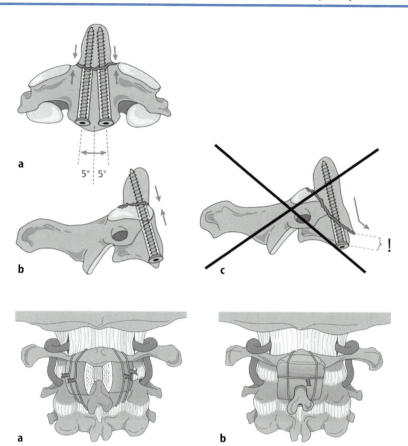

Fig. 12.3 a–c. Screw fixation of the dens only permissible for transverse fractures (from: Ulrich C. Verletzungen der Halswirbelsäule. Orthopädie und Unfallchirurgie update 2006; with permission of Thieme, Germany).

Fig. 12.4 a, b. Posterior C1/2 wire spondylodesis according to Brooks (**a**) and according to Gallie (**b**) (from: Ulrich C. Verletzungen der Halswirbelsäule. Orthopädie und Unfallchirurgie update 2006; with permission of Thieme, Germany).

Because of the very limited stability, sublaminar wire cerclage should nowadays only be an additional method applied after C1/2 screw fixation for fixation of the tricortical bone graft between the arches of C1 and C2. To this end, subperiosteal removal of the membrana atlantoaxialis and of the inner edge of the lamina of C2 is performed with fine, curved dissectors. It is important that this preparation on C1 is not performed further laterally than 1.5 cm from the center line, because the A. vertebralis is inevitably reached with the condyles. The technique according to Gallie (Fig. 12.4 b) is simpler than that of Brooks (Fig. 12.4 a), because the latter method involves preparation further laterally, with the associated risk for vascular injury.

▪ Screw placement C0

For fixation of the occipito-cervical region, screws can be inserted into the skull and will normally remain firmly in place in the region of the occiput even in the event of a very short length of run.

▪ Screw placement C1

Screw placement in C1, for restoration of an open atlas ring after a fracture, for example, is normally not indicated and would be an absolute exception because of the dimension of the C1 vertebral body.

▪ Posterior C1/2 fixation with transarticular screw fixation

The point of insertion for the screws is in the lower medial quadrant of the articular process C2, almost parallel to the intervertebral joints located underneath. To be on the safe side, the dissector should be used for exploration of the medial edge of the vertebral canal during drilling. Drilling is performed in ap-direction. Aim must be taken at the upper edge of the arch of the atlas, which can be made easily visible in a lateral radiograph (Fig. 12.5 a–c).

Before the screws are applied, CT must be performed for precise determination of the individual anatomy, since the course of the A. vertebralis can vary significantly between individ-

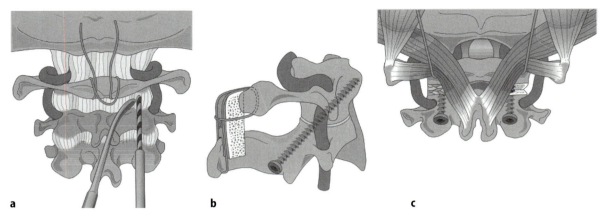

Fig. 12.5 a–c. Posterior C1/2 spondylodesis with transarticular screw fixation according to Magerl (from: Ulrich C. Verletzungen der Halswirbelsäule. Orthopädie und Unfallchirurgie update 2006; with permission of Thieme, Germany).

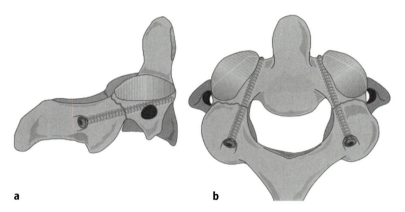

Fig. 12.6 a, b. Screw placement in C2 (from: Ulrich C. Verletzungen der Halswirbelsäule. Orthopädie und Unfallchirurgie update 2006; with permission of Thieme, Germany).

uals. Depending on whether osseous fusion is desired, the C1/2 joints will have to be imaged and removed.

Since the drill must be sunk very deeply in order to match the trajectory of the optimal screw position, it is recommended that two separate interscapular stab incisions are performed and that the soft tissue is perforated by means of a suitably long trocar.

Screw placement C2

Direct screw-fixed osteosynthesis of traumatic spondylolisthesis without comminution is technically demanding. Any decision in favor of this indication should be governed by the utmost reservation, especially because of the risk of injury to the A. vertebralis.

The point of insertion of the screw is the same as for atlanto-axial screw fixation, but the screw is applied at 25° converging antero-medially and parallel to the upper articular surface of C2. Here, too, it will be expedient to explore the inner edge of the spinal canal with a dissector and, as the case may be, to prefer to perforate the screw threads here instead of laterally, where the A. vertebralis passes (Fig. 12.6 a, b).

Lateral mass screws

The position of the screws is standardized, and the technique recommended by Magerl should be used as it permits a long osseous passage. The screw insertion point is located nearly medially from the geometric center of the joint mass. The drilling direction is determined by the inclination of the joint surfaces and in the lateral projection runs parallel to it. In the ap-projection, the screws must diverge around 25° laterally. It is essential to make sure that the tip of the screw does not cut out from the cortical bone on the other side, because this is where the Ramus dorsalis of the spinal ganglia passes, which may cause persistent headache (Fig. 12.7).

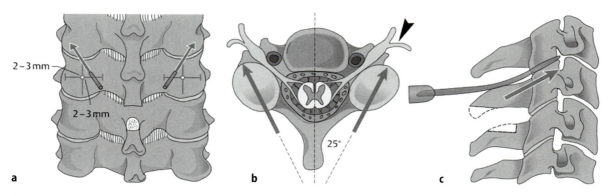

Fig. 12.7 a–c. Orientation lines for positioning massa lateralis screws (from: Ulrich C. Verletzungen der Halswirbelsäule. Orthopädie und Unfallchirurgie update 2006; with permission of Thieme, Germany).

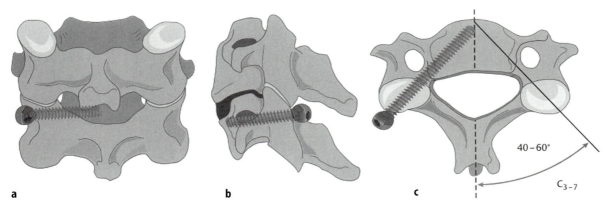

Fig. 12.8 a–c. Placement of transpedicular screws C3–C7 (from: Ulrich C. Verletzungen der Halswirbelsäule. Orthopädie und Unfallchirurgie update 2006; with permission of Thieme, Germany).

Transpedicular screws C3–C7

Transpedicular screw placement requires very extensive lateral preparation. The point of insertion of the screw is located on the upper edge of the lateral mass of the vertebral body to be instrumented. The drilling direction is lowered in the lateral projection by around 10° and converges in the ap-projection between 40° and 60°. Safe placement of a maximally 4 mm-screw is possible with a minimal-invasive method and proper drill gages under fluoroscopic monitoring.

Decompression should be performed after application of the screws and before the longitudinal rods are mounted. For definitive fusion, the cartilage of the intervertebral joints to be fused must be removed and autologous cancellous bone transplanted (Fig. 12.8 a–c).

Upper cervical spine injuries

Fractures of the occipital condyles

They are caused by severe trauma, in a traffic accident at a very high speed, for example; or by a fall on the head, with direct axial trauma being involved. Owing to the close anatomic vicinity of the N. hypoglossus, which exits from a bone canal in the area of the condyles and which in fractures of the condyles can easily be injured, radiological diagnostics must be followed by neurological examination.

Jeanneret presented a comprehensive classification in 1994 (Fig. 12.9 a–d):

- Type I: Fracture of the skull base originating in the foramen magnum and propagating through an occipital condyle.

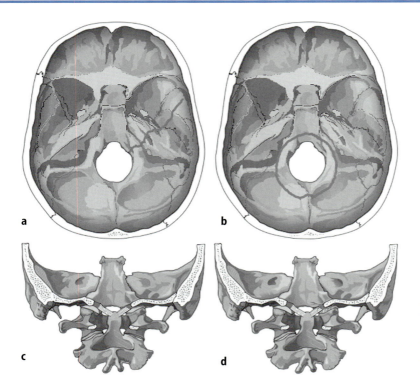

Fig. 12.9 a–d. Fractures of the occipital condyles type I (**a**), II (**b**), III (**c**), and IV (**d**) (from: Ulrich C. Verletzungen der Halswirbelsäule. Orthopädie und Unfallchirurgie update 2006; with permission of Thieme, Germany).

- Type II: Circular fracture of the skull base, so far only found during autopsies of traffic fatalities.
- Type III: (Unilateral) compression fracture of an occipital condyle.
- Type IV: (Unilateral) avulsion fracture of the ligamenta alaria in about one fourth of the cases, together with complete or incomplete atlanto-occipital dislocation.

The choice of therapy is determined by concomitant neurological injuries. Being an osseous injury, it is a domain for conservative treatment (type I injury: soft cervical support (Schanz collar), type II–IV without atlanto-occipital dislocation: soft cervical support for six weeks). However, type II–IV injuries with atlanto-occipital dislocation require stabilization, usually with a posterior spondylodesis C0–C2.

Atlanto-occipital dislocation (AOD)

This injury is normally fatal or is survived for a few hours only. It is characterized by a higher-than-average incidence in children, since their occipital condyles are smaller in relation to the joint masses of the atlas than is the case in adults, and because the joint surfaces are more oriented towards the horizontal plane.

Traynelis and co-workers presented the following classification in 1986, with classification being determined by the dislocation of the head relative to the cervical spine (Fig. 12.10 a–c):

- Type I: Anterior dislocation (most frequent form of luxation).
- Type II: Posterior dislocation.
- Type III: Axial dislocation, which is mostly combined with anterior dislocation.

Immediate trauma death is caused by brain stem and spinal cord injuries, which may include complete shearing-off, as well as lesions of the A. vertebralis. Owing to a perfected emergency service, there have been more and more survivors of such atlanto-occipital dislocations in recent years, with an astonishing age-dependent regeneration tendency found in children.

The conservative therapy consists of closed repositioning and immobilization in the Halo fixateur in adults and in the Minerva plaster in children. In any case, extension must be avoided. Alternatively, posterior atlanto-occipital fusion across the shortest-possible distance can be performed in adults whereas in children also

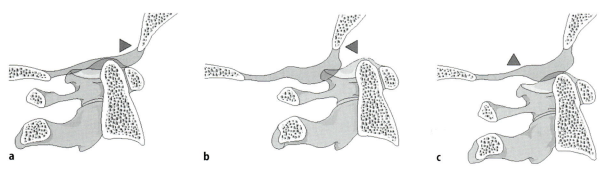

Fig. 12.10 a–c. Anterior (**a**), posterior (**b**), and axial (**c**) atlanto-occipital dislocation (from: Ulrich C. Verletzungen der Halswirbelsäule. Orthopädie und Unfallchirurgie update 2006; with permission of Thieme, Germany).

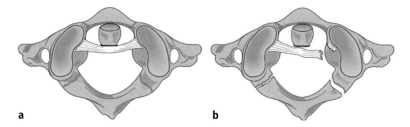

Fig. 12.11 a, b. Stable (**a**) and unstable (**b**) atlas fracture (from: Ulrich C. Verletzungen der Halswirbelsäule. Orthopädie und Unfallchirurgie update 2006; with permission of Thieme, Germany).

a temporary stabilization of the occipito-cervical transition without osseous fusion is possible.

Atlas factures

They are caused by a combination of axial compression and hyperextension, with the posterior atlas base being incarcerated/wedged between the occiput und the spinous process of C2.

Five fracture types are differentiated:
- Type I: Isolated fracture of the anterior atlas arch, stable.
- Type II: Isolated fracture of the posterior atlas arch, stable, always bilateral, similar to the frequent combination with other cervical-spine lesions preferably in the region of the sulcus arteriae vertebralis.
- Type III: Combined fractures of anterior and posterior atlas arch (Jefferson fracture); with intact ligamentum transversum: stable; with rupture or avulsion of the ligamentum transversum: unstable, partially dislocated lateral mass.
- Type IV: Isolated fracture of one lateral mass.
- Type V: Isolated fracture of the processus transversus.

As with the fractures of the condyles, it is necessary to check for concomitant neurological injuries. The N. glossopharyngeus, N. occipitalis major and minor and the chorda tympani are at risk. Differentiation between a stable and an unstable fracture is decisive for determination of the therapy.

An unstable fracture is always involved if in ap-projection one lateral mass extends or both of them extend laterally beyond the upper joints of the axis (Fig. 12.11 a, b).

Fractures, which are not dislocated, represent pure osseous injuries, and therefore conservative treatment in the Halo vest or a hard cervical support (stiff neck) can be initiated. Dislocated fractures can also be treated with Halo vest under extension, but if this fails, one should consider surgery. If repositioning of an unstable fracture is possible under longitudinal traction, C1/2 screw fixation under extension can be performed, with atlanto-occipital mobility being maintained. If this is not possible, occipito-cervical fixation must be considered.

Atlanto-axial dislocation (AAD)

Dislocations between atlas and axis may involve both translatory and rotatory components. Translatory atlanto-axial dislocation, which occurs much more seldom, results more frequently in severe neurological disturbances because of the shearing mechanism involved, so that the diagnosis of a translatory instability is often established post mortem. Rotatory instability is found rather often in adolescents. It causes the typical Cock Robin sign. Based on its intensity, four types are differentiated:

- Type I: Rotatory dislocation without forward dislocation of the atlas; there is still no complete luxation but a painful subluxation, which is the cause of the typical posture of the head; the ligamentum transversum is intact, and the atlanto-dental distance is normal.
- Type II: Rotatory dislocation with dislocation of the atlas by 3 to 5 mm caused by the rupture of the ligamentum transversum.
- Type III: Rotatory dislocation with dislocation of the atlas by more than 5 mm; all atlanto-axial ligamentous connections are ruptured and rotation is additionally associated with translatory displacement and loss of neurological function.
- Type IV: Rotatory dislocation with posterior dislocation of the atlas; this type is often associated with a persistent os odontoideum or dysplasia of the dens.

Diagnosis is easy and based on the typical posture of the head in the CT.

It must be expected that translatory atlanto-axial dislocations will not heal because of ligamentous insufficiency (missing ligamentum transversum). C1/2 screw fixation in anatomical position with osseous fusion is therefore to be aimed at in patients surviving this trauma. As regards the much more frequently occurring rotatory atlanto-axial dislocation, ligamentous injuries – especially in the event of subluxation – are not of primary concern.

The sooner a diagnosis is available after the event, the easier will repositioning be performed successfully. Ligamentous insufficiency will require a period of immobilization of several weeks only. As children are involved in most cases, prognosis is very favorable. Repositioning is performed on the supine child, with the aid of medical relaxation if required, through extension and by turning the head to the opposite side. In the event of a relaxed child, digital repositioning assistance may be performed on the posterior wall of the larynx by the surgeon's finger in the child's mouth applying additional pressure. If there is a reluxation tendency, reposition will be retained through fixation of the head in opposite direction. It is important to make sure in this process that the head only rotates and that it is not at same time flexed. Especially for children, we prefer the Minerva plaster to Halo fixation, because children get used to a Minerva plaster as quickly as they get used to a Halo fixateur. Moreover, the Minerva plaster is more suited to prevent partial removal by the children or their family, which for various reasons is a temptation.

If rupture of the ligamentum transversum is established by MRI, surgical C1/2 transfixation must be considered.

Odontoid fractures

Above the age of 70, fracture of the odontoid is the most common isolated cervical spine injury. On account of the typical accident mechanism, bruises on the forehead of these patients must draw the physician's attention to the dens.

Division of these fractures into three types according to Anderson and D'Alonzo is common. This is a morphological-anatomical classification, which at the same time has a certain predicative value with regard to the development of pseudarthrosis. Meanwhile it has be-

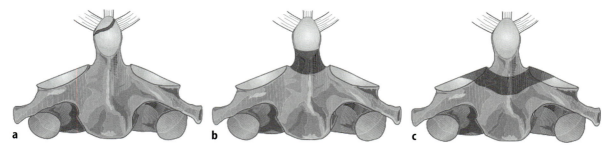

Fig. 12.12 a–c. Dens fracture type I (**a**), type II (**b**), and type III (**c**) (from: Ulrich C. Verletzungen der Halswirbelsäule. Orthopädie und Unfallchirurgie update 2006; with permission of Thieme, Germany).

come safe knowledge that it is less the type of fracture but much more the degree of dislocation, which is decisive for the development of any pseudarthrosis (Fig. 12.12 a–c).

- Type I: Fracture of the tip of the odontoid: Even though this fracture is located on the dens, it corresponds more to an avulsion of the ligamenta alaria and thus does not represent an isolated injury in the strictest sense; if dislocation is below 1 mm, external immobilization, i.e. a conservative approach, is the therapy to choose.
- Type II: Fracture of the odontoid process above its base: This is the most frequent type, and it is just as often associated with pseudarthrosis because of its dislocation tendency (67%); depending on the dislocation of the atlas, which "carries along" the broken-off tip of the dens, we talk about an extension fracture if the atlas with the dens fragment is dislocated posteriorly and about a flexion fracture if the atlas with the dens tip is dislocated anteriorly.
- Type III: Fracture course in the axis body: Fractures of this type directly turn into corpus fractures or traumatic C2 spondylolisthesis and require very precise analysis by means of multiplanar CT scans.

Regarding type II injuries, therapy is determined by the degree of dislocation: If we are dealing with a primarily non-displaced fracture, conservative therapy will be justified, either via Halo fixation or via the stiff neck, for at least eight weeks. After that, external immobilization is to be removed and mobility monitored via lateral image intensifier. Extension or flexion injuries are repositioned under lateral image intensifier monitoring and immobilized after repositioning is completed. Surgical stabilization (direct screw fixation) is indicated for a primary dislocation exceeding 1 mm, or if closed repositioning is not possible.

In type III fractures, if no spondylolisthesis is diagnosed, we are mostly dealing with an osseous injury, thus the therapeutic approach (conservative) is defined.

Odontoid fractures are chiefly associated with old age and very often with osteoporosis. Surgical therapy, in particular of dislocated type II fractures, with a direct lag screw is not always possible because of rarified bone. Posterior C1/2 fixation, however, is always possible, and provides the patient with a high degree of safety as well as it is easy to perform. If the fracture course is visible on functional radiographs for a long time without instability being identifiable, clinical checks at six-month intervals will be justified without further surgical measures being indicated.

Traumatic spondylolisthesis of the axis

The classification according to Effendi, which has been slightly modified and made more precise in the later years, is most frequently applied (Fig. 12.13 a–c):

- Type I: Most frequent type: Non-dislocated or only slightly dislocated traumatic spondylolysis with minimal dislocation of the corpus vertebrae of C2, but without injury to the disc; a fracture line width of 3 mm constitutes the borderline for the transition to an unstable type; interestingly, type I may within a few days turn into a type II or III if disc

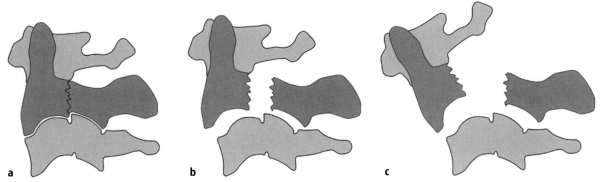

Fig. 12.13 a–c. Traumatic spondylolisthesis of the axis type I (**a**), type II (**b**), and type III (**c**) (from: Ulrich C. Verletzungen der Halswirbelsäule. Orthopädie und Unfallchirurgie update 2006; with permission of Thieme, Germany).

instability does not primarily lead to dislocation.

- Type II: The vertebral body of C2 is dislocated anteriorly and the intervertebral disc space is obviously injured; the joints, however, are not affected; depending on the position of the dens axis in flexion or in extension, this fracture type can be differentiated further; since the disc is injured, growing instability will have to be expected, so that surgical treatment is to be recommended.
- Type III: Combination of a spondylolisthesis with interlocked dislocation of the small vertebral joints, with the vertebral body being permanently under flexion; if this type, which actually corresponds to the historical Hangman injury, primarily occurs as a consequence of an accident, lethality must be expected to be high.

If we are dealing with a purely osseous type I injury without significant dislocation, conservative treatment via stiff neck or Halo fixateur will always be possible. The limits of the stiff neck are defined by the subjective symptoms of the patient in this case. With regard to type II injuries, therapy will consist either of closed repositioning with direct screw fixation of the broken-off pedicle on the vertebral body or of an anterior C2/3 spondylodesis, through which the slipped vertebral body can be re-attached to the arch. In case of an interlocked luxation, which means a type III injury, primary closed reduction is necessitated. If this can be achieved, anterior C2/3 fixation may be performed. If closed reduction is not possible, a posterior approach will as rule have to be implemented, with reduction being followed by direct translaminar screw fixation, as here, too, anterior spondylodesis with removal of the damaged disc is required.

However, there is no standardized surgical therapy for this type of injury; therapy will thus be determined by the individual case. If the posterior elements are intact, posterior C2/3 stabilization with screw fixation on the lateral mass and mounting of short longitudinal rods between the screws may represent a practicable surgical option. In an individual case it might be necessary to include C1 in this fixation via cerclage, without a definitive fusion with bone transplantation C1/2 being performed at the same time, or even to perform extension further cranially with inclusion of the occiput, i.e. a so-called occipito-cervical fixation. Especially in juveniles, this does not necessarily have to be associated with osseous fusion, so that after six to nine months the metal can be removed after osseous healing of the affected C2 or C1, with the prospect of restored mobility in the respective joints.

As with corpus fractures of C2, traumatic spondylolisthesis also requires exclusion of additional injury of the Arteria vertebralis, which takes a special course in C2.

Lower cervical spine injuries

The uniform anatomy of the lower cervical spine from C3 to C7 permits summarized classification of the types of injury, even though the size of the vertebral bodies increases between C3 and C7 by 20% to 30%.

In contrast to the thoraco-lumbar spine, there is no generally accepted classification for the lower cervical spine. However, the AO classification according to Magerl et al., originally developed for the thoraco-lumbar spine, is emerging as a classification that can also used for the cervical spine.

Table 12.1. Type A injuries of the lower cervical spine.

A1 Impact	A2 Split	A3 Burst
A1.1 Incomplete fracture of the upper endplate	A2.1 Split in the frontal plane without dislocation	A3.1 Incomplete burst fracture
A1.2 Wedge-shaped vertebral body	A2.2 Split in the frontal plane with dislocation	A3.2 Complete burst fracture
A1.3 Collapse of the vertebral body	A2.3 Split in the sagittal plane with/without split in the frontal plane	

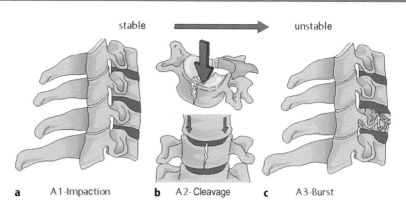

Fig. 12.14 a–c. Classification of A injuries of the lower cervical spine (with permission of Thieme, Germany).

a A1-Impaction
b A2-Cleavage
c A3-Burst

Table 12.2. Type B injuries of the lower cervical spine.

B1 Ligamentous injury of the posterior elements	B2 Osseous injury of the posterior elements	B3 Hyperextension with anterior dislocation through the disc
B1.1 Rupture of the posterior ligament complex with subluxation of the facet joints – bilateral	B2.1 Transverse fracture through the arch	B3.1 Rupture of the disc with osseous detachment/avulsion of base and upper endplate
B1.2 Rupture of the posterior ligament complex with luxation of the facet joints – bilateral (interlocking joints)	B2.2 Fracture through the facet joints – bilateral	B3.2 Rupture of the disc with facet joint fracture
B1.3 Rupture of the posterior ligament complex with luxation and/or fracture of the facet joints – bilateral – and anterior translation	B2.3 Fracture through the pedicles	B3.3 Rupture of the disc with facet joint fracture and posterior dislocation

Blauth suggested modification in 1998, which has been confirmed by Magerl in cooperation with Blauth in the meantime.

According to this classification, type A injuries (Table 12.1) are the result of compression (Fig. 12.14 a–c).

Type B injuries (Table 12.2) are always characterized as ruptures of posterior structures caused by excessive distraction. Originally, Blauth described osseous injuries in B1 and ligamentous injuries in B2. Magerl proposed to classify ligamentous injuries as B1 and osseous additional injuries as B2, because instability clearly increases between B1 and B2, as a result of which a classification criterion "increasing injury severity with higher numerical number" is fulfilled. Ligamentous injuries can be completely stable in the state of luxation, but they may under certain circumstances become unstable through repositioning (Fig. 12.15 a–c). Owing to the injury mechanism, neurological concomitant injuries occur much more frequently with the cervical type B than with the thoraco-lumbar type B, and even more often than with the type C of the cervical spine classification.

As regards this type of injury, particular attention must be paid to a possible indication for closed repositioning, as this has resulted in dramatic neurological deterioration in certain cases. A primarily posteriorly dislocated disc part, which in the absence of adequate extension during repositioning is pressed into the spinal canal, was identified as the cause. The procedure for such luxations is therefore as follows: If the indispensable CT shows a posteriorly dislocated disc part, this fragment will have to be surgically removed through (partial) vertebrectomy before repositioning and spondylodesis are performed.

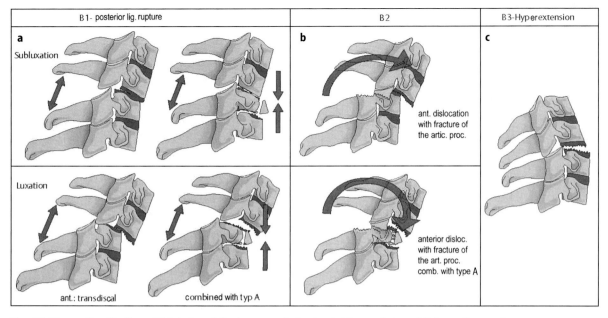

Fig. 12.15 a–c. Classification of B injuries of the lower cervical spine (with permission of Thieme, Germany).

Table 12.3. Type C injuries of the lower cervical spine.

C1 Combined with Type A injury	C2 Combined with Type B injury	C3 Specific injuries
Unifacetal fracture	C2.2 Unifacetal subluxation	C3.1 Unilateral fracture dislocation of the lateral mass
	C2.3 Unifacetal luxation with interlocking	C3.2 Slice fracture
		C3.3 Separating of the vertebral bodies from the arches across several segments

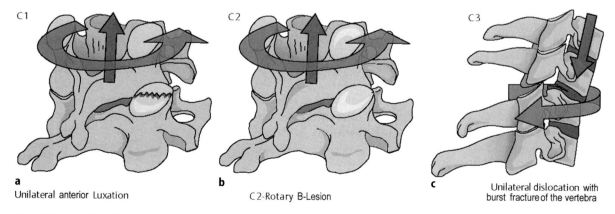

Fig. 12.16 a–c. Classification of C injuries of the lower cervical spine (with permission of Thieme, Germany).

Type C injuries (Table 12.3) involve both the anterior and posterior elements through rotation (Fig. 12.16 a–c).

In addition to the above-mentioned three main criteria for assessing surgery indication, and with special regard to a potentially posteriorly dislocated disc fragment, injuries on the lower cervical spine demand that the question is put as to whether or not functional treatment of the injury is possible without the risk of displacement or further dislocation.

As this question can be answered in the affirmative only for A1 injury types, the lower cervical spine is a domain for surgical stabilization as classical spondylodesis for all other types of injury besides the surgical indications applying to the entire spinal column; and, of course, performed preferably anteriorly because of the biologically favorable situation.

References

1. Blauth M (1998) Grundlagen der Wirbelsäulentraumatologie, Obere HWS, Untere HWS. In: Tscherne H, Blauth M (eds) Unfallchirurgie – Wirbelsäule. Springer, Berlin, S 2–238
2. Castro W, Lemcke H, Schilgen M, Lemcke L (1998) Das sogenannte „HWS-Schleudertrauma" – haftungsrechtliche und medizinische Überlegungen. Chirurg 37:176–184
3. Ebraheim NA, Haman ST, Xu R, Yeasting RA (1998) The anatomic location of the dorsal ramus of the cervical nerve and its relation to the superior articular process of the lateral mass. Spine 23:1968–1971
4. Glaser JA, Jaworks BA, Cuddy BG, Albert TJ, Hollowell JP, McLain RF, Bozzette SA (1998) Variation in surgical opinion regarding management of selected cervical spine injuries – a preliminary study. Spine 23:975–984
5. Graham JJ (1989) Complications of cervical spine surgery. A five-year report on a survey of the membership of the Cervical Spine Research Society by the morbity and mortality committee. Spine 14:1046–1050
6. Hofmeister M, Potulski M, Späth K, Jaksche H, Bühren V (1998) Klinische Ergebnisse der ventralen Fixation von HWS-Verletzungen. Osteosynthese International 6:112–120
7. Jónsson J, Bring G, Rauschning W, Sahlstedt B (1991) Hidden cervical spine injuries in traffic accident victims with skull fractures. J Spinal Disord 4:251–263
8. Kast E, Mohr K, Richter HP, Börm W (2006) Complications of transpedicular screw fixation in the cervical spine. Eur Spine J 15:327–334
9. Ulrich C, Nothwang J (1999) Biomechanik und Klinik der Spondylodese an der unteren HWS – Technik und Implantate. Orthopäde 28:637–650
10. Ulrich C, Nothwang J, Arand M (2001) Injuries of the lower cervical spine. Eur Spine J 10:88–100
11. Vecsei V, Fuchs M, Gäbler C (1998) Indikationen zum kombinierten dorso-ventralen Vorgehen bei HWS-Verletzungen. Osteosynthese International 6:121–128
12. White 3rd AA, Panjabi MM (1990) Clinical biomechanics of the spine. Lippincott, Philadelphia
13. Whitehill R, Stowers SF, Fechner RE, Ruch WW, Drucker S, Gibson LR, McKernan DJ, Widmeyer JH (1987) Posterior cervical fusions using cerclage wires, methacrylate cement and autogenous bone graft. An experimental study of a canine model. Spine 12:12–22

13 Thoracic spine injuries – open versus endoscopic procedures

Markus Arand and Markus Schultheiss

Introduction

Minimally invasive techniques are becoming more widespread in different surgical fields. Standard open surgical procedures were modified to become less invasive, with the intention to reduce recovery time, morbidity, and ultimately expenditures. Improvements in technology allow the surgeon to enter body cavities and create potential spaces such as the retroperitoneum by diaphragm splitting. Improved fiber optics, light sources, and use of 30° angled optic cameras result in improved visualization of the structures surrounding the spine [1–4, 6, 7, 14–18, 22]. Indications for endoscopic spinal surgery are degenerative diseases, infection, tumor, fracture, and ventral release for scoliosis and kyphosis. This minimally invasive technique seems to provide a feasible alternative to thoracotomy or posterolateral approaches for decompression and vertebral body reconstruction. Especially in fracture treatment with the necessity of spinal decompression, sometimes of several segments, long distance bridging by strut graft and stabilization play an important role. However, there is a lack of adequate instrumentation systems. It has been concluded that the limiting factor in the wide application of the endoscopic technique is the absence of a commercially available internal fixation system for this endoscopical approach [5]. This system has been developed during the last ten years and has been proven well concerning its biomechanical stability.

Beside this, the endoscopic procedure has been standardized and now is clinically well established [1–4, 19–21, 24, 25].

The endoscopic technique and the instrumentation system are described in the following part as well as an overview about advantages and disadvantages of this method is given.

Fracture classification, clinical examination and the pathway for indications are described in the following chapter "Surgical treatment of fractures of the lumbar spine".

Instrumentation system

A endoscopically implantable system for the treatment of fractures from T4 to L3 was developed. This modular anterior construct system (MACS TL, Modular Anterior Construct System Thoracic Lumbar, Aesculap, Tuttlingen, Germany (Fig. 13.1)) allows an endoscopic approach and thoracoscopic instrumentation from T4 to L1, endoscopic diaphragm splitting and thoracoscopic instrumentation to L2, and a minimally invasive retroperitoneal approach to L3/L4 for fracture stabilization [1–4, 19–21, 24, 25]. As a twin screw concept it consists of a rigid angle-stable monocortical anchorage due to two convergent polyaxial screws in each vertebral body and a low-profile plate (< 10 mm) or rods. The system is conceived for mono- and multisegmental stabilization. The self-cutting screws are both connected

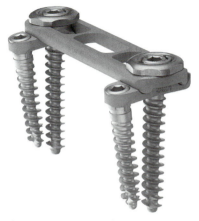

Fig. 13.1. MACS TL stabilization system.

with the fracture overbridging plate by means of a polyaxial clamping element. The cannulated posterior polyaxial screw can be inserted over a K-wire, its length ranges from 25 to 50 mm, the diameter is 7.0 mm and the angle of rotation is 14°. The direction of the anterior stabilization screw is given by the clamping element, its length ranges from 25 to 50 mm and the diameter is 6.5 mm. A locking mechanism in the clamp prevents the anterior screw from backing out. Plates are available in lengths from 45–100 mm, rods up to 200 mm. Locking nuts and screws guarantee a rigid fixation between over-bridging plate, clamping elements, and screws. Additionally a bone graft clamp can be used to fixate the bone graft with a screw.

Operative technique [1–3, 5, 22]

Due to the organs in the thoracic (heart, vascular situation) and upper abdominal cavity (liver) a left-sided position is preferred for the treatment of lesions from T4 to T8, whereas for the approach to the thoraco-lumbar junction (T9-L2), right-sided positioning is preferred with a minimal incision of the diaphragm which allows for a retroperitoneal approach down to the level of L2. Lesions affecting the spine below L2 are approached through a minimal retroperitoneal access from the left side, as described in the chapter 14: "Surgical treatment of fractures of the lumbar spine". The decision for the approach is taken in each individual case based on the preoperative CT scans. Double lung intubation is checked bronchoscopically, but no other specific anesthesiological monitoring is needed is case of thoracoscopic approach. In all our cases, except tumor and infection, blood saving techniques by cell saver were used. A single dose of a second-generation cephalosporin was given prior to surgery.

The whole operative endoscopic procedure is performed in a stable lateral position via three intercostal working channels and one optical channel in general anesthesia with one-lung ventilation. The surgeon and the camera assistant stand behind the patient, the first assistant on the opposite side. An image intensifier is positioned between the surgeon and the camera assistant.

Before operation the position and free tilt of the C-arm is checked and the projection of the target area as well as the optical and working channels are marked under fluoroscopic control on the skin with a water-resistant pen. This is important, because an incorrectly positioned port can become a hindrance during the following procedure.

The operation starts directly over the target area with a 1.5 cm skin incision followed by a mini-thoracotomy. The muscle layers of the thoracic wall are divided following the directions of the fibers with a zigzag incision, and the opening is gradually widened by the insertion of Langenbeck hooks. The pleura is perforated after collapsing of the lung and a spreader or frame needs to be placed.

Afterwards the optical channel (10 mm black trocar) is placed two to three intercostal spaces cranial to the injured vertebra in the spinal axis under video-visualization by the thoracoscope installed in the working channel. The channels for suction/irrigation (10 mm black trocar) and retractor for lung or diaphragm (10 mm black trocar) are placed about 5–10 cm anterior to the working and optical channel under videoscopic control. The operating field is identified after illumination by the thoracoscope and diaphragm and lung tissue are retracted with the help of endoretractors (Endo Paddle Retract, Auto Suture, Norwalk, USA). After orientation and identification of the exact level of the spine by an image intensifier, diaphragm splitting is performed with monopolar cauterization if necessary. Overlying muscles or retroperitoneal fat tissue are dissected bluntly from the lateral side of the vertebral body with preservation of the segmental blood vessels. Those vessels of the fractured vertebra – and if necessary also those of the adjacent vertebrae – need to be mobilized and clipped. The branches of the sympathetic chains are identified and, if possible, preserved.

As the next step, it is important to create landmarks via K-wires to maintain proper alignment and surgical trajectories. K-wires have to be positioned into the vertebral bodies above and below of the level of corporectomy in case of a bisegmental stabilization, and in case of a monosegmental stabilization in the non-fractured caudal zone of the affected vertebral body. The K-wires have to be positioned approximately 10 mm from the dorsal edge and 10–13 mm from the cranial or caudal end plate to a maximal depth of 20 mm in case of bisegmental stabilization. Figure 13.2 a–g illustrates this K-wire insertion as well as the whole procedure (Fig. 13.2 a–g).

a Insertion of the K-wires approximately 10 mm from the dorsal edge and 10–13 mm from the cranial or caudal end plate.

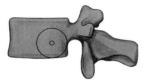

b Preparation of screw insertion point by opening the cortex.

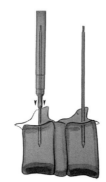

c Connection of the centralizer to the insertion sleeve.

d Implantation of the posterior polyaxial screw driven in via K-wire.

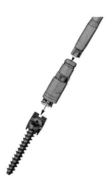

e Removal of the screw driver and insertion sleeve; both clamping elements now serve as landmarks for the alignment.

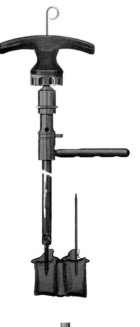

f Insertion of the stabilizing screw: The polyaxial screw is now driven into the final depth to ensure optimum form fit with the spinal anatomy followed by placement of the anterior stabilization screw.

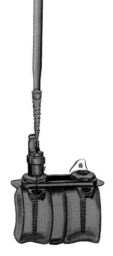

g Locking the polyaxiality.

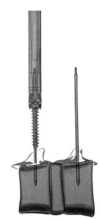

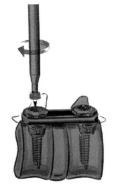

Fig. 13.2 a–g. Step by step description of the endoscopic implantation of MACS TL (with permission of Aesculap, Germany).

The K-wire placement is followed by insertion of the dorsal polyaxial screws in the adjacent vertebrae in case of a bisegmental stabilization. The K-wire has to be removed at this stage because jamming in the cannulated screw can lead to perforation of the opposite cortex. The clamping element needs to be orientated in a way that the hole for the anterior stabilization screw lies anterior. The two screws and the clamping element in the adjacent vertebrae are landmarks for the following decompression and corporectomy. With the help of these markers orientation of the spinal axis and distance to the spinal canal is possible. Using a long osteotome the extent of the planned corporectomy is defined. The next step is the resection of the adjacent discs and the careful removal of fragmented parts under video assistance with long rongeurs. With the help of video magnification, posterior fragments of the vertebral body which compromise the spinal canal can be carefully resected. Finally, measurement of the graft bed and strut grafting are performed. Autologous tricortical bone graft from the iliac crest or bovine bone cages (Tutogen, Tutogen Medical GmbH, Neunkirchen, Germany) are inserted in adequate lengths in a press-fit technique through the working channel. Afterwards a slight reduction is performed manually with pressurizing on the spinous processes in case of single anterior approach. If more correction of the spinal alignment is necessary, expandable cages (Synex, Stratec Medical, Oberdorf, Switzerland) are implanted.

Measuring the distance between the connecting elements and adding 25 mm establishes the exact length of the plate. Afterwards this fitting plate can be laid onto the connecting elements

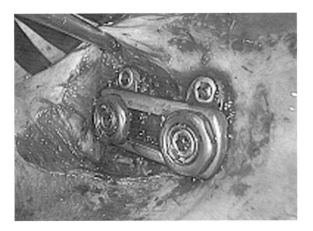

Fig. 13.3. Final fixation with MACS TL system.

by introducing it lengthwise into the chest cavity and connecting it by its fixation nuts. Tightening of the polyaxial screws will bring the assembly into the final position directly onto the surface of the vertebral bodies. Finally the anterior screws are fixed in the connecting element being part of the rigid four-point stabilization mechanism (Fig. 13.3). Locking nuts have to be tightened with a torque of 15 Nm, locking screws with 10 Nm using an appropriate torque wrench.

If necessary the diaphragm is closed with sutures in common endoscopic technique. A 24-Charriere chest tube is placed in the costo-diaphragmatic recess. All portals are closed with sutures after removal of the trocars.

Postoperatively, patients with chest tube normally are monitored for one day on the intermediate care unit and afterwards on the normal unit. Mobilization and ventilation training

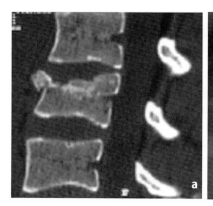 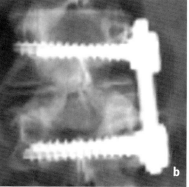 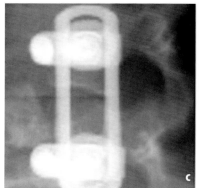

Fig. 13.4 a–c. Case example of a monosegmental stabilization of an A 3.1 fracture using the MACS TL system.

started on the first postoperative day without orthosis with the help of a physiotherapist.

Figure 13.4 illustrates a typical case of monosegmental stabilization in case of an A 3.1 fracture with the MACS TL system (Fig. 13.4 a–c).

Special considerations

Corporectomy and spinal decompression of the dorsal rim

The most common technique for the reconstruction of the load-bearing anterior column is a lesion bridging fusion between the neighboring intact vertebral bodies.

Autologous bone from the iliac crest is considered the gold standard. However, several vertebral body replacement systems are increasingly used, predominantly titanium cages (Synex, Synthes, Umkirch, Switzerland or Obelisc, Ulrich medical, Ulm, Germany) [1, 11, 23].

The corporectomy requires long-shaft resection instruments like chisels, rongeurs, punches and curettes with a scale controlling the working depth. The instruments should be controlled with both hands. A long-shaft milling cutter is not recommendable in our opinion, since it bears a considerable risk of damaging adjacent vessels.

Before starting the corporectomy, segmental vessels need to be clipped. After mobilization and ligation with double clips, the vessels are divided with endoscopic scissors.

Then the boundaries of the planned bone graft bed, parallel to the anterior and posterior walls, are marked with an osteotome. A safe working corridor needs to be established by the positioning of the clamping elements. The bony material of the fractured vertebral body and the adjacent discs are ablated with the rongeur or punch. The endplates of the adjacent discs can be roughened with a curette.

Indications for spinal decompression are undoubtedly given in case of neurological symptoms. A relative indication for posterior wall resection is a remaining dislocated posterior wall fragment without neurological deficits, for example after dorsal laminectomy and stabilization. Depending on the extent of stenosis, anterior decompression should be considered, to reduce the risk of subsequent myelopathy.

If spinal decompression of the dorsal rim is necessary, a partial corporectomy should initially be carried out with a safe zone of approximately 5 mm from the posterior wall. The lower boundary of the pedicle is probed with a nerve hook. Then the pedicle of the vertebral arch can be resected step by step in a cranial direction using a punch in order to visualize the dura. After this, the posterior dislocated fragment can be removed through mobilization of the fragment into the created cavity following partial corporectomy.

A hemorrhage or a little dura leak can be covered by a hemostypticum.

Open versus endoscopic procedures

Minimally invasive techniques avoid part of the access related morbidity of conventional open approaches, especially with regard to postoperative pain, bleeding and surgical trauma. In addition, postoperative morbidity is reduced and rehabilitation time is shortened [1, 2, 8–10].

However, many orthopedic surgeons might not be familiar with minimally invasive endoscopic techniques. For example, most surgeons are used to a conventional open view on a surgical field and the ability to physically verify events whereas they are not used to a magnified two-dimensional image like in pure endoscopic procedures. Even in the presence of specially designed instrumentation systems prolonged learning curves may be the result. Therefore both surgeons and scrub nurses need some extensive training in order to acquire the necessitated skills.

In the beginning of thoracoscopic spinal surgery there was a lack of specially adapted systems. As a consequence, devices, which were designed for an open implantation technique, had been used. However, disadvantages resulting from the use of such devices have been eliminated by the implementation of new systems like the MACS TL system.

Table 13.1 summarizes the advantages and disadvantages of endoscopic procedures in contrast to open techniques, which have been evaluated during clinical application (Table 13.1) [1, 2, 9–11, 22].

Meanwhile the initial enthusiasm for endoscopic techniques was replaced by a more realistic approach with regard to practicability and safety of this new technique. We prefer a mini-

Table 13.1. Advantages and disadvantages of thoracoscopic spine surgery.

Advantages of the thoracoscopic technique
- Tissue preserving procedure; no rib resection or retraction is needed for the approach
- Excellent visualization within the thoracic cavity due to modern 30° optics
- Reduced blood loss
- Efficient and safe anterior decompression and stabilization
- Reduced postoperative morbidity
- Reduced pain and accelerated rehabilitation
- Improved cosmetic result

Disadvantages of the thoracoscopic technique
- Complexity of anesthesia (double-lumen intubation)
- Learning curve for intraoperative endoscopical handling
- Two-dimensional view
- Bleeding control in case of major complications
- Reposition of larger deformities is limited

mally open, but still less invasive endoscopically assisted approach in contrast to Bühren and coworkers [5]. In all cases of strut grafting or implantation of an extendable cage, a larger incision of the working channel must be performed. Therefore we use this "enlarged" working channel from the beginning of the operation with a spreader frame which facilitates the whole procedure [22]. An intermediate direct three-dimensional view in contrast to the two-dimensional screen view prevents disorientation of the surgeon and overestimation of the real situation, which might be caused by magnification. Consequently, this might increase the safety of the procedure. Besides this, the repeated installation of a speculum to enlarge the small skin incision of the working channel during the whole procedure is time consuming and may cause infection. Finally this "open window" makes it easier to manage complications, especially in tumor cases [12–14].

A comparison of endoscopic spine surgeries to open procedures with regard to operation duration, blood loss, pain relief, and hospitalization time revealed superiority of the minimally invasive procedure. However, the complication rate of endoscopic procedure is equal to that known from open techniques [1].

In conclusion, endoscopic procedures on the spine have become an alternative to open standard procedures. Nevertheless, the indication for any anterior thoracic spine surgery should be set very careful and independent from the assumed feasibility of the procedure (open versus endoscopic).

Summary

Endoscopic procedures on the spine have become an alternative to standard spine surgeries in the last ten years.

In times of technical remodeling minimally invasive procedures like endoscopic spine surgery are in favour to open procedures with regard to operation duration, blood loss, pain relief and overall hospitalization time.

However, such endoscopic procedures are technically demanding and, even in the presence of specially adapted instrumentation systems, spine surgeons need time to become familiar with these procedures.

References

1. Beisse R (2006) Endoscopic surgery on the thoracolumbar junction of the spine. Eur Spine J 15: 687–704
2. Beisse R, Potulski M, Beger J, Bühren V (2002) Entwicklung und klinischer Einsatz einer thorakoskopisch implantierbaren Rahmenplatte zur Behandlung thorakolumbaler Frakturen und Instabilitäten. Orthopäde 31:413–422
3. Beisse R, Potulski M, Temme C, Bühren V (1998) Das endoskopisch kontrollierte Zwerchfellspitting. Ein minimal-invasiver Zugang zur ventralen Versorgung thorakolumbaler Frakturen der Wirbelsäule. Unfallchirurg 101:619–627
4. Bühren V (1998) Thorakoskopische Versorgung von Frakturen der Brust- und Lendenwirbelsäule. Langenbecks Arch Chir Suppl Kongressbd 115: 108–112
5. Bühren V, Beisse R, Potulski M (1997) Minimalinvasive ventrale Spondylodesen bei Verletzungen der Brust- und Lendenwirbelsäule. Chirurg 68: 1076–1084
6. Connelly CS, Manges PA (1998) Video-assisted thoracoscopic discectomy and fusion. Aorn J 67: 940–945
7. Cunningham BW, Kotani Y, McNulty PS, Cappucino A, Kanayama M, Fedder IL (1998) Video-assisted thoracoscopic surgery versus open thora-

cotomy for anterior thoracic spinal fusion. A comparative radiographic, biomechanical, and histologic analysis in a sheep model. Spine 23: 1333–1340
8. Knop C, Blauth M, Bühren V, Arand M, Egbers HJ, Hax PM, Nothwang J, Oestern HJ, Pizanis A, Roth R, Weckbach A, Wentzensen A (2001) Operative Behandlung von Verletzungen des thorakolumbalen Übergangs – Teil 3: Nachuntersuchung. Ergebnisse einer prospektiven multizentrischen Studie der Arbeitsgemeinschaft „Wirbelsäule" der Deutschen Gesellschaft für Unfallchirurgie. Unfallchirurg 104:583–600
9. Knop C, Blauth M, Bühren V, Hax PM, Kinzl L, Mutschler W, Pommer A, Ulrich C, Wagner S, Weckbach A, Wentzensen A, Wörsdorfer O (1999) Operative Behandlung von Verletzungen des thorakolumbalen Übergangs. Teil 1: Epidemiologie. Unfallchirurg 102:924–935
10. Knop C, Blauth M, Bühren V, Hax PM, Kinzl L, Mutschler W, Pommer A, Ulrich C, Wagner S, Weckbach A, Wentzensen A, Wörsdorfer O (2000) Operative Behandlung von Verletzungen des thorakolumbalen Übergangs. Teil 2: Operation und röntgenologische Befunde. Unfallchirurg 103: 1032–1047
11. Knop C, Lange U, Bastian L, Blauth M (2000) Three-dimensional motion analysis with Synex. Comparative biomechanical test series with a new vertebral body replacement for the thoracolumbar spine. Eur Spine J 9:472–485
12. Kossmann T, Jakobi D, Trentz O (2001) The use of a retractor system (SynFrame) for open, minimal invasive reconstruction of the anterior column of thoracic and lumbar spine. Eur Spine J 10:396–402
13. Mayer HM (1997) A new microsurgical technique for minimally invasive anterior lumbar interbody fusion. Spine 22:691–699
14. Mayer HM (2000) Minimally invasive spine surgery. A surgical manual. Springer, Berlin
15. Regan JJ, Ben-Yishay A, Mack MJ (1998) Video-assisted thoracoscopic excision of herniated thoracic disc: description of technique and preliminary experience in the first 29 cases. J Spinal Disord 11:183–191
16. Regan JJ, Guyer RD (1997) Endoscopic techniques in spinal surgery. Clin Orthop 335:122–139
17. Regan JJ, Mack MJ, Picetti GD 3rd (1995) A technical report on video-assisted thoracoscopy in thoracic spinal surgery. Preliminary description. Spine 20:831–837
18. Rosenthal D, Dickman CA (1998) Thoracoscopic microsurgical excision of herniated thoracic discs. J Neurosurg 89:224–235
19. Schultheiss M, Claes L, Wilke HJ, Kinzl L, Hartwig E (2003) Enhanced primary stability through additional cementable cannulated rescue screw for anterior thoracolumbar plate application. J Neurosurg 98 (Suppl):50–55
20. Schultheiss M, Hartwig E, Kinzl L, Claes L, Wilke HJ (2004) Thoracolumbar fracture stabilization: comparative biomechanical evaluation of a new video-assisted implantable system. Eur Spine J 13:93–100
21. Schultheiss M, Hartwig E, Sarkar M, Kinzl L, Claes L, Wilke HJ (2006) Biomechanical in vitro comparison of different mono- and bisegmental anterior procedures with regard to the strategy for fracture stabilization using minimally invasive techniques. Eur Spine J 15:82–89
22. Schultheiss M, Kinzl L, Claes L, Wilke HJ, Hartwig E (2003) Minimally invasive ventral spondylodesis for thoracolumbar fracture treatment: surgical technique and first clinical outcome. Eur Spine J 12:618–624
23. Schultheiss M, Sarkar M, Arand M, Kramer M, Wilke HJ, Kinzl L (2005) Solvent preserved, bovine cancellous bone blocks used for reconstruction of thoracolumbar fractures in minimally invasive spinal surgery – first clinical results. Eur Spine J 14:192–196
24. Schultheiss M, Wilke HJ, Claes L, Kinzl L, Hartwig E (2002) MACS-TL-Polyaxialscrew XL. Ein neues Konzept zur Stabilitätserhöhung ventraler Spondylodesen in Anwesenheit dorsaler Verletzungen. Orthopäde 31:397–401
25. Schultheiss M, Wilke HJ, Claes L, Kinzl L, Hartwig E (2002) MACS-TL-twin-screw. Ein neues thorakoskopisch implantierbares Stabilisationssystem zur Behandlung von Wirbelfrakturen – Implantatdesign, Implantationstechnik und In-vitro-Testung. Orthopäde 31:362–367

14 Surgical treatment of fractures of the lumbar spine

FLORIAN GEBHARD and MARKUS SCHULTHEISS

Introduction

Fractures of the lumbar spine are common and often result in significant disability. They are mostly the result of high-energy trauma (a fall from a height or a road accident). The mechanism, which causes the lesion should be investigated as this will provide useful clues to the injury pattern that may be encountered [13, 17]. However, such as in elderly people, patients with metabolic bone disorders and in people with cancer, affected vertebrae fracture with little or no force. Most commonly broken are those in the lower back [7].

The goals of surgery are decompression of the spinal canal if necessary, reduction of the deformity and a stable fixation of the spine to permit early mobilization.

When intervention is indicated, the choice of surgical technique, beginning with the approach, remains a point of discussion [14–16].

Biomechanical factors play an important role in deciding whether an anterior, a posterior or a combined approach is the best option [25, 27].

Specially adapted to the specific characteristics of lumbar spine fractures an overview of treatment options is summarized in this chapter.

Anatomy, pathophysiology and fracture classification

The lumbar spine consists of five free vertebrae. The thoracic spine is stabilized by the attached rib cage and intercostal musculature, whereas the sacral segments are fused. Between the thoracic spine and the sacrum, the relatively mobile segments of the lumbar spine must transmit all of the compressive, bending, and rotational forces generated between the upper and the lower part of the body. Therefore the lumbar spine is enclosed in strong muscles and ligaments.

The forces responsible for spinal fractures are compression, rotation, shear, or distraction forces or a combination of these mechanisms. The most common acute fractures are compression fractures or vertebral endplate fractures caused by sudden axial loading.

Fractures of the spine have been classified by Magerl and co-workers [17]. According to this classification there are three basic injury patterns:
- compression fractures (type A),
- distraction injuries (type B),
- and type A or B injuries with rotation (type C).

Clinical findings

Patients with lumbo-sacral fractures may present with severe pain, deformity, and neurological deficits related to compression of neural structures. Caused by lesions of the conus medullaris and lumbar nerve roots a mixture of cord and root syndromes can be produced by fractures below the thoraco-lumbar junction. Complete damage of the conus medullaris manifests as no motor function or sensation below L1. Complete damage to the sacral portion of the cord leads to partial movement of the lower extremities and loss of control of bladder and bowel function. Fractures in the lumbar region also can cause a cauda equina syndrome. This includes variable paraparesis, asymmetrical saddle anesthesia, radiating pain, and sphincter disturbance. A rectal examination to check for rectal tone and voluntary sphincter function is mandatory. The physical examination of a patient with an acute lumbar fracture usually is limited by severe pain. However, a detailed neurological evaluation should include assessment of sensory level, posterior column function, normal and abnormal reflexes, and examination of rectal tone and perianal sensation. Documentation of any neurological deficit according to the American Spinal Injury Association (ASIA) impairment scale should be done.

In presence of a neurological deficit steroids according to the NASCIS III protocol are no longer recommendable in our opinion because no level C evidence based data are available and side effects are obvious.

Spinal stabilization techniques

Several instrumentation systems and operative techniques for the surgical treatment of fractures of the spine have been developed and marketed in the past.

Recent biomechanical studies have reported the mechanical characteristics and the primary stability of several anterior, posterior and combined instrumentation systems in worst-case models [20–23].

Bone grafting and single ventral instrumentation have been shown to be more effective in restoring acute stability than single dorsal instrumentation [27].

Considering the results of a load cell representing a bone strut graft, the axial compression force without loading of an anterior system was more than doubled in comparison to a posterior system. This inadequate load-sharing of a posterior construct may lead to delayed bony ingrowth, pseudarthrosis or mechanical failure [27].

Despite this, dorsal implants have become a standard in the treatment of fractures without neurological deficit due to their decided advantages. In the treatment of fractures with spinal cord compression, posterior instrumentation may provide indirect decompression of retropulsed intracanal bone fragments via ligamentotaxis, which is effected by distraction. However, such a reduction of intracanal bone fragments by indirect decompression depends on the degree of ligamentous continuity to the fragment, retropulsion of the fragment, and the displacement pattern of the fragment. These criteria are difficult to assess preoperatively and may result in variable degrees of reduction. Short segment pedicle instrumentation techniques also have been associated with loss of reduction and instrumentation failures.

Often a second anterior intervention is necessary and is associated with an extensive approach-related trauma, increased blood loss, a higher risk of infection and the problem of reduced screw purchase in the vertebral body. In addition, anterior surgery is technically demanding and therefore not all orthopaedic surgeons might be familiar with this procedure, especially under emergency conditions.

However, suitable anterior instrumentation systems have demonstrated their biomechanical in-vitro superiority compared to single dorsal devices [27]. Also direct anterior approaches may provide an optimal exposition for decompression of neural structures and enable the reconstruction, alignment, and immediate stabilization of the anterior load-bearing column through strut grafting [6, 9, 10, 28].

The decision for the approach is chosen in each individual case based on the preoperative computed tomography (CT)-scans and the amount of the neurological deficit.

Clinical pathway (Fig. 14.1)

- Endplate fractures or apophyseal avulsion fractures (A1) generally are stable and heal with conservative and non-surgical management.
- In all cases of a neurological deficit a dorsal laminectomy and stabilization has to be done immediately under emergency conditions. There is no linear correlation between the percentage of canal compromise and the degree of neurological deficit.
- Split fractures (A2) or compression fractures (A3) have to be stabilized from posterior

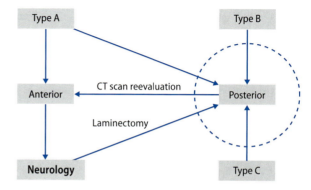

Fig. 14.1. Clinical Pathway.

first, which is also true for all type B and C fractures.
- After postoperative re-evaluation with a CT-scan total split fractures or compression fractures with posterior wall involvement and remaining spinal canal stenosis of more than 30% or kyphotic deformity of more than 20° have to be additionally stabilized from anterior (bisegmental reconstruction of the anterior load bearing column), which also enables further decompression of neural elements. Anterior monosegmental stabilization can be performed in type A 3.1 fractures, only.
- Type B and C fractures with circumferential instability always have to be treated by a combined anterior and posterior approach, usually with internal instrumentation from anterior as the second step.

Operative technique

Posterior stabilization

The incision is in the posterior midline. The fascia is detached from the spinous processes using cutting diathermy, and the muscles are stripped first from the spinous processes and then from the laminae using a very wide elevator, which is too big to pass between two transverse processes. Retractors are inserted and haemostasis is obtained with bipolar diathermy. The entry points for the transpedicular screws will depend on the section of spine involved. Computer navigation systems for screw placement are helpful if available [2, 3]. The vertebral canal can be decompressed depending on the specific requirements of the situation, after correct level identification by image intensifier.

Instrumentation mostly is done using screw-rod fixations devices. Short instrumentation with one level above and one level below the affected vertebra is recommended. Due to the variety of available systems, a detailed description can not be given here, but the surgeon should be familiar with the system he uses. The muscles, fascia, subcutaneous tissue and the skin are closed with interrupted sutures. Additionally two deep and one superficial drain are inserted.

Especially when dorsal stabilization combined with laminectomy is done under emergency conditions, CT-scan re-evaluation of the patient with regard to remaining intracanal fragments is required in order to decide about the necessity of an additional anterior instrumentation and decompression.

Anterior procedures

Several minimally invasive anterior approaches have been developed in the past and have become a standard in spinal surgery.

The essential advantages of minimally invasive surgery include the reduction of postoperative pain, the accelerated functional recovery, and the reduction in duration and intensity of analgesics. Furthermore the improved cosmesis compared to conventional surgical procedures may also be important.

Therefore a minimally invasive retroperitoneal approach to the lumbar spine is now described in detail.

Preoperative conventional X-rays in two planes and a CT-scan are mandatory for vertebral broad and height measurement. This information is necessary for preoperative planning of screw and plate length, as well as the length of a strut graft/spacer. Starting 24 hours prior the surgery, the patients are treated with routine procedures to empty the colon.

Lesions affecting the spine below L2 were approached through a minimal retroperitoneal access from the left side. The affected vertebra is identified with the image intensifier and its projection is marked laterally on the flank with a water-resistant pen.

A video-assisted minimally invasive retroperitoneal open procedure is recommended. The length of the skin incision is up to 6–8 cm. Blunt preparation of the retroperitoneal tissue with a wet sponge mounted on a stick and dissection of the muscles in the direction of their fiber orientation (external oblique, internal oblique, transverse abdominal, and psoas muscle) follows, taking care not to harm the ilio-hypogastric and ilio-inguinal nerves and the ureter.

The created space is kept open with a self-retaining frame retractor (such as Miaspas Retroperitoneal Retractor System, Aesculap, Tuttlingen, Germany or SynFrame, Synthes, Umkirch, Switzerland) and illuminated under video assistance with the 30° angled optic [18, 19].

The psoas muscle is mobilized along its fibers to enable the surgeon to reach the lateral aspect of the affected vertebral body. After that, orientation landmarks have to be set under fluoroscopic control. To do this, K-wires are placed above and below the lesion approximately on the transition from the rear to the central third of the vertebrae with reference to the anterior and posterior edges. The overlaying segmental vessels need to be clipped. The adjacent discs are removed and the corresponding endplate is cleaned with curettes carefully, not to penetrate the endplates. The fractured vertebral body is then removed using long osteotomes and rongeurs. Anterior spinal decompression follows in case of spinal canal narrowing of more than 30%. For bisegmental reconstruction various materials such as autologous iliac crest bone grafts or cages are available. Stand-alone implantation of anterior cages with or without supplemental bone but without additional anterior instrumentation is not recommendable as described above even in presence of a dorsal pedicle screw system.

Instrumentation is than performed with special adapted instruments and an angle-stable anterior plate system like the MACS TL stabilization system for example, which is described in detail in the chapter about endoscopic spinal surgery of the thoracolumbar spine [5, 6, 10, 28]. As prementioned in case of type A 3.1 fracture a monosegmental anterior stabilization is possible.

Mobilization is possible immediately after surgery without any restriction.

Treatment modalities of osteoporotic fractures

According to the International Osteoporosis Foundation (IOF) 40% of all middle-aged women and 15% of middle-aged men in Europe will suffer one or more osteoporotic fractures during their remaining lifetime.

Vertebral compression fractures that are secondary to osteoporosis can occur either spontaneously or after a minor trauma.

Due to reduced bone quality there are several newly developed techniques for stabilization:

- The neurological deficit separates patients with the necessity for an open stabilization with decompression from patients suited for percutaneous, transpedicular procedures, like kyphoplasty [8].
- In case without neurological deficit we favour kyphoplasty for transpedicular reduction and cement augmentation.
- Contrary, in case of neurological deficit we prefer decompression and dorsal stabilization with specially designed screw-rod systems, which allow for cement augmentation.

Kyphoplasty

Best results concerning the amount of fracture reduction have been seen in fresh fractures. Magnetic resonance imaging (MRI) is the best way of predicting the age of a fracture. We routinely perform a STIR MRI scan to identify fresh fractures.

We always perform kyphoplasty under general anesthesia with the patient in prone position, using bi-plane fluoroscopic control. The total procedure time is about one hour per patient and generally requires a very short hospital stay.

Table 14.1 describes the procedure of balloon kyphoplasty more in detail (Table 14.1).

After removal of the instruments we always wait with the turnover of the patient until total cement hardening to guarantee a good reduction result. Post-operatively, most patients experience immediate pain relief and early remobilization. After the procedure, the patient requires long-term follow-up and medical management.

Cement augmented instrumentation systems

In case of neurological deficit we advocate decompression and dorsal stabilization with specially designed implants, which allow for cement augmentation [24, 26, 28, 29].

These new anterior and posterior stabilization systems have specific anchorage characteristics, adapted by geometric optimization and the option of additional cement augmentation after screw insertion to compensate for poor bone quality.

Table 14.1. Balloon kyphoplasty (with permission of Kyphon, Germany).

Stage 1	Bilateral transpedicular insertion of the deflated balloons into the vertebral body.	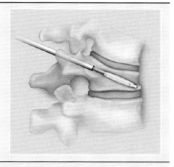
Stage 2	Gentle inflation of both balloons in the collapsed area of the vertebral body, leading to fracture reduction and elevation of the endplate.	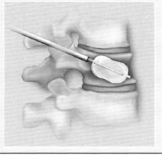
Stage 3	Following maximum fracture reduction, removal of both balloons and filling of the cavity under low, manual pressure with high viscosity, radiopaque, bone cement.	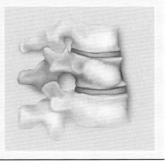

For anterior procedures the polyaxial screw XL (MACS TL system, Aesculap, Tuttlingen, Germany) and for posterior instrumentations the Socon CS (SOCON system, Aesculap, Tuttlingen, Germany) are available (Fig. 14.2) [24, 26, 28, 29].

In both cases additional cementation after implantation of the screws is possible through three slots along the longitudinal axis of the inserted screws. Exactly 2 ml of Osteopal V bone cement is used (Merk Biomaterial, Darmstadt, Germany); a larger volume is not permitted by the cement applicator. Only this small amount of cement is needed to enhance the screw base, therefore potential problems with flowing off or cement heating do not appear to be of concern.

For patients with poor bone quality due to osteoporosis or metastatic disease involving vertebral bodies, these new anchorage devices achieve rigid anterior or posterior stabilization initially or can serve as rescue screws in case of poor screw stability. Some clinical examples are shown in Fig. 14.3 and Fig. 14.4 a, b.

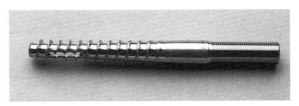

Fig. 14.2. SOCON CS cementable pedicle screw (Aesculap, Tuttlingen, Germany).

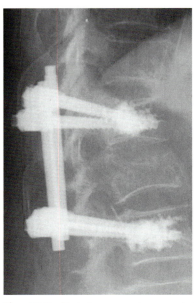

Fig. 14.3. Posterior cement-augmented stabilization with SOCON CS system (Aesculap, Tuttlingen, Germany) in case of osteoporotic L1 fracture.

Evidence-based spine surgery

AO Spine International performed a Medline search to identify comparative studies on the treatment of thoraco-lumbar fractures via open anterior or posterior approach [1]. Common outcome measures were total clinical complications, kyphosis at last follow-up, intraoperative blood loss, Frankel grade improvement and length of hospital stay. Of 23 articles (more than ten patients and follow-up rate of more than 60%) only two randomized controlled trials were found (class of evidence II). One trial included patients with stable burst fractures without neurological deficit and the other one included patients without describing their stability status [11, 30]. Another two cohort studies were identified (class of evidence III) [12, 31].

Fractures and the following interventions were divided according to stability criteria into stable and unstable fractures. Within the first group anterior instrumentation was done with allograft or autograft placement and fixation with Kaneda or Isola plate. Additional posterior fusion was done without any attempts at decompression, but three to four level instrumentation with cephaled claws/hooks or caudal pedicle screws one vertebra below the fracture, supplemented with infralaminar hooks at the same vertebra. In the second group, decompression was followed by anterior fusion with autograft placement and fixation by Kaneda or Z-plate or Kostuik-Harrington instrumentation.

Posterior fusion following decompression and stabilization was done with Steffee plate, pedicle screws or Cotrel-Dubousset hook and claws,

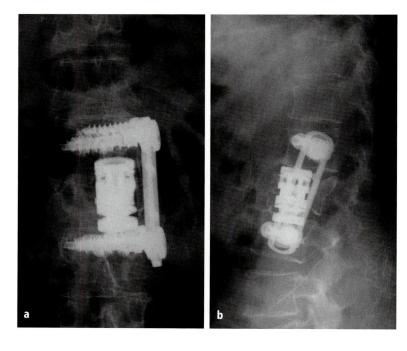

Fig. 14.4 a, b. Anterior stabilization L1–L3 with MACS TL system with cemented polyaxial screws XL (Aesculap, Tuttlingen, Germany) and L2 vertebral body replacement with Obelisc (Ulrich medical, Ulm, Germany) in case of osteoporotic L2 fracture.

Harrington distraction rods with hook or Luque ring with sublaminar wiring or Synthes Fixateur interne. Also semi-rigid fixation with a combination of hook rod and pedicle screws was done.

The total complication rates were slightly lower in the posterior fixation group in the unstable or stability unknown fracture group. Significant fewer complications were associated with anterior fixation compared with posterior fixation in the stable fracture group. No significant differences were found concerning the kyphosis at last follow-up. Anterior fixation was associated with significant greater blood loss.

A higher percentage of patients receiving posterior stabilization improved one or more Frankel Grades compared with anterior stabilization. Finally anterior fixation appears to result in longer hospital stay.

Critical evaluation

Even although evidence based studies still are missing in the new field of minimally invasive spine surgery, such techniques are becoming more widespread in spinal fracture treatment. At the thoracic spine and the thoraco-lumbar junction they are performed endoscopically meanwhile as a standard procedure. Also at the lumbar spine a minimally invasive retroperitoneal approach is possible as described. In addition, new methods of transpedicular cement augmentation and stabilization systems with the option of supplemental cement application are available now.

The existing evidence with regard to spine surgery is based on studies on conventional open procedures. However, recent publications also demonstrated the feasibility of the minimally invasive techniques and their good clinical results [4]. Therefore, traditional recommendations concerning the approach have to be re-evaluated under the specific consideration of well-designed prospective studies on minimally invasive techniques.

Until such studies are performed, decisions whether to perform an anterior, posterior or combined approach should be based especially on the surgeon's personal skills. Anterior minimally invasive surgery is a demanding procedure, especially under emergency conditions, and a learning curve is mandatory. Therefore, indications for anterior procedures should be carefully chosen.

Summary

Most fractures of the lumbar spine are found on the thoraco-lumbar junction. The aim of therapy is to achieve stable fixation in order to prevent secondary kyphosis and sufficient spinal decompression.

Type A fractures are usually stabilized from posterior alone. For higher degree of instability there is still discussion about anterior and/or posterior procedures.

For unstable thoraco-lumbar and lumbar burst fractures, there is some evidence that posterior fixation results in fewer complications, shorter hospital stays, and less operative blood loss compared with anterior fixation.

However, minimally invasive anterior procedures have been introduced and therefore the discussion whether anterior, posterior or combined procedures are sufficient is still going on.

Also osteoporotic fractures are more in the field of interest, because patient's age increases. These fractures may need special fixation devices like kyphoplasty or instrumentation with cement-augmented screws.

References

1. AO S (2005) Evidence-based spine surgery. Excellence in Spine 1:17–25
2. Arand M, Hartwig E, Hebold D, Kinzl L, Gebhard F (2001) Präzisionsanalyse navigationsgestützt implantierter thorakaler und lumbaler Pedikelschrauben. Eine prospektive klinische Studie. Unfallchirurg 104:1076–1081
3. Arand M, Kinzl L, Gebhard F (2002) Fehlerquellen und Gefahren der CT-basierten Navigation. Orthopäde 31:378–384
4. Beisse R (2006) Endoscopic surgery on the thoracolumbar junction of the spine. Eur Spine J 15: 687–704
5. Beisse R, Potulski M, Beger J, Bühren V (2002) Entwicklung und klinischer Einsatz einer thorakoskopisch implantierbaren Rahmenplatte zur Behandlung thorakolumbaler Frakturen und Instabilitäten. Orthopäde 31:413–422

6. Beisse R, Potulski M, Temme C, Bühren V (1998) Das endoskopisch kontrollierte Zwerchfellsplitting. Ein minimal-invasiver Zugang zur ventralen Versorgung thorakolumbaler Frakturen der Wirbelsäule. Unfallchirurg 101:619–627
7. Berlemann U, Müller CW, Krettek C (2004) Perkutane Augmentierungstechniken der Wirbelsäule – Möglichkeiten und Grenzen. Orthopäde 33:6–12
8. Broszcyk BM, Bierschneider M, Hauck S, Vastmanns J, Potulski M, Beisse R, Robert B, Jaschke H (2004) Kyphoplastie im konventionellen und halboffenen Verfahren. Orthopäde 33:13–21
9. Bühren V (1998) Thorakoskopische Versorgung von Frakturen der Brust- und Lendenwirbelsäule. Langenbecks Arch Chir 115(suppl):108–112
10. Bühren V, Beisse R, Potulski M (1997) Minimal-invasive ventrale Spondylodesen bei Verletzungen der Brust- und Lendenwirbelsäule. Chirurg 68:1076–1084
11. Danisa O, Shaffrey C (1990) Surgical approaches for the correction of unstable thoracolumbar burts fractures: a retrospective analysis of treatment outcomes 1977–1983. J Neurosurg 83:977–983
12. Esses S, Botsford D, Kostuik J (1990) Evaluation of surgical treatment for burst fractures. Spine 15:667–673
13. Kaneda K, Taneichi H, Abumi K, Hashimoto T, Satoh S, Fujiya M (1997) Anterior decompression and stabilization with the Kaneda device for thoracolumbar burst fractures associated with neurological deficits. J Bone Joint Surg Am 79:69–83
14. Knop C, Blauth M, Bühren V, Arand M, Egbers HJ, Hax PM, Nothwang J, Oestern HJ, Pizanis A, Roth R, Weckbach A, Wentzensen A (2001) Operative Behandlung von Verletzungen des thorakolumbalen Übergangs – Teil 3: Nachuntersuchung. Ergebnisse einer prospektiven multizentrischen Studie der „Wirbelsäule" der Deutschen Gesellschaft für Unfallchirurgie. Unfallchirurg 104:583–600
15. Knop C, Blauth M, Buhren V, Hax PM, Kinzl L, Mutschler W, Pommer A, Ulrich C, Wagner S, Weckbach A, Wentzensen A, Wörsdorfer O (1999) Operative Behandlung von Verletzungen des thorakolumbalen Übergangs. Teil 1: Epidemiologie. Unfallchirurg 102:924–935
16. Knop C, Blauth M, Buhren V, Hax PM, Kinzl L, Mutschler W, Pommer A, Ulrich C, Wagner S, Weckbach A, Wentzensen A, Wörsdorfer O (2000) Operative Behandlung von Verletzungen des thorakolumbalen Übergangs. Teil 2: Operation und röntgenologische Befunde. Unfallchirurg 103:1032–1047
17. Magerl F, Aebi M, Gretzbein SD, Harms J, Nazarian S (1994) A comprehensive cassification of thoracic and lumbar injuries. Eur Spine J 3:184–201
18. Mayer HM (1997) A new microsurgical technique for minimally invasive anterior lumbar interbody fusion. Spine 22:691–699
19. Mayer HM (2000) Minimally Invasive Spine Surgery. A surgical manual. Springer, Berlin
20. Panjabi MM (1988) Biomechanical evaluation of spinal fixation devices: I. A conceptual framework. Spine 13:1129–1134
21. Panjabi MM (1992) The stabilizing system of the spine. Part I. Function, dysfunction, adaptation, and enhancement. J Spinal Disord 5:383–389
22. Panjabi MM (1992) The stabilizing system of the spine. Part II. Neutral zone and instability hypothesis. J Spinal Disord 5:390–396
23. Panjabi MM, Kato Y, Hoffman H, Cholewicki J (2001) Canal and intervertebral foramen encroachments of a burst fracture: effects from the center of rotation. Spine 26:1231–1237
24. Schultheiss M, Claes L, Wilke HJ, Kinzl L, Hartwig E (2003) Enhanced primary stability through additional cementable cannulated rescue screw for anterior thoracolumbar plate application. J Neurosurg 98(suppl):50–55
25. Schultheiss M, Hartwig E, Kinzl L, Claes L, Wilke HJ (2004) Thoracolumbar fracture stabilization: comparative biomechanical evaluation of a new video-assisted implantable system. Eur Spine J 13:93–100
26. Schultheiss M, Hartwig E, Kinzl L, Claes L, Wilke HJ (2004) Influence of screw cement enhancement on the stability of anterior thoracolumbar fracture stabilization with circumferential instability. Eur Spine J 13:598–604
27. Schultheiss M, Hartwig E, Kinzl L, Claes L, Wilke HJ (2003) Axial compression force measurement acting across the strut graft in thoracolumbar instrumentation testing. Clin Biomech 18:631–636
28. Schultheiss M, Kinzl L, Claes L, Wilke HJ, Hartwig E (2003) Minimally invasive ventral spondylodesis for thoracolumbar fracture treatment: surgical technique and first clinical outcome. Eur Spine J 12:618–624
29. Schultheiss M, Wilke HJ, Claes L, Kinzl L, Hartwig E (2002) MACS-TL-Polyaxialscrew XL. Ein neues Konzept zur Stabilitätserhöhung ventraler Spondylodesen in Anwesenheit dorsaler Verletzungen. Orthopäde 31:397–401
30. Stancic M, Gregorovic E, Nozica E, Penezic L (2001) Anterior decompression and fixation versus posterior reposition and semirigid fixation in the treatment of unstable burst thoracolumbar fracture: prospective clinical trial. Croat Med J 42:49–53
31. Wood K, Bohn D, Mehbod A (2005) Anterior versus posterior treatment of stable thoracolumbar burst fractures without neurologic deficit: a prospective, randomized study. J Spinal Disord Tech 18(suppl):15–23

15 The role of vertebroplasty and kyphoplasty in the management of osteoporotic vertebral compression fractures

René Schmidt

Introduction

Osteoporosis is the most common metabolic bone disorder, affecting more than 200 million people worldwide [44]. Despite the fact that osteoporosis gains more and more recognition and that today there is less undertreatment [17], there are still an estimated 1.5 million osteoporotic fractures each year in the United States [60]. 700 000 of these fractures affect the spine, which makes the vertebra the most frequent and the earliest complication of osteoporosis. Although only up to one third of the individuals have symptoms severe enough to seek medical treatment [6, 45], these patients are a challenge for the treating physician. Conventional surgery such as fusion with or without instrumentation or vertebral body replacement has high complication rates [10] due to the underlying osteoporosis with poor bone quality and the general status of the older patients [15]. Open surgical treatment was therefore mainly restricted to patients with neurological deficits. However this condition is rare with less than 5% of patients requiring decompression [39]. Out of these reasons the treatment of symptomatic patients with osteoporotic vertebral compression fractures was for a long time mainly of conservative nature. In 1984 Galibert and Deramond [16] invented vertebroplasty as a treatment for vertebral hemangiomas. The procedure was quite fast also adopted for myelomas, malignomas and osteoporotic fractures. Currently the osteoporotic fractures make up for most of the indications. On the basis of vertebroplasty in 1998 the kyphoplasty procedure was invented. Both of the procedures are now available as minimal invasive percutaneous alternatives for the treatment of osteoporotic spine fractures.

Diagnostical work-up

Patients with a symptomatic osteoporotic vertebral compression fracture typically present with back pain, which usually follows minor trauma. Pain is often postural, with worsening by standing errect and often shows a wide variability, which can eventually be debilitating to the point of confining the patient to a wheelchair or bed. On inspection a thoracic hyperkyphosis, often called a dowagers hump or lumbar flattening can be found and is dependent on the amount of compression and also the number of levels involved. On palpation many of the fractures show a reproducible pain over the fracture site on deep pressure of the spine. Nevertheless this is not a must and may eventually be missing without affecting the result [19].

Besides the history and clinical examination, which also must include a neurologic examination, it is important to filter out patients with a risk for osteoporosis. Risk factors are amongst others higher age, female sex, early menopause, history of minor trauma with hip, radius or vertebral fracture, smoking, and excessive alcohol intake. In these patients an early x-ray should be taken, which is the primary radiographic tool for diagnosing a vertebral compression fracture (Fig. 15.1). This is in contrast to younger patients presenting with low back pain of unspecific origin, without red flags, where an x-ray can be postponed up to six to twelve weeks. The x-ray can display the vertebral deformation, although this may be difficult in small deformity and on the background of limited visibility due to the osteoporotic bone and frequently seen concomitant degeneration or scoliotic deformity. Furthermore x-ray cannot determine the age of the fracture, which is important against the background that only one third of patients with osteoporotic vertebral fractures have severe symptoms and seek medical treat-

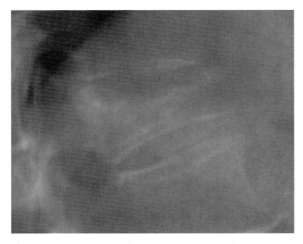

Fig. 15.1. Lateral x-ray of an osteoporotic vertebral compression wedge fracture Th12.

ment. Especially in patients presenting with multiple fractures and back pain, the distinction between previous unrecognized and acute fractures is essential (Fig. 15.2 a, b). The main challenge for the physician is therefore to correlate the fracture with actual pain and to discriminate it from unspecific low back pain on the basis of multi-level degeneration. This is important as we nowadays know that unspecific low back pain is not obligatory decreasing in older patients, as it was thought for a long time [69]. Therefore, the only direct therapeutical consequence of an osteoporotic vertebral fracture seen on x-ray is further evaluation and treatment of the osteoporosis, not a surgical intervention. Also the type of fracture does not give information about the amount of pain, as back pain is equally likely with all fracture types [28]. To better correlate actual pain with an osteoporotic fracture, many authors think that the age of the fracture can give the important information for surgical indication. In x-ray only sclerotic changes or a spontaneous fusion may suggest a chronic fracture (Fig. 15.2 a). Bone scans have been used to detect acute fractures, but the increased bone turn-over can persist over two years [48] and does not differ between an acute or healing fracture or bone remodelling. Magnetic resonance imaging (MRI) is nowadays thought to be the most important single tool for determining fracture age. In the acute phase MRI shows a geographic low intensity signal in T1 weighted and high intensity in T2 weighted images (Fig. 15.3). Additional

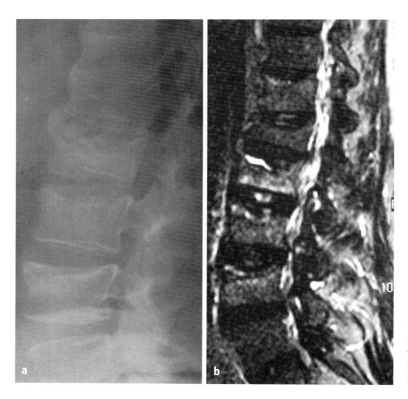

Fig. 15.2 a, b. Lateral x-ray of multiple lumbar fractures and anterior spontaneous fusion Th12/L1 (**a**). MRI (STIR) of patient in (**a**) with edema Th12, L2, L3, L4 but not L1, fluid sign L2 (**b**).

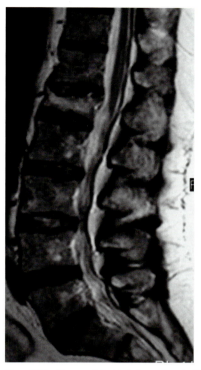

Fig. 15.3. Geographic high intensity in T2 weighted MRI of an L1 fracture.

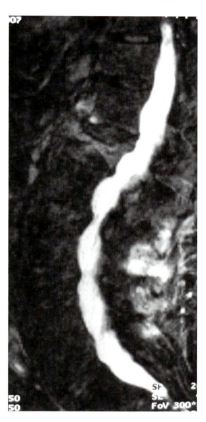

Fig. 15.4. Geographic high intensity in Th12 fracture (STIR).

sequences, such as the short tau inversion recovery (STIR) are used (Fig. 15.2 b and Fig. 15.4). In some cases a linear enhancement is found, which is referred to as the "fluid sign" or intravertebral cleft (Fig. 15.2 b and Fig. 15.5), and which is accompanied by an intravertebral vacuum phenomenon (Fig. 15.6 a). This was thought to be a sign of ischemic vertebral necrosis (Kümmels disease), but there are also findings which suggest that this is a sign of pseudarthrosis [24, 36]. MRI can also help to rule out malignant tumors, although it may not be feasible in all patients. Possible hints of malignancy are the affection of pedicles or posterior elements and fractures in the upper thoracic spine, which are not typical for osteoporotic fractures and should eventually lead to a biopsy. Summarizing the diagnosis of an acute painful osteoporotic vertebral compression fracture is based upon a combination of clinical and radiographic examinations. The major difficulty thereby is the discrimination from unspecific back pain and old prevalent fractures.

Indication

After the diagnosis of an acute and painful osteoporotic vertebral fracture the main problem is the indication for either a conservative or an operative treatment. Besides clear indications for surgery, such as a significant neurologic deficit, there are no real evidence-based recommendations. Randomized trials comparing augmentation and conservative therapy are missing, and existing non-randomized studies show a short-term benefit for vertebroplasty and kyphoplasty which disappears between three and six months postoperatively or after onset of conservative therapy, respectively [11, 12]. Nevertheless, some authors advocate these procedures already as the standard of care [52], whereas others are less optimistic [4, 5]. The existing studies probably do not allow general recommendations for or against these procedures. What reasons may then make sense to indicate surgery, although they might not be evidence-based? As mentioned above, a questionable ma-

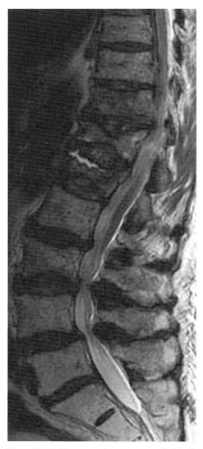

Fig. 15.5. Linear enhancement (fluid sign) L1, no enhancement Th11 and Th12 in T2 weighted MRI.

lignancy can lead to an early augmentation and biopsy, which then combines a diagnostic and therapeutic approach. The amount of initial pain alone is probably no indication for early surgery, except if the patient does not sufficiently benefit from pain medication. We feel that a fracture in a patient who is consequently bed ridden or wheel chair bound due to pain and who is unable to be mobilized under adequate pain medication is an indication for early surgery. The reason therefore is that these patients often have multiple comorbidities, especially heart and pulmonary diseases, which are negatively affected by a prolonged time of restricted mobility and can lead to further deconditioning of the patient. Bed rest should also be avoided for these reasons and because bed rest may also aggravate bone loss as found in younger individuals [22, 35, 37]. For these reasons we do not feel that bed rest is an adequate therapy in these patients.

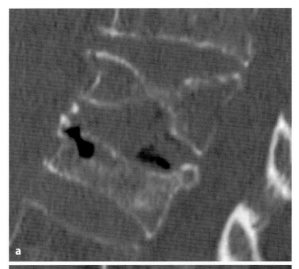

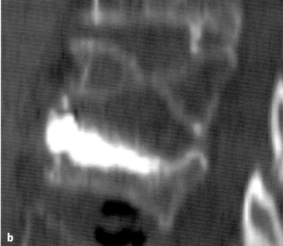

Fig. 15.6a, b. CT-scan of patient in Fig. 15.5 with intravertebral vacuum phenomenon (**a**). Vertebra after augmentation of the cleft (**b**).

Another indication for surgery might be severe side effects due to the pain medication, e.g. dizziness with recurrent falls due to narcotics. This also emphasizes that the patients with painful osteoportic vertebral fractures have to be followed-up by their physicians. The treatment is not a one-time prescription of analgetics. Follow-up does also include a radiographic follow-up. Lyritis et al. could divide their patients into two groups [46]. One of them had a single severe pain attack and a short duration of pain, whereas in the other group subsequent pain attacks with a prolonged time of pain were found. They attributed this to subsequent compression of the fractured vertebra with new pain

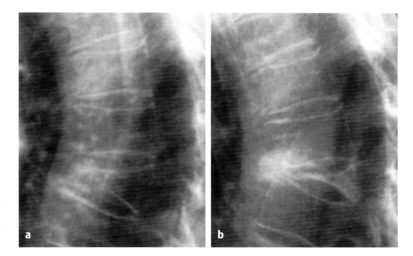

Fig. 15.7 a, b. Lateral x-ray of an acute compression fracture Th9 (**a**). Progressive collapse over a four month period under conservative therapy (**b**).

attacks and a gradually developing deformity (Fig. 15.7 a, b). As the duration of pain reached on average 49 weeks in the latter group, these patients pose an indication for early surgical therapy. In these circumstances another point has to be considered. Altough studies show the possibility of filling a vertebra plana with cement [56], it is from a surgical point of view more difficult to get a sufficient trajectory for needle placement as well as the rate of cement leak and of persisting kyphotic deformity is higher. Therefore, a radiographic follow-up in conservatively treated patients seems important, not to miss a level of deformity where a safe augmentation is possible and where the consecutive kyphosis is acceptable. The time period therefore could e.g. be one to two, four to six and twelve weeks after onset of pain. However, this recommendation is not evidence-based.

The amount of deformity (kyphosis) leads to another point, which has to be considered. It is known that an increasing thoracic kyphosis or lumbar kyphosis can lead e.g. to a flexed posture with gait disturbance and recurrent falls, a protuberant abdomen with abdominal compression and early satiety and weight loss [65] or decreased lung function [40, 63] which can also lead to an increased mortality rate [30]. Moreover osteoporotic vertebral fractures can lead to mental affection with depression, decreased quality of life and chronic pain, with the risk increasing with the number of levels fractured [26, 53]. On the other hand there seems to be no linear dependency of quality of life and radiographic deformation [41]. This makes an evidence-based decision with the aim to prevent physiologic and psychologic consequences of osteoporotic vertebral fractures very difficult. Multiple acute fractures may be better adressed early to prevent a pronounced deformation with potential sequelae. The same could be true for patients with one acute fracture and multiple old fractures to prevent an aggravation of the existing deformity. Nevertheless, the aim to prevent these long-term sequelae is hypothetical, as even in cases with good reposition of height and sagittal balance, we usually do not reach the prefracture state and in up to 40% of cases we do not reach any measurable restoration of height or alignment at all [27]. For the patient with only one acute fracture the prevention of kyphosis seems questionable, as we can neither predict the developing deformity, nor whether this patient will suffer further fractures.

The indication for vertebroplasty or kyphoplasty seems to be the most challenging aspect of these new procedures and besides medical points as mentioned here, also the economic consequences for the health care systems have to be considered. The costs for osteoporotic related fractures in the United States in 2001 were estimated to be 17 billion dollars or 47 million a day. As an increase of osteoporotic fractures is expected in the next decades [60] and the population over 50 years of age grows, an increase of costs up to 60 billion a year or 164 million a day is estimated in 2030, only for the United States [59]. As this estimated explosion of expenditures is a threat to every health care system worldwide, further studies have to consider the cost-benefit relation for these procedures. Summarized it seems to be a long way until we will have evidence-based guidelines, considering all the above-mentioned and not mentioned facts, for the indication to vertebroplasty or kyphoplasty in osteoporotic vertebral fractures.

Technique

After the indication is set, the next question is whether a vertebroplasty or kyphoplasty is used. Both procedures are percutaneous, can be performed in local or general anaesthesia and use a trans- or extrapedicular approach. The difference between the two techniques is that in vertebroplasty the cement is directly injected into the vertebral body, whereas in kyphoplasty prior to cement injection a balloon tamp is inserted, which is then inflated (Fig. 15.8 a–c) in an attempt to at least partially restore vertebral body height and reduce kyphotic deformity.

The leading clinical symptom and hence the cardinal criteria of a successful surgery for the patient is pain. The majority of studies about vertebroplasty and kyphoplasty addresses this topic revealing at least some pain relief. The achieved pain reduction varies somewhat between 60% to 100% for vertebroplasty [2, 7, 9, 20, 25, 34, 47, 50, 62] even over a longer time period [20, 70]. Similar results are reported for kyphoplasty [3, 14, 42, 57, 66]. Difficulties in the comparison arise out of different measurement methods and levels of relevant pain relief. Furthermore the techniques used differ amongst others for the type and amount of cement applicated and uni- or bipedicular administration. Although this may not have an effect on the clinical outcome [32] it complicates the comparison of results. Currently there seems to be no clearly evident benefit concerning pain relief between both procedures based on the existing studies. The same is true for the improvement of mobility and physical function of the patients [1, 7, 13, 18, 21, 31, 49, 54].

For the correction of the vertebral height and alignment one major point seems to be whether a mobile fracture with intravertebral cleft is present, because in these patients positioning alone seems to be able to partially restore the height independent of the used technique [51]. Moreover the age of the fracture may have an impact on the amount of reduction [3, 8]. Overall it seems that with both procedures in up to 40% a reduction is not possible [27]. Hence it is important to evaluate predictors for a good reposition, before recommendations can be made in which cases the cheaper vertebroplasty or the more expensive kyphoplasty are indicated. After these biomechanical and technical points are cleared, the clinical outcome has to be considered. As clincal results concerning pain and physical function on short term are comparable, further questions have to be studied by long-term follow-up. These are which patients could benefit more from a restoration of height and alignment, which amount of reduction has to be achieved and whether at all we can avoid or lessen some of the above mentioned physiologic consequences? Currently these aspects are mainly hypothetical.

One point which seems clear is that the amount of cement leaks is higher with vertebroplasty, although this is not found in all cases [21]. Theoretically this is because a higher pressure is needed to inject the cement when no

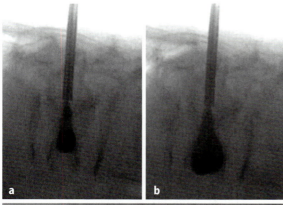
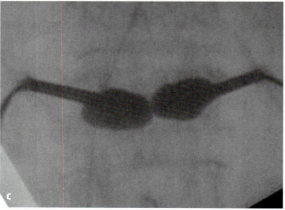

Fig. 15.8 a–c. Lateral fluoroscopy of inserted balloon in kyphoplasty (**a**). Inflation of the balloon (**b**). A-P fluoroscopy after bipedicular balloon insertion and inflation (**c**).

preformed cavity exists. This highlights the effect of the amount of cement injected. If with kyphoplasty a filling of the whole vertebra is aimed for, this means a filling beyond the preformed cavity, the rate of leaks might increase to rates comparable to vertebroplasty [3]. This emphasizes how important it would be, from a clinical as well as from a biomechanical point of view, to have evidence-based recommendations for the amount of cement to be injected. Otherwise one runs the risk of determining the confounding factors rather than the procedures themselves [27]. Although the rate of leaks might be higher for vertebroplasty, the amount of clinically symptomatic leaks is low for both procedures. The consequences of clinical symptomatic leaks nevertheless might be high as they can include paraplegia, radiculopathy or pulmonary embolism [23, 29, 38, 55, 58, 64, 67]. Whether the leak into the adjacent disc increases the risk of subsequent fractures [43, 68] or whether the augmentation itself does enhance the risk for new fractures by changing vertebral stiffness [33], alignment or patients physical activity cannot be definitely answered yet. The problem here is to distinguish between fractures due to augmentation and fractures due to the natural history of osteoporosis, which comprises a much higher risk for subsequent fractures if the patients have already a prevalent fracture [45, 61]. In fact this is of crucial importance, as this would be the first known severe negative consequence of these procedures, besides complications by cement leaks or general complications by the surgery or anaesthesia.

From a technical point and considering the existing studies there might be a benefit for kyphoplasty concerning leakage rate. Nevertheless, many open questions such as amount of cement and the type of cement have to be cleared and economical aspects have to be considered before a recommendation for one of the procedures can be made. Summarizing, the choice of procedure seems currently be negligible compared to the indication.

Conclusion

Vertebroplasty and kyphoplasty play an important role in the management of osteoporotic compression fractures of the spine as they pose a minimal invasive procedure with a high efficacy concerning pain relief and improvement of mobility and physical activity. The perioperative and anaesthesiological complications are low, which makes these procedures a real alternative to conventional surgery in these aged and multimorbid patients. Even though symptomatic complications are rare, we should not underplay them, as they can be catastrophic for the patient. In addition, we cannot rule out that these procedures negatively affect the adjacent fracture rate and besides these points, we should not forget the positive results we have achieved by conservative therapy. Hence, despite our surgical enthusiasm for these procedures, a general recommendation for augmentation is currently not possible. Therefore, we must now make the next step with randomized and controlled clinical studies to answer the open questions, which will enable us to finally assess the role of vertebroplasty and kyphoplasty in the mangement of osteoporotic vertebral compression fractures.

References

1. Amar AP, Larsen DW, Esnaashari N, Albuquerque FC, Lavine SD, Teitelbaum GP (2001) Percutaneous Transpedicular Polymethyl methacrylate Vertebroplasty for the Treatment of Spinal Compression Fractures. Neurosurgery 49:1105–1115
2. Barr JD, Barr MS, Lemley TJ, McCann RM (2000) Percutaneous vertebroplasty for pain relief and spinal stabilization. Spine 25:923–928
3. Berlemann U, Franz T, Orler R, Heini PF (2004) Kyphoplasty for treatment of osteoporotic vertebral fractures: A prospective non-randomized study. Eur Spine J 13:496–501
4. Bono CM (2006) Point of View: The honest truth about vertebroplasty. Spine 31:11–19
5. Boswell MV, Trescot AM, Datta S, Schultz DM, Hansen HC, Abdi S, Sehgal N, Shah RV, Singh V, Benyamin RM, Patel VB, Buenaventura RM, Colson JD, Cordner HJ, Epter RS, Jasper JF, Dunbar EE, Atluri SL, Bowman RC, Deer TR, Swicegood JR, Staats PS, Smith HS, Burton AW, Kloth DS, Giordano J, Manchikanti L, Pyhsicians ASoIP (2007) Interventional techniques: evidence-based practice guidelines in the management of chronic spinal pain. Pain Physician 10:7–111
6. Cooper C, Atkinson EJ, O'Fallon WM, Melton 3rd LJ (1992) Incidence of clinically diagnosed vertebral fractures: a population based study in Rochester, Minnesota, 1985–1989. J Bone Miner Res 7:221–227

7. Cortet B, Cotton A, Boutry N, Flipo RM, Duquesnoy B, Chatsanet P, Delcambre B (1999) Percutaneous vertebroplasty in the treatment of osteoporotic vertebral compression fractures: an open prospective study. J Rheumatol 26:2222–2228
8. Crandall D, Slaughter D, Hankins PJ, Moore C, Jerman J (2004) Acute versus chronic vertebral compression fractures treated with kyphoplasty: early results. Spine J 4:418–424
9. Cyteval C, Sarrabere MP, Roux JO, Thomas E, Jorgensen C, Blotman F, Sany J, Taourel P (1999) Acute osteoporotic vertebral collapse: open study on percutaneous injection of acrylic surgical cement in 20 patients. Am J Roentgenol 173:1685–1690
10. DeWald CJ, Stanley T (2006) Instrumentation-related complications of multilevel fusions for adult spinal deformity patients over age 65: surgical considerations and treatment options in patients with poor bone quality. Spine 31:144–151
11. Diamond TH, Bryant C, Browne L, Clark WA (2006) Clinical outcomes after acute osteoporotic vertebral fractures: a 2-year non-randomised trial comparing percutaneous vertebroplasty with conservative therapy. Med J Aust 184:113–117
12. Diamond TH, Champion B, Clark WA (2003) Management of acute osteoporotic vertebral fractures: a nonrandomized trial comparing percutaneous vertebroplasty with conservative therapy. Am J Med 114:257–265
13. Evans AJ, Jensen ME, Kip KE, DeNardo AJ, Lawler GJ, Negin GA, Remley KB, Boutin SM, Dunnagan SA (2003) Vertebral compression fractures: pain reduction and improvement in functional mobility after percutaneous polymethyl methacrylate vertebroplasty retrospective report of 245 cases. Radiology 226:366–372
14. Fourney DR, Schomer DF, Nader R, Chlan Fourney J, Suki D, Ahrar K, Rhines LD, Gokaslan ZL (2003) Percutaneous vertebroplasty and kyphoplasty for painful vertebral body fractures in cancer patients. J Neurosurg 98:21–30
15. Fujita T, Kostuik JP, Huckell CB, Sieber AN (1998) Complications of spinal fusion in adults more than 60 years of age. Orthop Clin North Am 29:669–678
16. Galibert P, Deramond H, Rosat P, Le Gars D (1987) Note preliminaire sur le traitement des angiomes vertebraux par vertebroplastie acrylique percutanee. Neurochirurgie 33:166–168
17. Gardner MJ, Flik KR, Mooar P, Lane JM (2002) Improvement in the undertreatment of osteoporosis following hip fracture. J Bone Joint Surg [Am] 84:1342–1348
18. Gaughen JR, Jensen ME, Schweickert PA, Kaufmann TJ, Marx WF, Kallmes DF (2002) Relevance of antecedent venography in percutaneous vertebroplasty for the treatment of osteoporotic compression fractures. Am J Neuroradiol 23:594–600
19. Gaughen JR, Jensen ME, Schweikert PA, Kaufmann TJ, Marx WF, Kallmes DF (2002) Lack of preoperative spinous process tenderness does not affect clinical success of percutaneous vertebroplasty. J Vasc Interv Radiol 13:1135–1138
20. Grados F, Depriester C, Cayrolle G, Hardy N, Deramond H, Fardellone P (2000) Long-term observations of vertebral osteoporotic fractures treated by percutaneous vertebroplasty. Rheumatology (Oxford) 39:1410–1414
21. Grohs JG, Matzner M, Trieb K, Krepler P (2005) Minimal invasive stabilization of osteoporotic vertebral fractures: a prospective nonrandomized comparison of vertebroplasty and balloon kyphoplasty. J Spinal Disord Tech 18:238–242
22. Hansson TH, Roos BO, Nachemson A (1975) Development of osteopenia in the fourth lumbar vertebra during prolonged bed rest after operation for scoliosis. Acta Orthop Scand 46:621–630
23. Harrington KD (2001) Major neurological complications following percutaneous vertebroplasty with polymethyl methacrylate: a case report. J Bone Joint Surg [Am] 83:1070–1073
24. Hasegawa K, Homma T, Uchiyama S, Takahashi HE (1998) Vertebral pseudarthrosis in the osteoporotic spine. Spine 23:2201–2206
25. Heini PF, Walchli B, Berlemann U (2000) Percutaneous transpedicular vertebroplasty with PMMA: operative technique and early results. A prospective study for the treatment of osteoporotic compression fractures. Eur Spine J 9:445–450
26. Huang C, Ross PD, Wasnich RD (1996) Vertebral fractures and other predictors of physical impairment and health care utilization. Arch Intern Med 156:2469–2475
27. Hulme PA, Krebs J, Ferguson SJ, Berlemann U (2006) Vertebroplasty and kyphoplasty: A systematic review of 69 clinical studies. Spine 31:1983–2001
28. Ismail AA, Cooper C, Felsenberg D, Varlow J, Kanis JA, Silman AJ, O'Neill TW (1999) Number and type of vertebral deformities: epidemiological characteristics and relation to back pain and height loss. European Vertebral Osteoporosis Study Group. Osteoporos Int 9:206–213
29. Jang JS, Lee SH, Jung SK (2002) Pulmonary embolism of polymethyl methacrylate after percutaneous vertebroplasty: a report of three cases. Spine 27:416–418
30. Kado DM, Browner WS, Palermo L, Nevitt MC, Genant HK, Cummings SR (1999) Vertebral fractures and mortality in older women: a prospective study. Study of Osteoporotic Fractures Research Group. Arch Intern Med 159:1215–1220
31. Kaufmann TJ, Jensen ME, Schweickert PA, Marx WF, Kallmes DF (2001) Age of fracture and clinical outcomes of percutaneous vertebroplasty. Am J Neuroradiol 22:1860–1863

32. Kim AK, Jensen ME, Dion JE, Schweickert PA, Kaufmann TJ, Kallmes DF (2002) Unilateral transpedicular percutaneous vertebroplasty: initial experience. Radiology 222:737–741
33. Kim SH, Kang HS, Choi JA, Ahn JM (2004) Risk factors of new compression fractures in adjacent vertebrae after percutaneous vertebroplasty. Acta Radiol 45:440–445
34. Kobayashi K, Shimoyama K, Nakamura K, Murata K (2005) Percutaneous vertebroplasty immediately relieves pain of osteoporotic vertebral compression fractures and prevents prolonged immobilization of patients. Eur Radiol 15:360–367
35. Krolner B, Toft B (1983) Vertebral bone loss: an unheeded side effect of therapeutic bed rest. Clin Sci (Lond) 64:537–540
36. Lane JI, Maus TP, Wald JT, Thielen KR, Bobra S, Luetmer PH (2002) Intravertebral clefts opacified during vertebroplasty: pathogenesis, technical implications, and prognostic significance. Am J Neuroradiol 23:1642–1646
37. Leblanc AD, Schneider VS, Evans HJ, Engelbretson DA, Krebs JM (1990) Bone mineral loss and recovery after 17 weeks of bed rest. J Bone Miner Res 5:843–850
38. Lee BJ, Lee SR, Yoo TY (2002) Paraplegia as a complication of percutaneous vertebroplasty with polymethylmethacrylate: a case report. Spine 27:419–422
39. Lee YL, Yip KM (1996) The osteoporotic spine. Clin Orthop 323:91–97
40. Leech JA, Dulberg C, Kellie S, Pattee L, Gay J (1990) Relationship of lung function to severity of osteoporosis in women. Am Rev Respir Dis 141:68–71
41. Leidig-Bruckner G, Minne HW, Schlaich C, Wagner G, Scheidt-Nave C, Bruckner T, Gebest HJ, Ziegler R (1997) Clinical grading of spinal osteoporosis: quality of life components and spinal deformity in women with chronic low back pain and women with vertebral osteoporosis. J Bone Miner Res 12:663–675
42. Lieberman IH, Dudeney S, Reinhardt MK, Bell G (2001) Initial outcome and efficacy of "kyphoplasty" in the treatment of painful osteoporotic vertebral compression fractures. Spine 26:1631–1638
43. Lin EP, Ekholm S, Hiwatashi A, Westesson PL (2004) Vertebroplasty: Cement leakage into the disc increases the risk of new fracture of adjacent vertebral body. Am J Neuroradiol 25:175–180
44. Lin JT, Lane JM (2004) Osteoporosis: A review. Clin Orthop 425:126–134
45. Lindsay R, Silverman SL, Cooper C, Hanley DA, Barton I, Broy SB, Licata A, Benhamou L, Geusens P, Flowers K, Stracke H, Seeman E (2001) Risk of New Vertebral Fracture in the Year Following a Fracture. JAMA 285:320–323
46. Lyritis GP, Mayasis B, Tsakalakos N, Lambropoulos A, Gazi S, Karachalios T, Tsekoura M, Yiatzides A (1989) The natural history of the osteoporotic vertebral fracture. Clin Rheumatol 8 (suppl 2):66–69
47. Martin JB, Jean B, Sugiu K, San Millan Ruiz D, Piotin M, Murphy K, Rufenacht B, Muster M, Rufenacht DA (1999) Vertebroplasty: clinical experience and follow-up results. Bone 25:11–15
48. Maynard AS, Jensen ME, Schweickert PA, Marx WF, Short JG, Kallmes DF (2000) Value of bone scan imaging in predicting pain relief from percutaneous vertebroplasty in osteoporotic vertebral fractures. Am J Neuroradiol 21:1807–1812
49. McGraw JK, Lippert JA, Minkus KD, Rami PM, Davis TM, Budzik RF (2002) Prospective evaluation of pain relief in 100 patients undergoing percutaneous vertebroplasty. Results and follow-up. J Vasc Interv Radiol 13:883–886
50. McKiernan F, Faciszewski T, Jensen R (2004) Quality of life following vertebroplasty. J Bone Joint Surg [Am] 86:2600–2606
51. McKiernan F, Jensen R, Faciszewski T (2003) The dynamic mobility of vertebral compression fractures. J Bone Miner Res 18:24–29
52. Nevasier A, Toro-Arbelaez JB, Lane JM (2005) Is kyphoplasty the standard of care for compression fractures in the spine, especially in the elderly? Am J Orthop 34:425–429
53. Oleksik A, Lips P, Dawson A, Minshall ME, Shen W, Cooper C, Kanis JA (2000) Health-related quality of life in postmenopausal women with low BMD with or without prevalent fractures. J Bone Miner Res 15:1384–1392
54. O'Brien JP, Sims JT, Evans AJ (2000) Vertebroplasty in patients with severe vertebral compression fractures: a technical report. Am J Neuroradiol 21:1555–1558
55. Padovani B, Kasriel O, Brunner P, Peretti Viton P (1999) Pulmonary embolism caused by acrylic cement: a rare complication of percutaneous vertebroplasty. Am J Neuroradiol 20:375–377
56. Peh WC, Gilula LA, Peck DD (2002) Percutaneous vertebroplasty for severe osteoporotic vertebral body compression fractures. Radiology 223:121–126
57. Phillips FM, Ho E, Campbell-Hupp RN, McNally T, Wetzel FT, Gupta P (2003) Early Radiographic and Clinical Results of Balloon Kyphoplasty for the Treatment of Osteoporotic Vertebral Compression Fractures. Spine 28:2260–2267
58. Ratliff J, Nguyen T, Heiss J (2001) Root and spinal cord compression from methyl methacrylate vertebroplasty. Spine 26:300–302
59. Ray NF, Chan JK, Thamer M, Melton L Jr (1997) Medical expenditures for the treatment of osteoporotic fractures in the United States in 1995: report from the National Osteoporosis Foundation. J Bone Miner Res 12:24–35

60. Riggs BL, Melton LJ, 3rd (1995) The worldwide problem of osteoporosis: insights afforded by epidemiology. Bone 17:505–511
61. Ross PD, Davis JW, Epstein RS, Wasnich RD (1991) Pre-existing fractures and bone mass predict vertebral fracture incidence in women. Ann Intern Med 114:19–23
62. Ryu KS, Park CK, Kim MC, Kang JK (2002) Dose-dependent epidural leakage of polymethyl methacrylate after percutaneous vertebroplasty in patients with osteoporotic vertebral compression fractures. J Neurosurg 96:56–61
63. Schlaich C, Minne HW, Bruckner T, Wagner G, Gebest HJ, Grunze M, Ziegler R, Leidg-Bruckner G (1998) Reduced pulmonary function in patients with spinal osteoporotic fractures. Osteoporos Int 8:261–267
64. Shapiro S, Abel T, Purvines S (2003) Surgical removal of epidural and intradural polymethyl methacrylate extravasation complicating percutaneous vertebroplasty for an osteoporotic lumbar compression fracture. Case report. J Neurosurg 98:90–92
65. Silverman SL (1992) The clinical consequences of vertebral compression fracture. Bone 13 (suppl 2):27–31
66. Theodorou DJ, Theodorou SJ, Duncan TD, Garfin SR, Wong WH (2002) Percutaneous balloon kyphoplasty for the correction of spinal deformity in painful vertebral body compression fractures. Clin Imaging 26:1–5
67. Tozzi P, Abdelmoumene Y, Corno AF, Gersbach PA, Hoogewoud HM, von Segesser LK (2002) Management of pulmonary embolism during acrylic vertebroplasty. Ann Thorac Surg 74:1706–1708
68. Vasconcelos C, Gailloud P, Beauchamp NJ, Heck DV, Murphy KJ (2002) Is percutaneous vertebroplasty without pretreatment venography safe? Evaluation of 205 consecutives procedures. Am J Neuroradiol 23:913–917
69. Weiner DK, Haggerty CL, Kritchevsky SB, Harris T, Simonsick EM, Nevitt M, Newman A (2003) How does low back pain impact physical function in independent, well functioning older adults? Evidence from the Health ABC cohort and implications for the future. Pain Med 4:311–320
70. Zoarski GH, Snow P, Olan WJ, Stallmeyer MJ, Dick BW, Hebel JR, De Deyne M (2002) Percutaneous vertebroplasty for osteoporotic compression fractures: quantitative prospective evaluation of long-term outcomes. J Vasc Interv Radiol 13:139–148

Tumor and infection

16 Tumor lesions of the cervical spine – pitfalls and their solution

Klaus Huch

Introduction

Several entities can cause symptomatic and asymptomatic lesions of the cervical spine (Table 16.1). This article will focus on benign and malignant tumor lesions.

Primary bone tumors represent only 0.4% of all tumors. Of these about 4% are seen in the spine [1]. In contrast, spinal metastases develop in 5% of all cancer patients. Between 8% and 20% of the spinal metastases are located in the cervical spine. In women, over 50% of all metastatic lesions of the spine are caused by breast cancer. Neurologic dysfunction complicates the disease in 5% to 10%. The average age at diagnosis is about 60 years [15].

Table 16.1. Differential diagnosis of lesions of the cervical spine.

Entity	Remarks
Osteoporosis	Rare, in the elderly more often
Spondylodiscitis	Rare
Rheumatic disease	See article by Kocak and Huch in this book
Gorham's disease	Massive osteolysis of unknown etiology (Foult et al. 1995)
Tumor like lesions	E.g. aneurismal bone cyst
Benign primary bone tumors	Rare
Paget's disease	
Chordoma	Semi-malignant
Eosinophilic granuloma	Especially in children
Multiple myeloma (plasmocytoma)	Single myeloma is very rare
Malignant primary bone tumors	Rare, e.g. osteosarcoma
Bone metastases	Relative frequent
Others	Lipoma, haemangioma

It seems that different primary tumors cause different metastatic distribution patterns in the spine. In hypernephroma a only cervical involvement is described in 5% of the spinal metastases [34], whereas in mamma carcinoma 20% of the spinal metastases are found in cervical vertebrae [35].

Due to small numbers there is convincing evidence just for the treatment of tumor lesions of the cervical spine.

Imaging

Lesions of the cervical spine, especially with neurological dysfunction, demand for a professional work-up. After clinical examination of the patient radiographs have to be taken in at least two planes including a special anterior-posterior projection of the dens. In addition, functional radiographs of the cervical spine are recommended. Magnetic resonance imaging (MRI) including sequences with contrast media is indicated in neurological deficits and suspected or evident osteolysis. It allows to detect relative small lesions and to distinguish between different entities. It also presents the spinal cord with its nerve roots. Computed tomography (CT)-scans help to estimate the stability of the cervical spine and to detect lesions like osteoidosteoma.

A bone scan may help to detect bone lesions in the thoracic and lumbar spine as well as in the peripheral skeleton. The fusion technology of positron emission tomography (PET) in combination with a CT-scan offers the opportunity to correlate an increased tracer up-take (soft-tissue or bone) with morphologic changes in the CT-scan of the entire body.

Treatment options

After completion of the imaging it has to be decided, whether a biopsy of a specific alteration of the cervical spine (or elsewhere, if the access is easier) is indicated. In spinal cord compression or imminent compression instant decompression and stabilization can lead to neurological improvement [10, 13], and simultaneously a biopsy can be performed. However, Rades et al. found an improvement of motor function in 33% and no further progression in 53% of prostate cancer patients with metastatic spinal cord compression following radiotherapy [22]. 33% of the nonambulatory patients regained the ability to walk. The faster the motor deficits developed the worse was the outcome in this study. Hill et al. observed 45% reambulation in patients unable to walk due to spinal cord compression by breast cancer metastasis [10]. They observed no significant difference between the surgical and the radiotherapy group either for survival (median of four months) or neurological improvement in advanced breast carcinoma.

In tumor lesions of the cervical spine age, general medical condition and overall life expectancy, degree of instability and presence of neurologic compromise, location, type, and radio-, chemo- and anti-hormon-sensitivity of the tumor are very important in the process of decision-making for the surgical management. This aims not only for the prophylaxis or the reduction of neurological deficiencies, but also for the improvement of biomechanical stability and reduction of pain as well as the promotion of quality of life [4, 37].

Anterior decompression, restoration of the anterior column with cage, polymethyl metacrylat (PMMA) or bone blocks combined with anterior plate instrumentation can be considered as the general routine procedure [20]. Abumi et al. [2] and Olerud et al. [21] described the first angle stable internal fixators for the dorsal instrumentation of the cervical spine. Recently, our group [11, 12] evaluated a modular angle-stable rod-screw implant system with a high biomechanical stability [25, 26] for tumor lesions of the cervical and cervico-thoracic spine in analogy to our established algorithm for the thoracic and lumbar spine [17]. Since the posterior approach avoids the tumor masses, which are regularly found in the anterior half of the spinal column, it helps to reduce the risk of bleeding, especially in highly vascularized metastases like in hypernephroma [11]. In addition, it is technically less demanding, especially in cases with tumor in-growth in the vertebral artery or the esophagus. Computernavigation can help to position the transarticular C1–2 screws or the cervical pedicle screws [24].

Pitfalls

Pitfalls are imminent for diagnostic evaluation and for therapeutic procedures and it is evident that the right diagnosis of the responsible pathology will be crucial for the optimal treatment strategy.

Awareness of tumors in children

The diagnostic strategy for patients suffering from local or segmental pain or limited motion in the cervical spine should not only include a clinical examination but also radiographs. In radiographs without pathologic findings and persisting symptoms, MRI has to be considered as the next diagnostic step.

Tumor lesions of the cervical spine can be seen even in children. In young children eosinophilic granuloma is a very important differential diagnosis (Fig. 16.1). The therapy should start

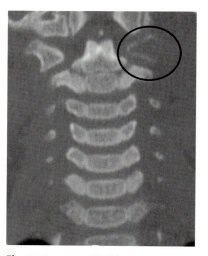

Fig. 16.1. 18-month-old girl presenting with acute torticollis: CT-scan revealed osteolysis of the right atlas; biopsy was performed and histology demonstrated eosinophilic granuloma; due to multilocular disease chemotherapy was initiated and performed without need for subsequent surgery.

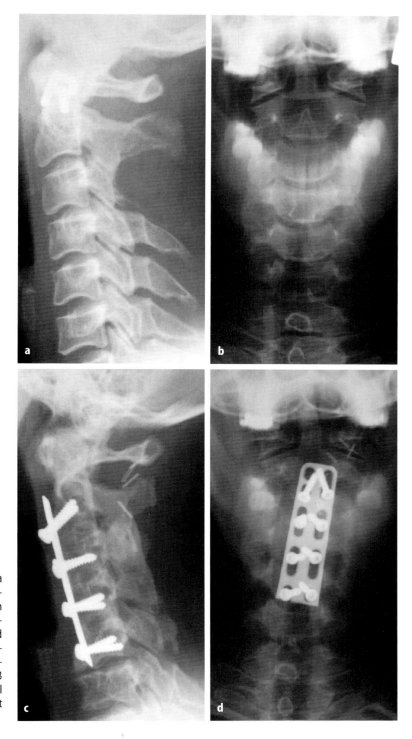

Fig. 16.2 a–d. Low-grade osteosarcoma of the dorsal structures of C3 in a 26-year-old woman, who was operated on with posterior tumor resection and combined anterior-posterior fusion C2–5 and still is free of disease ten years after surgery: Preoperative biplanar X-rays showing the dorsal destruction at the level C3 (**a, b**); biplanar X-rays of the cervical spine five years postoperatively without evidence for tumor recurrence (**c, d**).

early to avoid further destruction of the involved structures. Depending on the distribution and localization (singular versus multiple form) local steroids or chemotherapy should be administered.

Examples for other possible lesions in young patients are aneurismal bone cysts and osteosarcoma (Fig. 16.2 a–d). As many as 10% of all aneurismal bone cysts are found in the vertebral column, about 3.5% in the cervical spine.

Treatment options include resection und curettage, embolization, radiation therapy, injection with calcitonin and corticosteroids [3, 5, 6]. 4.1% of all osteosarcomas are detected in the spine, 0.5% in the cervical spine. In 17% two spinal levels are involved [14]. Metastasis is very rare in children. The most frequent primary tumors are neuroblastomas, rhabdomyosarcomas, and Wilm's tumors [5].

Atypical lesions in adults

In adults, metastasis has to be considered as the most frequent tumor lesion in the cervical spine. However, spondylodiscitis (Fig. 16.3 a, b) can also lead to bone destruction and in combination with a pathological fracture or epidural abscess formation to neurological dysfunction.

In patients with tetraplegia tumors can be asymptomatic since pain does not serve as the main symptom. Therefore, the diagnosis of a tumor can be significantly delayed. Recently, we have seen an advanced multiple myeloma of the spine with massive cervical and thoracic involvement, stage III according to Durie and Salmon [7], in a pain-free but cachectic patient with tetraplegia (Fig. 16.4 a, b).

Therapy

To avoid failure of the instrumentation for cervical lesions it is very important to use the optimal technique (ventral/dorsal approach) for the given lesion. It is also crucial to estimate a realistic prognosis of the individual patient to decide about the length of the instrumentation (number of fixed segments) and the choice of implant (e.g. possible extension of an anterior plate by additional pedicle screws). Since different primary tumors in different stages imply a different prognosis, the score described by Tokuhashi et al. [30] was very helpful in our patients with spine metastasis [34, 35]. The score accounts for the general condition, the number of extraspinal bone metastases foci, number of metastases in the vertebral bodies, metastases to the major internal organs, primary site of cancer, and spinal cord palsy.

Tatsui et al. described a one-year survival of 83% for patients with metastases by prostatic cancer, 78% for breast cancer, 51% for renal cancer, 22% for lung cancer and 0% for gastric cancer, respectively [29].

Spinal metastases have to be seen as a sign of spread of tumor disease with no realistic cure option. In late single metastasis of hypernephroma a vertebrectomy can be discussed as the attempt to achieve a wide resection [28]. In general, a resection of metastasis does not appear to be necessary and a dorsal approach appears to be

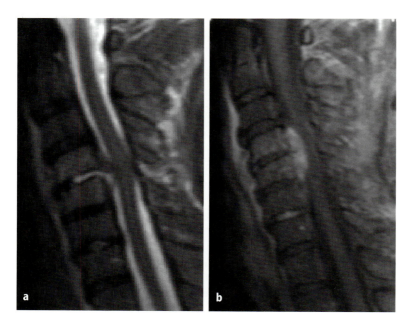

Fig. 16.3 a, b. 73-year-old patient with spondylodiscitis C4/5: Sagittal MRI reveals a fistula in the vertebral disc (**a**) as well as epidural abscess formation (**b**); patient was treated conservatively with spontaneous bony healing.

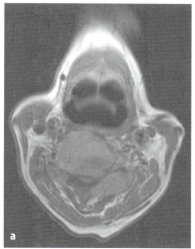
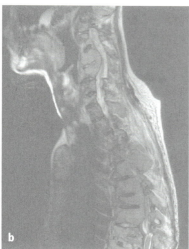

Fig. 16.4 a, b. 43-year-old male patient with high tetraplegia due to advanced multiple myeloma (Durie stage III, prefinal): Transversal (**a**) and sagittal (**b**) MRI revealing both the considerable size and the multiple spread of the tumor; patient died before treatment could be initiated.

suitable. The posterior approach has the advantage to avoid the preparation through the tumor masses, which are frequently located at the anterior aspect of the vertebrae and to allow for a notable decompression. To avoid an injury of the vertebral artery and to keep away from the spinal canal, careful preoperative planning is essential. We routinely perform a CT-scan of the region of interest including multi-planar reconstructions to have a clear impression of the individual anatomy (e.g. aberrant course of the vertebral artery in about 20% of the patients) and to receive a net of landmarks. To reduce the risk of screw misplacement we often use a computer-assisted surgery system (CAS-system) [18, 24]. Ma et al. described the placement of pedicle screws in C1 (50 cadavers and five patients) using the lateral mass of C2 as a landmark [19]. Harms et al. published their posterior fusion technique for the segment C1/2 with polyaxial screws and rod fixation performing a bilateral instrumentation of the lateral mass of C1 and the pedicle of C2 [9]. This reduces the risk of a damage of the vertebral artery and allows in selected cases – like young patients with a fracture or a subluxation – a removal of the fixator.

In the subaxial spine pedicle screws allow significantly improved biomechanical stability and offer better reposition possibilities compared to lateral mass screws. After probing the pedicle a blunt 1.5 mm K-wire is installed to direct the cannulated screw reducing the risk of a screw breakout. For C1/2 instrumentation we use transarticular screws in the Magerl technique [23]. Especially in long instrumentations a cross-linking device helps to improve rotational stability.

For patients with osteolysis below the C2-level and a life expectancy of more than 18 months we mostly perform an additional anterior approach with corporectomy for tumor reduction and reconstruction of the anterior column with an expandable cage, since this can prevent spinal cord or nerve root compression. In addition, this extended approach allows for a durable stabilization of the spine preventing screw loosening or instrumentation failure.

In cases of high perfusion (e.g. hypernephroma) as visualized by MRI with gadolinium we consider preoperative embolization [8, 16, 27, 36].

Conclusion

In unclear cervical pain and suspected tumor disease radiographs and MRI have to be considered as the gold standard for diagnosis, both in children and in adults. Depending on the primary tumor, lesions of the cervical spine need to be treated specifically.

The management of cervical tumor lesions remains challenging especially due to several difficulties in the decision-making process. This is mainly influenced by the prognosticated life expectancy, which depends mainly from the en-

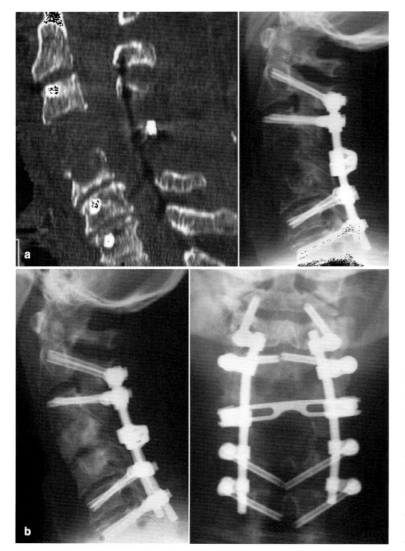

Fig. 16.5 a, b. 58-year-old male patient with bronchial carcinoma and cervical spine metastases at the level C4 and C5: Initial postoperative CT-scan with sagittal reconstruction and lateral radiograph showing the osteolysis of C4 and C5 and the posterior instrumentation C2/3–C6/7 (**a**); biplanar radiographic control eight months after surgery revealing sclerotic reaction of C4 and C5 after radiation with 40 Gy, chemotherapy and application of bisphosphonates (**b**) [11] (with permission of Springer, Heidelberg, Germany).

tity and supportive treatment options. The survival of lung tumors with bone metastases is on average close to eight months, the survival of breast carcinoma with skeletal metastasis about 30 months.

Due to the final stage of disease a resection of spinal metastases is generally not indicated. Therefore, a dorsal instrumentation with decompression appears to be a good alternative (Fig. 16.5 a, b) allowing a rigid fixation of the cervical spine including the cranio-cervical and the cervico-thoracic junction. A careful preoperative planning helps to avoid technical problems during the instrumentation of the cervical spine. A navigation system offers additional advantages with regard to screw positioning.

In anterior approaches to the cervical spine tumor bleeding has to be considered as a main problem, whereas in posterior instrumentations the vertebral artery has to be respected.

References

1. Abdu WA, Provencher M (1998) Primary bone and metastatic tumors of the spine. Spine 23: 2767–2777
2. Abumi K, Itoh H, Taneichi H, Kaneda K (1994) Transpedicular screw fixation for traumatic lesions of the middle and lower cervical spine: description of the techniques and preliminary report. J Spinal Disord 7:19–28
3. Beiner JM, Sastry A, Berchuck M, Grauer JN, Kwon BK, Ratliff JK, Stock GH, Brown AK, Vaccaro AR (2006) An aneurysmal bone cyst in the cervical spine of a 10-year-old girl: a case report. Spine 31:475–479
4. Böhm P, Huber J (2002) The surgical treatment of bony metastases of the spine and limbs. J Bone Joint Surg Br 84:521–529
5. Campanacci M, Enneking WF (1999) Bone and soft tissue tumors. Springer, Berlin
6. Dekeuwer P, Odent T, Cadilhac C, Journeau P, Langlais J, Padovani JP, Glorion C, Pouliquen JC (2003) Kyste anévrysmal du rachis chez l'enfant. Sept cas avec un recul moyen de 9 ans et revue de la littérature. Rev Chir Orthop Reparatrice Appar Mot 89:97–106
7. Durie BG, Salmon SE (1975) A clinical staging system for multiple myeloma. Correlation of measured myeloma cell mass with presenting clinical features, response to treatment, and survival. Cancer 36:842–854
8. Gellad FE, Sadato N, Numaguchi Y, Levine AM (1990) Vascular metastatic lesions of the spine: preoperative embolization. Radiology 176:683–686
9. Harms J, Melcher RP (2001) Posterior C1–C2 fusion with polyaxial screw and rod fixation. Spine 26:2467–2471
10. Hill ME, Richards MA, Gregory WM, Smith P, Rubens RD (1993) Spinal cord compression in breast cancer: a review of 70 cases. Br J Cancer 68:969–973
11. Huch K, Cakir B, Dreinhöfer KE, Puhl W, Richter M (2004) A new dorsal modular fixation device allows a modified approach in cervical and cervicothoracic neoplastic lesions. Eur Spine J 13: 222–228
12. Huch K, Cakir B, Ulmar B, Schmidt R, Puhl W, Richter M (2005) Prognose, operative Therapie und Verlauf bei zervikalen und hochthorakalen Tumorosteolysen. Z Orthop 143:213–218
13. Huddart RA, Rajan B, Law M, Meyer L, Dearnaley DP (1997) Spinal cord compression in prostate cancer: treatment outcome and prognostic factors. Radiother Oncol 44:229–236
14. Ilaslan H, Sundaram M, Unni KK, Shives TC (2004) Primary vertebral osteosarcoma: imaging findings. Radiology 230:697–702
15. Jenis LG, Dunn EJ, An HS (1999) Metastatic disease of the cervical spine. A review. Clin Orthop 359:89–103
16. King GJ, Kostuik JP, McBroom RJ, Richardson W (1991) Surgical management of metastatic renal carcinoma of the spine. Spine 16:265–271
17. Kluger P, Korge A, Scharf HP (1997) Strategy for the treatment of patients with spinal neoplasms. Spinal Cord 35:429–436
18. Ludwig SC, Kramer DL, Balderston RA, Vaccaro AR, Foley KF, Albert TJ (2000) Placement of pedicle screws in the human cadaveric cervical spine: comparative accuracy of three techniques. Spine 25:1655–1667
19. Ma XY, Yin QS, Wu ZH, Xia H, Liu JF, Zhong SZ (2005) Anatomic considerations for the pedicle screw placement in the first cervical vertebra. Spine 30:1519–1523
20. Marchesi DG, Boos N, Aebi M (1993) Surgical treatment of tumors of the cervical spine and first two thoracic vertebrae. J Spinal Disord 6:489–496
21. Olerud C, Lind B, Sahlstedt B (1999) The Olerud Cervical Fixation System: a study of safety and efficacy. Ups J Med Sci 104:131–143
22. Rades D, Stalpers LJ, Veninga T, Rudat V, Schulte R, Hoskin PJ (2006) Evaluation of functional outcome and local control after radiotherapy for metastatic spinal cord compression in patients with prostate cancer. J Urol 175:552–556
23. Richter M (2003) Posterior instrumentation of the cervical spine for instability using the "neon occipito-cervical system". Operat Orthop Traumatol 15:70–89
24. Richter M, Amiot LP, Neller S, Kluger P, Puhl W (2000) Computer-assisted surgery in posterior instrumentation of the cervical spine: an in-vitro feasibility study. Eur Spine J 9(Suppl):65–70
25. Richter M, Wilke HJ, Kluger P, Neller S, Claes L, Puhl W (2000) Biomechanical evaluation of a new modular rod-screw implant system for posterior instrumentation of the occipito-cervical spine: in-vitro comparison with two established implant systems. Eur Spine J 9:417–425
26. Richter M, Wilke HJ, Neller S, Claes L, Puhl W (2002) Neon – ein neues winkelstabiles Implantatsystem für die dorsale okzipitozervikale Instrumentierung. Biomechanischer Vergleich mit etablierten Systemen. Orthopäde 31:346–355
27. Roscoe MW, McBroom RJ, St-Louis E, Grossman H, Perrin R (1989) Preoperative embolization in the treatment of osseous metastases from renal cell carcinoma. Clin Orthop 238:302–307
28. Russo P (2000) Renal cell carcinoma: presentation, staging, and surgical treatment. Semin Oncol 27:160–176
29. Tatsui H, Onomura T, Morishita S, Oketa M, Inoue T (1996) Survival rates of patients with metastatic spinal cancer after scintigraphic detection

of abnormal radioactive accumulation. Spine 18:2143–2148
30. Tokuhashi Y, Matsuzaki H, Toriyama S, Kawano H, Ohsaka S (1990) Scoring system for the preoperative evaluation of metastatic spine tumor prognosis. Spine 15:1110–1113
31. Ulmar B, Catalkaya S, Naumann U, Cakir B, Schmidt R, Reichel H, Huch K (2006) Chirurgische Therapie und Evaluation von Prognosefaktoren bei Wirbelsäulenmetastasen durch Nieren-Zell-Karzinome. Z Orthop 144:58–67
32. Ulmar B, Huch K, Kocak T, Catalkaya S, Naumann U, Gerstner S, Reichel H (2007) Der prognostische Einfluss von Primarius und Höhe des befallenen Wirbelsäulenabschnitts bei 217 operativen Patienten mit Wirbelsäulenmetastasen unterschiedlicher Entität. Z Orthop 145:31–38
33. Ulmar B, Huch K, Naumann U, Catalkaya S, Cakir B, Gerstner S, Reichel H (2007) Evaluation of the Tokuhashi prognosis score in 217 patients with vertebral metastases. Eur J Surg Oncol [Epub ahead of print]
34. Ulmar B, Naumann U, Catalkaya S, Muche R, Cakir B, Schmidt R, Reichel H, Huch K (2007) Prognosis scores of Tokuhashi and Tomita for patients with spinal metastases of renal cancer. Ann Surg Oncol 14:998–1004
35. Ulmar B, Richter M, Cakir B, Muche R, Puhl W, Huch K (2005) The Tokuhashi score: significant predictive value for the life expectancy of breast cancer patients with spinal metastases. Spine 30:2222–2226
36. Vetter SC, Strecker EP, Ackermann LW, Harms J (1997) Preoperative embolization of cervical spine tumors. Cardiovasc Intervent Radiol 20:343–347
37. Vieweg U, Rao G, Meyer B (2000) Tumorchirurgie an der oberen Halswirbelsäule. Chirurg 71:1144–1151

17 Tumorous diseases of the thoracic and lumbar spine

Jürgen Nothwang and Christoph Ulrich

Introduction

Due to improved oncological care and increased survival rate of many malignant tumors, surgeons are confronted with a rising number of metastases of the spine. With further progress of vertebral metastases the patient is threatened by segmental instability, mechanical pain, deformity, pathological fracture and/or neurological deficits.

While primary malignant tumors of the skeletal axis are rarely found, osseous spinal metastases occur much more frequently. In any case, the patient experiences tumor invasion of the spine as extremely alarming because of the possibility of sudden paraplegia is associated with it. When this ominous threat to the patient is related to the total figure of merely 3% of vertebral tumors compared to the total number of tumor patients [7], the therapy of such tumors will appear in a different light. The physician is faced with high demands, which is due to the necessity of a patient-orientated individual therapy with consideration of tumor-biological, homeostatic, and economic aspects.

Incidence

Little is known about the incidence of tumor metastases in the thoraco-lumbar spine due to the absence of systematical analysis of vertebral tumor spread in autopsies. Even primary tumors are a rare pathologic entity in the spine. Only 1.5% of all primary tumors of the bone involve the vertebral column [9].

In spine, primary tumors have to be distinguished in benign and primary malignant tumors and those with potential malignancy. Most frequent malignant tumors in the spine are tumor metastases with 62% [9] to 85% [1]. Usually they do not extravagate the borders of a intervertebral disc. If these tumors penetrate the posterior wall of the vertebral body, spinal cord compression can be observed in 5% to 10% of patients [10].

Localization

Basically any type of tumor may occur in the vertebral column, but it is a striking fact that some anatomical structures of this motion segment are not affected by tumors. This is especially true for the intervertebral disc, which may be related to its specific nutritional method via diffusion. Vertebral joints are rarely affected [23]. This means that in contrast to traumatic lesions of the spine, we do not find segmental but osseous tumor invasion of the spine. The avalvular veins of the vertebral venous system play an important role. The core of this system is made up of three venous ring systems, which are concentrically arranged. They constitute a separate entity and are connected to the valvular veins of the thoraco-abdominal space via the central vertebral venous plexus [1]. Through this vascular system, all tumors with a preference to metastasize in bones, such as bronchial, thyroid and renal carcinomas as well as carcinomas of the breast and prostate, have access to the spine [26]. This explains the exposed role of the spinal column as a location of secondary osseous spread of cancer. As a rule, spinal metastasis occurs along the anterior vertebral column and much less frequently at the posterior elements [3]. Again, the cause is the vertebral venous plexus, which has the effect that in 80% the vertebral body [12] and only in 20% the posterior elements and the spinal cord are affected [5].

Classification

In contrary to tumors of the long bones, the spine does not have a typical compartmental structure with anatomical (muscular) borders. This leads to limitations in the application of the Enneking classification. With regard to prognostic aspects it seems helpful to cover the spine with a comparable classification system, which might favor decision making with regard to the therapeutic management. Tomita and co-workers suggested a classification system according to the tumor spread and the extent of the tumor [28]. According to this scoring system, treatment goals and surgical strategy can be defined.

Biomechanics

Basically, various forms of instability can be expected to affect the spinal column. Component instability [29] reflects an alteration process of the anatomical components of the "functional spine unit" (FSU) as it can be caused not only by trauma or tumor but also by degenerative changes. This is to be distinguished from kinematic instability, which is characterized by altered quality of motion, and from combined instability (kinematic and component instability). While trauma, as an incident having an external impact on the body, usually has an indirect effect on the spinal column, tumor invasion of a vertebral body can directly result in a slowly progressing instability. In contrast to traumatic impacts, tumor-induced component instability is restricted to the bone. Ligamentous structures are only secondarily affected by infiltration.

Silva and co-workers [25] performed an experimental study on thoracic vertebral bodies to investigate to what extent transcortical defects result in reduced stability, and they compared their results with pedicular destruction. Total defect size was calculated on the basis of the relationship between defect size and total section at the center of the body; cortical defect size on the basis of the relationship between defect width and defect circumference. It was shown that transcortical defects significantly weaken the resistance of the vertebral body while isolated pedicel destruction does not have this capability [25].

Differential diagnosis

In the light of the 80- to 85-percentage of metastases of all spinal tumors, tumor surgery on the spinal column is essentially metastases surgery. This is especially true, since lymphomas and multiple myelomas also belong to this group due to their classification as systemic diseases [22]. For differentiation from metastases the location of the lesion, its growth pattern, as well as co-existing soft tissue reactions and the evidence of atypical calcifications are important. Giant cell tumors and chordomata prefer the sacral region whereas osteoblastomata can mainly be found in the vertebral arches and the spinal processes. Osteosarcomata, chondrosarcomata but chordoma as well typically produce calcifications and bone formations [14].

While malignant neoplasms are predominantly diagnosed in adults, differential diagnosis of benign bone tumors and tumor-like lesions is more frequent in children and adolescents [13]. However, only 8% to 10% of all spinal tumors can be classified as belonging to this group [1]. Their distribution in the various segments of the spinal column, 20% cervical, 30% thoracic and 50% lumbar, follows a cranio-caudal pattern, whereas the distribution of spinal metastases between cervical, thoracic, and lumbar spine is about 1 to 6 to 4, with an increase in cervical spine metastases [19].

Diagnostic work-up

History and physical examination

Pain is the principal sign of vertebral body destruction. In view of the large number of patients with functional and degenerative back pain, early diagnosis is often delayed. In the patient's history there is mostly evidence of a traumatized back due to the lifting of an object or a fall, leading the physician performing the initial assessment to wrong diagnosis, especially if radiographs do not show vertebral destruction. Especially radiography of the thoracic spinal column involves the possibility of erroneous interpretation due to overlap and quality problems. Discrete radicular symptoms can easily be misinterpreted if thorough anamnesis does not take place. But it is exactly this symptom that is prevalent on the mechanically not much stressed cervical spine and on the radiographically poorly accessible cervico-thoracic transition.

Radiography

According to standard protocols, conventional X-ray examination is performed in two planes. Satisfactory exposure provided, it will permit assessment of form and structure of the vertebral bodies. By means of non-radiolucent marking, the center of the main pain can be more precisely marked and the X-ray path centered. Osteolytic or osteoblastic growth processes are differentiated on the basis of the X-ray.

Computed tomography (CT)

CT is of central importance when clarification of defined osseous vertebral lesions is required. By adding contrast media, a higher-contrast outline of tumor tissue and better assessment of tumor extension is possible. Sagittal and coronar planes of section permit three-dimensional reconstruction. A drawback of CT is the high radiation exposure. This is aggravated by the considerable time required, especially if CT involves several vertebral regions. Metal artefacts in patients having had prior surgery also influence interpretation of the CT.

Magnetic resonance imaging (MRI)

MRI is the diagnostic tool to gain insight into potential compromise of spinal cord or nerve roots without having to take recourse to invasive methods such as myelography or myelo-CT. Furthermore, good visibility of larger vessels without contrast medium permits conclusions as to the vascularization of a tumor. However, assessment of the actual extension of a tumor might be influenced by the high sensitivity of MRI.

Bone scintigraphy/Positron emission tomography (PET)

If conventional X-rays do not show clear pathological changes, highly sensitive though minimally specific skeletal scintigraphy is a diagnostic means that may show pathological bone processes with raised osteoblastic activity [15]. Apart from so-called hot spots as signs of raised local osteoblastic activity, osteolytically growing malignomas often show cold spots, which correspond to areas of reduced activity. Nevertheless one should keep in mind that in case of highly proliferative metastases the bone scintigraphy can be without representative result. A further improvement with regard to specificity represents positron emission tomography (PET) and the fusion technology PET-CT, which also enables an improved areal mapping of lesions.

Angiography

In case of a vascular tumor, spinal angiography (if applicable, with subsequent tumor embolization) serves not only as a diagnostical, but also as a therapeutical tool. Knowledge of the vascularity of the spinal cord and selective examination of the tumor-supplying vessels may help to prevent permanent neurological damage. For example, it is essential to find out to what extent the arteria radicularis magna ("Adamkiewicz") communicates with the tumor-supplying vessels. In 75% of cases it is located between Th9 and Th12, predominantly on the left side. Ischemic reactions can be recognized in adequate time only in non-anesthetized patients. Occlusion of tributary vessels is performed during a second, interventional session. Embolization might be helpful in the vascular hemangioblastomas and in metastases of a hypernephroma, since intraoperative bleeding can be significantly reduced [21].

Surgical management

Absolute indications

A pathological fracture and sudden neurological symptoms are absolute indications for surgery. The latter can easily be diagnosed during clinical examination. As the prognosis with regard to complete restoration deteriorates 24 hours after onset of symptoms, this represents a genuine emergency indication.

Protocols of prophylactic stabilization

While pathological fractures and neurological symptoms can be more precisely defined through additional diagnostics, we are faced with problems when rating and assessing tumor-induced instability and the issue of prophylactic stabilization.

In literature there are some attempts at diagnostic systematization: Cybulski, based on the 3-column model of Denis, sees the indication for a surgical intervention if anterior and middle column are damaged, and with corpus collapse exceeding 50% [6]. DeWald and co-workers [8] as well as Siegel et al. [24] are in favor of surgical stabilization if more than 50% of the vertebral body is destroyed or a pedicel is affected. Moreover, surgery has been recommended if two neighboring vertebrae are tumor-invaded, anterior and posterior elements are destroyed, or progressive vertebral body collapse can be seen, especially with regard of the relationship between absorbed trabecular mass and stability reduction [18]. Asdourian showed that in the early stage of tumorous vertebral body deformity, the base plate or the upper vertebra collapses first, followed by progressive vertebral body collapse [2]. According to a study by Taneichi and co-workers, invasion of the costo-vertebral joints in case of metastases of the thoracic spine (Th1 to Th10) seems to be a decisive factor for vertebral body collapse [27]. In addition, increased instability risk for the thoracic spine exists with a tumor extension in the vertebral body of 50% to 60%, and in the thoraco-lumbar and lumbar region of 35% to 40%. This allows the conclusion that the thoracic spine will tolerate a more extensive intracorporal tumor invasion compared to the lumbar spine. These findings are supported by studies of White and Panjabi, who attribute the stabilizing effect of the bony thorax to the role of costovertebral joints with additional, stabilizing ligamentous structures and a considerable increase of the surface of the thoracic spine in the transversal plane, which strengthens resistance to rotational forces [29].

In contrast to the thoracic spine, intracorporal tumor invasion of the thoraco-lumbar and the lumbar spine seems to be the decisive factor for the development of vertebral body collapse and the resulting instability. However, if pedicel infiltration is added, the risk for the development of a vertebral body collapse is heightened further.

In all cases of vertebral body metastases without relevant vertebral canal narrowing and without relevant instability, alternative methods of treatment must be discussed in close cooperation with oncologists and radiotherapists. Radiation therapy is particularly indicated for the treatment of pain. Compared to the peripheral skeleton, the spinal column is capable of a higher rate of radiographically verifiable recalcification [20].

Contraindications for surgery

In moribund patients surgical intervention is contraindicated. All interventions should be preceded by a benefit-risk analysis and a line should be drawn between what is surgically feasible and what is surgically reasonable. Some authors consider rapid tumor progression and an expected survival time of less than four weeks as further contraindications.

Principles of tumor disease management

The general condition of the patient, tumor type and the pattern of tumor spread should be evaluated. Although prognosis cannot be an exclusive parameter for treatment strategies the estimated survival rates should be reflected. According to Kocialkowski and Webb [16], the average survival time for a bronchial carcinoma with osseus metastasis is 11.3 weeks and for a hypernephroma it is 27.3 weeks. However the minimum survival time can be as low as one to two weeks in individual cases. Proof of visceral metastatic spread is an essential decision criterion because as a result prognosis is even worse. Radiation should be considered, and the same is true for neo-adjuvant or adjuvant chemotherapy.

Technical aspects of surgical treatment

Once the decision for surgical intervention is set, the individually best matching method needs to be chosen among the multitude of operative procedures.

While the surgical concept for primary tumors with a potentially curative therapeutic approach comprises a 360° stabilization, palliative treatment aims at providing a reliable sta-

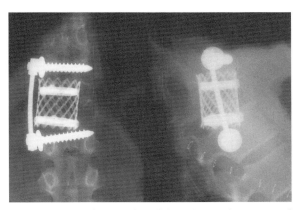

Fig. 17.1. Secondary implant failure (VDS-rod system and Harms cage).

bility through restoration of the anterior column and reconstruction of the posterior traction band. A stabilization device must possess longitudinal and transverse rigidity so that the implant can resist the load in all six degrees of freedom. In addition it should be biologically compatible, and it must not impede progress checks (titanium implants).

The Fixateur interne has proven successful for posterior stabilization with or without decompression, and it is typically used with transverse rods to increase rotatory stability. Additional cement augmentation might improve anchorage in osteoporotic bone.

Anterior implants are directly exposed to the influence of sagittal rotation, which makes angular rigidity mandatory for these implants. If the implant does not fulfill this requirement, which is generally possible for a single-rod system, dislocation of the vertebral body replacement is very likely to happen (Fig. 17.1). According to our experience, fixation systems capable of exerting pressure on the spacer and providing a four-point fixation are particularly suited for the thoraco-lumbar transition and the lumbar spine (Fig. 17.2 a, b), if there is no extensive invasion of the vertebral arch.

The type of spacer used after corporectomy is another crucial issue. In vertebral metastases autologous or homologous bone material cannot be recommended for vertebral body replacement. In such a situation, they are often made of bone cement. Combined with osteosynthesis material it works as compound osteosynthesis. Titanium spacers as load-bearing anterior column replacement particularly suited for the thoraco-lumbar transition and the lumbar spine (Fig. 17.2 b) are widely used.

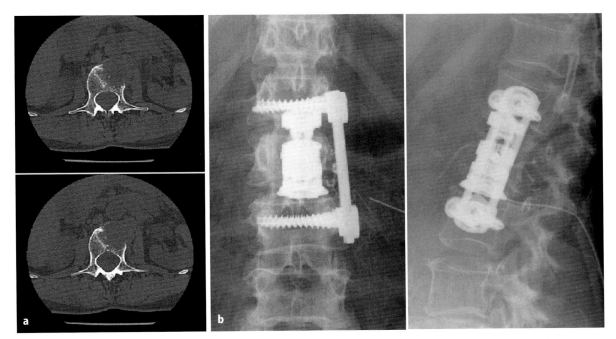

Fig. 17.2 a, b. 64-year-old woman with colon carcinoma and solitary bone metastasis of L2 with imminent vertebral collapse (**a**); pure anterior procedure after preoperative embolization: minimal invasive antero-lateral approach, subtotal corporectomy, interposition of a distractible vertebral body replacement and additional anterior plate stabilization (**b**).

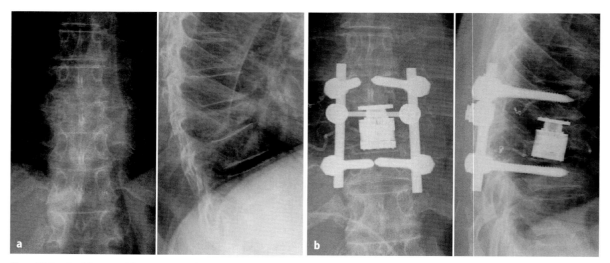

Fig. 17.3 a, b. 70-year-old woman with solitary metastasis Th9 with spinal canal infiltration (**a**); 360° stabilization as a single-stage posterior procedure: posterior instrumentation, fixation with a longitudinal rod on the right side, extended laminectomy, tumor resection and spinal canal clearance, corporectomy after resection of the pedicles Th9, posterior positioning of a distractible spacer, and fixation with a left-lateral longitudinal rod with transverse rod for increased rotatory stability (**b**).

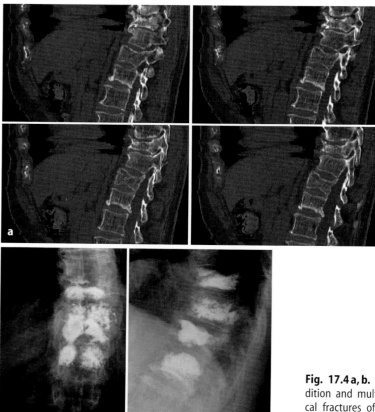

Fig. 17.4 a, b. 61-year-old woman with limited general condition and multiple myeloma with multisegmental pathological fractures of Th11 (old), L2 (subacute), and Th12 and L1 (acute) without spinal canal compromise, but severe back pain (**a**); kyphoplasty Th12, L1 and L2 and vertebroplasty Th11 (**b**).

Tumors with long survival time should be treated with regard to long-term stability. It needs to be considered that with solely posterior four-point stabilization the implant will be subject to fatigue due to the absence of anterior support. Maximum stability can only be attained by 360° instrumentation, if possible by an exclusively posterior approach (Fig. 17.3 a, b). When performing such a single-stage procedure it is recommendable to first instrument the pedicels, to mount the longitudinal rod on one side, to perform corporectomy with subsequent positioning of the vertebral body replacement and then to complete the posterior rod construction.

Alternatively, such 360° instrumentations can be performed in a combined two-stage procedure, when additional anterior stabilization by means of a plate or a rod system follows primary posterior stabilization.

There is general agreement that the technically simple laminectomy should no longer be performed without stabilization, particularly not below the level of Th10, as it aggravates instability and neurological disturbances. In the case of unisegmental spinal canal invasion above Th10, laminectomy may be sufficient for acute paraplegia and a very progressed tumor stage, provided the vertebral body is not threatened by collapse and the costovertebral joints are not affected. However, such a palliative measure will certainly remain an exception.

If no spinal canal invasion is detected and pathological fracture has not yet let to a total vertebral collapse, but imminent or already occurred pathological painful fracture is demonstrated, vertebro- or kyphoplasty are minimally invasive procedures with high effect on corporal stability (Fig. 17.4 a, b). Progressing vertebral fracture without extensive corporal bone defects is a good indication for vertebroplasty. Kyphotic deformity needs restoration of the vertebral alignment, which might be regained by kyphoplasty. The extent of vertebral wall destruction causes a limitation to these procedures although one may avoid perivertebral cement leakages by the "egg-shell technique".

Summary

Due to improved treatment modalities, an increasing number of patients will experience spinal metastases. Considering the tumor type and its prognosis as well as the individual condition and differences in anatomical regions, the physician planning surgical intervention can either choose a purely stabilizing and decompressing posterior method, or anterior decompression with vertebral body resection and replacement with or without supplemental posterior fixation. Generally, the latter can be performed as a single-stage or a two-stage posterior-anterior procedure.

In line with the guiding principle, "add life to years, not just years to life", restoration of function, which is pain-free mobility and maintenance of quality of life, is the objective of surgical treatment of spinal metastases. In addition, adjuvant therapy needs to be considered.

References

1. Adler CP (1983) Knochenkrankheiten. Thieme, Stuttgart
2. Asdourian PL (1991) Metastatic disease of the spine. In: Bridwell KH, DeWald RL (eds) The textbook of spinal surgery. Lippincott, Philadelphia, p 1187–1242
3. Black P (1979) Spinal metastases: current status and recommended guidelines for management. Neurosurgery 5:726–746
4. Bridwell KH, Jenny AB, Saul T, Rich KM, Grubb RL (1988) Posterior segmental spinal instrumentation (PSSI) with posterolateral decompression and debulking for metastatic thoracic and lumbar spine disease. Spine 13:1383–1394
5. Brihage J, Ectors P, Lenart M, van Houtte P (1988) The management of the spinal epidural metastases. Adv Tech Stand Neurosurg 16:121–176
6. Cybulski GR (1989) Methods of surgical stabilization for metastatic disease of the spine. Neurosurgery 25:240–252
7. Dahmen G, Bernbeck R (1987) Entzündungen und Tumoren der Wirbelsäule. Thieme, Stuttgart
8. DeWald RL, Bridwell KH, Prodromas C, Rodts MF (1985) Reconstructive spinal surgery as palliation for metastatic malignancies of the spine. Spine 10:21–26
9. Dominok GW, Knoch HG (1971) Knochengeschwülste und geschwulstähnliche Erkrankungen. Fischer, Jena

10. Gilbert RW, Kim JH, Posner JB (1978) Epidural spinal cord compression from metastatic tumor: Diagnosis and treatment. Ann Neurol 3:40–51
11. Goltzmann D (1997) Mechanisms of the development of osteoblastic metastases. Cancer (Suppl): 1581–1587
12. Harrington KD (1984) Anterior cord decompression and spinal stabilization for patients with metastatic lesion of the spine. J Neurosurg 61:107–117
13. Hohmann D, Liebig KJ, Beyer W (1987) Gutartige Tumoren der Wirbelsäule. Orthopäde 16:402–414
14. Huk WJ, Schuierer G (1987) Bildgebende Diagnostik bei Wirbelsäulentumoren. Orthopäde 16:371–378
15. Immenkamp M, Weidner A (1984) Gutartige Wirbeltumoren. In: Schmitt E (ed) Tumoren der Wirbelsäule. Hippokrates, Stuttgart
16. Kocialkowski A, Webb JK (1992) Metastatic spinal tumours: survival after surgery. Eur Spine J 1:43–48
17. Manabe S, Tateishi A, Abe M, Ono T (1989) Surgical treatment of metastatic tumors of the spine. Spine 14:41–47
18. McGowan DP, Hipp JA, Takeichi T, White AA, Hayes WC (1993) Strength reduction from trabecular destruction within thoracic vertebrae. J Spinal Disord 6:130–136
19. Nottebaert M, Hochstetter AR, Exner GU, Schreiben A (1987) Metastatic carcinoma of the spine. A study of 92 cases. Int Orthop (SICOT) 11:345–348
20. Rieden K (1988) Knochenmetastasen – Radiologische Diagnostik, Therapie und Nachsorge. Springer, Berlin
21. Ritschl P, Eyb R, Samec P, Lack W, Kotz R (1987) Behandlungsstrategie maligner Knochentumoren der Wirbelsäule. Orthopäde 16:379–388
22. Rössner A, Bosse A, Erlemann R, Grundmann E (1987) Zur Pathologie der Wirbelsäulentumoren. Orthopäde 16:358–370
23. Schmitt E (1984) Tumoren der Wirbelsäule. Die Wirbelsäule in Forschung und Praxis. Hippokrates, Stuttgart
24. Siegel T, Tiqua P, Siegel T (1985) Vertebral body resection for epidural compression by malignant tumors. J Bone Joint Surg Am 67:375–382
25. Silva MJ, Hipp JA, McGowan DP, Takeuchi T, Hayes WC (1993) Strength reductions of thoracic vertebrae in the presence of transcortical osseous defects: effect of defect location, pedicel disruption and defect size. Eur Spine J 2:118–125
26. Sim FH (1988) Diagnosis and management of metastatic bone disease. A multidisciplinary approach. Raven Press, New York
27. Taneichi H, Kaneda K, Takeda N, Abumi K, Satoh S (1997) Risk factors and probability of vertebral body collapse in metastases of the thoracic and lumbar spine. Spine 22:239–245
28. Tomita K, Kawahara N, Kobayashi T, Yoshida A, Murakami H, Akamaru T (2001) Surgical strategies for spinal metastases. Spine 26:298–306
29. White AA, Panjabi MM (1990) Clinical biomechanics of the spine. Lippincott, Philadelphia

18 Epidemiology and prognosis in spinal metastasis

Klaus Huch

Introduction

Improved survival time of patients with cancer is most likely responsible for the increase of the incidence of spinal metastasis [11]. In addition, modern diagnostic tools such as magnetic resonance imaging (MRI) or positron emission tomography (PET) may detect metastatic lesions earlier. According to Campanacci nearly 30% of all bone metastases can be observed in the spine [1]. The data from Bologna reveal a small percentage of cervical metastases (12%), whereas the thoracic (36%) and the lumbar spine (52%) represent the major side for vertebral metastases. Klimo and Schmidt described 70% thoracic, 20% lumbar, and 10% cervical involvement in spinal cord compression [13]. A dorsal localization is a rare finding in spinal metastases, whereas the vertebral body and the peridural space are mostly involved [6].

About 75% of vertebral metastases originate from carcinomas of the breast, prostate, lung, thyroid gland, and kidney [7], whereas metastases of unknown primary tumors account for only 3% to 4% [9]. Gerszten and Welch observed differences in the frequency of epidural spinal cord compression by metastases of different primary tumors: 22% in breast cancer, 15% in lung cancer and 10% in prostate cancer [3].

Even if curative surgery for a single metastasis in renal cell carcinoma is a topic of current discussion, surgery for bone metastasis will commonly remain palliative. Therapy therefore has to strive for an optimal reduction of pain and the maintenance or restoration of function and stability of the spine, with a minimum of operative morbidity and mortality.

Radiotherapy is not only considered to be an adjuvant but also to be an important alternative treatment. The advantages are the non-surgical treatment and the highly effective relief of pain. The main disadvantage is the interval, which is necessary to achieve sclerosis and consequently stability of osteolysis. Klimo et al. observed in their meta-analysis of surgery versus conventional radiotherapy for the treatment of metastatic spinal epidural disease an overall ambulatory success rate of 85% for surgery versus 64% for radiation [14]. In this analysis it appears

Table 18.1. Tokuhashi score for the prognosis evaluation of metastatic spine tumors [17] and performance status according to Karnofsky [12].

Parameters	Score (points)
General condition (performance status)	
Poor (PS 10–40%)	0
Moderate (PS 50–70%)	1
Good (PS 60–100%)	2
Number of extraspinal bone metastases foci	
≥3	0
1–2	1
0	2
Number of metastases in the vertebral bodies	
≥3	0
2	1
1	2
Metastases to the major internal organs	
Unremovable	0
Removable	1
No metastases	2
Primary site of the cancer	
Lung, stomach	0
Kidney, liver, uterus, unidentified, other	1
Thyroid, prostate, breast, rectum	2
Spinal cord palsy	
Complete	0
Incomplete	1
None	2

that surgery is superior at relieving pain and recovering sphincter function. However, since this study is based on uncontrolled cohort studies the data have to be interpreted cautiously.

The decision for or against surgery should be strongly influenced by the predicted survival. Tatsui et al. have published 1-year survival rates for patients with spinal metastases due to different primary tumors: prostate cancer 83%, breast cancer 78%, kidney cancer 51%, uterus cancer 45%, bronchial carcinoma 22%, and stomach cancer 0% [16]. However, the primary tumor is not the only parameter to estimate the prognosis. In 1990, Tokuhashi and co-workers created a clear-cut scoring system (0 to 12 points) for the preoperative evaluation of the prognosis of patients with spinal metastases [17]. The six parameters are depicted in Table 18.1. For scores of 9 or more points Tokuhashi expects a survival of twelve months and more and recommends excisional surgery of the metastases.

The ideal score should predict long-term survival of individual patients with spine metastases as exact as possible. This would help to prevent mechanical complications in isolated dorsal instrumentations by means of additional reconstruction of the anterior column following corporectomy [2, 4, 5, 7, 8, 10, 15]. To validate the Tokuhashi score we performed a retrospective study with more than 200 surgical patients.

Results of our retrospective cohort study

We recently analyzed 217 patients (114 males, 103 females; mean age 57 ± 16.3 years) receiving surgery for spinal metastasis in our Department between 1984 and 2005 [18–24]. Spine metastases of mamma carcinoma were seen relatively often in the cervical spine, whereas those of re-

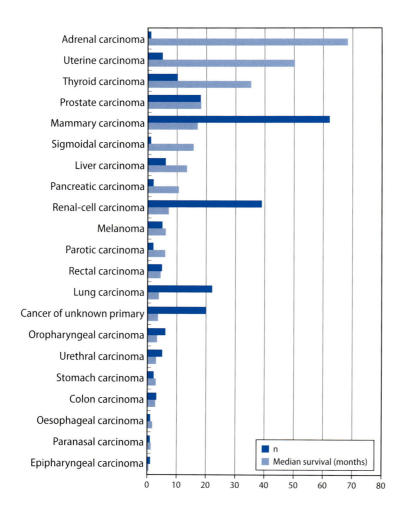

Fig. 18.1. Different primary tumor entities and median survival of 217 patients [19].

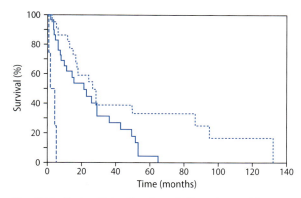

Fig. 18.2. Kaplan-Meier function of 55 patients with mamma carcinoma (represents Fig. 2B from [24], with permission of Lippincott, Williams & Wilkins) divided into the three prognostic groups [24]: long dashes = patients with a total number of ≤4 score points, solid line = patients with a total number of 5–8 score points, small dashes = patients with a total number of ≥9 points.

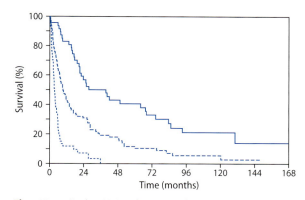

Fig. 18.4. Kaplan-Meier function of all 217 patients with various primary tumors (represents Fig. 1 from [20]; with permission of Elsevier Limited) divided into the three prognostic groups according to the Tokuhashi score [17]: small dashes = patients with a total number of ≤5 score points, medium dashes = patients with a total number of 6–8 score points, solid line = patients with a total number of ≥9 points.

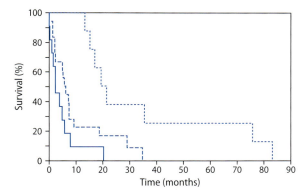

Fig. 18.3. Kaplan-Meier function of 37 patients with renal cell carcinoma (represents Fig. 1 from [21], with permission of Springer Science and Business Media) divided into the three prognostic groups according to the Tokuhashi score [17]: solid line = patients with a total number of ≤5 score points, long dashes = patients with a total number of 6–8 score points, small dashes = patients with a total number of ≥9 points.

nal-cell carcinoma were observed more often in the lumbar spine. The anatomic distribution of metastases for the complete study group was 12% at the cervical, 51% at the thoracic, and 37% at the lumbar spine.

The median survival of our study population was eight months (mean: 21.7 ± 31.8 months; range: 0 to 16 years). Figure 18.1 reveals the median survival for the different primary malignant tumors including the number of patients for each entity. The three most frequent tumors were mamma carcinoma (28.6%), renal-cell carcinoma (18%), and lung carcinoma (10.1%) [20]. Figures 18.2 and 18.3 demonstrate the prognostic groups (Kaplan-Meier-function) for patients with mamma [24] and renal cell carcinoma [21], whereas Figure 18.4 depicts the results of the total study group of 217 patients [20].

In all 217 patients the score result for group I (prognosis less than three months) was true for 40% of the patients, for group II (three to twelve months) the score correctly predicted 58% of the cases and for group III (predicted survival over twelve months) the prognosis came true in 84% [20].

Discussion

Patients with advanced spinal metastases frequently require immediate (acute neurologic dysfunction) or urgent (i.e. pathologic fracture) surgery. In these patients only limited diagnostic work-up can be performed preoperatively and the spinal tumor process often represents the first clinical manifestation of the disease.

Especially in the thoracic and lumbar spine we start in these cases with a dorsal approach for decompression and instrumentation. However, our surgical strategy considers the expected survival (interdisciplinary statement desirable) to avoid possible mechanical complications of an isolated dorsal instrumentation. If there is a survival of more than twelve months likely, we achieve additional stability by reconstruction of the anterior column. Therefore, the fact that the prediction of a 12-month-plus survival is true in 84% of the patients with a Tokuhashi score of nine or more points appears to be very helpful. However, this is statistical evaluation, whereas individual survival prediction remains a challenge since it may be influenced by various isolated patient- and tumor-based parameters [20].

Therefore, the interdisciplinary discussion of patients with spinal metastases is very important for the optimal treatment. In this context the Karnofsky index [12] and the primary tumor have to be considered also as important single factors for the estimation of life expectancy. However, both parameters are already represented in the Tokuhashi score [17].

Acknowledgments. The author thanks the co-authors of the following articles: [18–24].

References

1. Campanacci M, Enneking WF (1999) Bone and soft tissue tumors. Springer, Berlin, 780–787
2. Dick W (1992) Fixateur interne. State of the art reviews. Spine 6:147–172
3. Gerszten PC, Welch WC (2000) Current surgical management of metastatic spinal disease. Oncology 14:1013–1024
4. Gertzbein SD, Court-Brown CM, Marks P, Martin C, Fazel M, Schwartz M, Jacobs RR (1988) The neurological outcome following surgery for spinal fractures. Spine 13:641–644
5. Gertzbein SD (1994) Neurologic deterioration in patients with thoracic and lumbar fractures after admission to the hospital. Spine 19:1723–1729
6. Harrington KD (1997) Orthopedic surgical management of skeletal complications of malignancy. Cancer 80:1614–1627
7. Harrington KD (1981) The use of methylmethacrylate for vertebral body replacement and anterior stabilization of pathologic fracture dislocation of the spine due to metastatic malignant disease. J Bone Joint Surg Am 63:36–47
8. Hertlein H, Hartl WH, Dienemann H, Schurmann M, Lob G (1995) Thoracoscopic repair of thoracic spine trauma. Eur Spine J 1:142–151
9. Holmes FF, Fouts TL (1970) Metastatic cancer of unknown primary site. Cancer 26:816–820
10. Huch K, Cakir B, Dreinhöfer KE, Puhl W, Richter M (2004) A new dorsal modular fixation device allows a modified approach in cervical and cervicothoracic neoplastic lesions. Eur Spine J 13:222–228
11. Jacobs WB, Perrin RG (2001) Evaluation and treatment of spinal metastases: an overview. Neurosurg Focus 11:e10
12. Karnofsky DA (1967) Clinical evaluation of anticancer drugs: Cancer chemotherapy. GANN Monograph 22:223–231
13. Klimo P Jr, Schmidt MH (2004) Surgical management of spinal metastases. Oncologist 9:188–196
14. Klimo P Jr, Thompson CJ, Kestle JR, Schmidt MH (2005) A meta-analysis of surgery versus conventional radiotherapy for the treatment of metastatic spinal epidural disease. Neurol Oncol 7:64–76
15. Lord CF, Herndon JH (1986) Spinal cord compression secondary to kyphosis associated with radiation therapy for metastatic disease. Clin Orthop 210:120–127
16. Tatsui H, Onomura T, Morishita S, Oketa M, Inoue T (1996) Survival rates of patients with metastatic spinal cancer after scintigraphic detection of abnormal radioactive accumulation. Spine 18:2143–2148
17. Tokuhashi Y, Matsuzaki H, Toriyama S, Kawano H, Ohsaka S (1990) Scoring system for the preoperative evaluation of metastatic spine tumor prognosis. Spine 15:1110–1113
18. Ulmar B, Catalkaya S, Naumann U, Cakir B, Schmidt R, Reichel H, Huch K (2006) Chirurgische Therapie und Evaluation von Prognosefaktoren bei Wirbelsäulenmetastasen durch Nieren-Zell-Karzinome. Z Orthop 144:58–67
19. Ulmar B, Huch K, Kocak T, Catalkaya S, Naumann U, Gerstner S, Reichel H (2007) Der prognostische Einfluß von Primärtumor und Höhe des befallenen Wirbelsäulenabschnitts bei 217 operativen Patienten mit Wirbelsäulenmetastasen unterschiedlicher Entität. Z Orthop 145:31–38
20. Ulmar B, Huch K, Naumann U, Catalkaya S, Cakir B, Gerstner S, Reichel H (2007) Evaluation of the Tokuhashi prognosis score in 217 patients with vertebral metastases. Eur J Surg Oncol 33:914–919
21. Ulmar B, Naumann U, Catalkaya S, Muche R, Cakir B, Schmidt R, Reichel H, Huch K (2007) Prognosis scores of Tokuhashi and Tomita for patients with spinal metastases of renal cancer. Ann Surg Oncol 14:998–1004
22. Ulmar B, Reichel H, Catalkaya S, Naumann U, Schmidt R, Gerstner S, Huch K (2007) Evaluation and modification of the Tomita score in 217 patients with vertebral metastases. Onkologie 30:414–418
23. Ulmar B, Richter M, Cakir B, Brunner A, Puhl W, Huch K (2005) Chirurgische Behandlung und Prognosefaktoren von Wirbelsäulen-Metastasen bei Mamma-Ca. Z Orthop 143:186–194
24. Ulmar B, Richter M, Cakir B, Muche R, Puhl W, Huch K (2005) The Tokuhashi Score: Significant predictive value for the life expectancy of breast cancer patients with spinal metastases. Spine 30:2222–2226

19 Spondylitis and spondylodiscitis

ROLF SOBOTTKE and PEER EYSEL

Introduction

At the beginning of the 20th century, Smith and Ruffer, while examining an Egyptian mummy, found changes in its spinal column corresponding to spondylodiscitis [71]. The consequences of infectious destructions of the spinal column with a possible kyphotic deformity have often been described and illustrated in the history of medicine. The terms scoliosis, kyphosis, and lordosis, coined by van Galen in his writings dating from the 2nd century A.D. have remained well-established until today. In 1779, Percival Pott was first to describe the segmental destruction of the spinal column with kyphotic deviation caused by tuberculosis, today well known as Pott's disease. Until some decades ago, spondylodiscitis had a distinctly unfavourable prognosis, and even nowadays it can cause serious symptoms and become life threatening. In current studies the mean hospital stay is stated as being 30–49 days, with a hospital lethality of 2–17% [9, 21, 32, 49, 73, 83]. Infection of the spinal column is a rare disease, but clearly increasing in frequency, often recognized and treated too late [34, 35].

Spondylitis is an osteomyelitis of the spinal column. It is defined as a mostly bacterial infection with a destruction of the vertebral bodies starting from the endplates and secondarily spreading to the vertebral discs [11, 15, 17, 21, 41]. The term spondylodiscitis, on the other hand, describes the primary infection of a vertebral disc with propagation of the infection to the neighbouring vertebral bodies. At the time of diagnosis, however, inflammatory changes of both vertebral body and vertebral disc are already evident in radiographs, so that it becomes impossible to exactly determine the original location of the bacterial settlement. Both terms are therefore mostly used as synonyms.

As a general rule, in case of spondylitis the inflammation spreads within the anterior parts of the spinal column. Vertebral arches and vertebral joints are usually not involved.

Isolated discitis is found but rarely and is rather considered as an infantile disease [17, 60]. While the nucleus pulposus is never supplied with blood, regardless of the patient's age, the cartilaginous endplates of the vertebral bodies show vascularization approximately up to the seventh year of age, the anulus fibrosus even up to the twentieth year of age; thus it is possibly here that a haematogenous bacterial dissemination has its place of origin. The average age distribution curve of spondylodiscitis in infancy shows an amassment in the 1st–2nd and in the 10th–12th year of age [37, 39]. Isolated discites are also known to occur in old age or after surgery. Degenerative changes of the spinal column and vertebral fractures induce a blood supply of the vertebral disc and show a higher risk of spondylodiscitis [26, 60].

Infection path

There are two ways of infection to be distinguished: the endogenous and the exogenous transmission. When compared with osteomyelitis of the extremities, endogenous transmission is far more frequent in spondylodiscitis. Endogenously transmitted spondylodiscitis is often preceded by an infection totally different in origin, e.g. of the urogenital tract or the abdominal cavity; other possible sources are pulmonary infections or septicaemia. All of these can lead to a haematogeneous – either arterial or venous – bacterial spread with settlement in one or more vertebral bodies. The bacterial embolus settles particularly frequently in the complex and dense net of blood vessels in the subchondral region of the endplates, being fed by the paravertebral vessels [11, 17, 79, 82]. The spinal venous plexus, also known as Batson's plexus, is valveless. When abdominal pressure is increased, it can result in a reversal of the venous blood flow from the abdominal cavity toward the vertebral bodies. Because of this retrograde blood flow, in case of an infection of the abdominal cavity a local, or even a multilocular, bacterial settlement of the spinal column can take place [11, 17, 79, 82]. Frequently, the primary source of infection is no longer traceable when spondylodiscitis is eventually diagnosed.

Surgical intervention, injection therapy, or the very rarely found perforating injury of the spinal column, resulting in a bacterial inflammation, are possible exogenous causes of spondylodiscitis. Exogenous spondylodiscitis occurs much less frequently than the endogenous one; nevertheless, in recent years there has been an increase in this type of spondylodiscitis because of a higher occurrence of invasive therapies (e.g. spinal infiltrations and minimally invasive therapy procedures) [21]. Apart from exogenous and endogenous infections of the spinal column, lymphogenous ways of infection and spread per continuitatem are likewise possible [11, 21].

Pathogen spectrum

Possible pathogens responsible for spondylodiscitis include bacteria, fungus, and parasites (e.g. hydatidosus). In the majority of cases, however, the infection is of bacterial origin. Within this group one has to differentiate between the tuberculous (specific) and the non-tuberculous (non-specific) type of spondylodiscitis, depending on the pathogen involved [11, 17, 60]. The bacterial agent most frequent by far is the staphylococcus aureus, having an incidence rate of between 30 and 80% (as seen in Table 19.1) [9, 10, 11, 17-19, 32, 34, 45, 46, 50, 60, 73, 83]. The percentage of MRSA (methicillin resistant staphylococcus aureus) is reported as being 2-16% [9, 32, 45, 73]. The catheter-associated, nosocomial bacteraemia by MRSA is an important source of a spondylodiscitis caused by MRSA [23].

The specific type of spondylodiscitis always develops in an endogenous way. In HIV-negative patients with tuberculosis, the tuberculosis manifests itself in the skeleton in 3-5% of the cases, in patients infected with HIV in 60%

Table 19.1. Frequency distribution of pathogens of non-specific spondylodiscitis according to Nolla et al. [62].

Staphylococcae 39%
- Staphylococcus aureus 36%
- Staphylococcus epidermidis 3%

Gram-negative bacteria 39%
- Escherichia coli 23%
- Pseudomonas aeruginosa 5%
- Eikenella corrodens 3%
- Proteus mirabilis 3%

Streptococcae 19%
- Streptococcus sanguis 8%
- Streptococcus agalactiae 5%

[58]. 50% of all skeletal tuberculoses are to be found in the spinal column [58, 78]. The ratio of specific to non-specific spondylodiscitis strongly depends on the collective examined and varies in literature from 1:20 to 7:3 [17, 21, 41, 46, 49, 50]. The course of disease tends to be chronic in case of specific spondylodiscitis, whereas non-specific spondylodiscitis often takes a highly acute course, depending on the immunological status of the patient [11].

Mixed infections are rare, only to be found in up to 2.5% of the cases [32, 72].

Brucella spondylodiscitis affects almost exclusively people employed in agriculture, forestry and meat processing. Typically it occurs in the lower lumbar spine, but infections of the cervical spine have been described as well [50, 53, 67].

As a possible parasite causing spondylodiscitis echinococcus has been mentioned. Intraosseous hydatidosis is mostly found in the thoracic spine [8].

With the increasing incidence of HIV, mycotic infections of the spinal column and infections with atypical mycobacteria (MOTT – Mycobacteria Other Than Tuberculosis) gain greater significance [14, 22, 40, 54, 64, 81]. Within the opportunistic infections, the aspergillus is the most frequent cause of a skeletal mycotic infection, the spinal column being the most frequent localization of a mycotic osteomyelitis [40, 64]. While mycosis typically occurs in the lumbar spine and frequently affects several segments of it, the thoracic spine is often attacked by an infection of atypical mycobacteria. The probability of an infection with atypical mycobacteria depends strongly on the CD4 cell count; with a CD4 cell count lower than 40 cells/µl, the risk increases about 2.5 fold [5]. After the introduction of HAART (Highly Active Antiretroviral Therapy) in 1996, infections with MOTT and its mortality rate were fast declining [5]. The quick increase of CD4 cells by HAART caused a so-called "immune reconstitution syndrome" which led to atypical and decelerated courses of disease, partially even to spontaneous healings [5, 7]. It is by no means uncommon that many years pass by between the beginning of the patient's complaints and the eventual diagnosis [12, 44].

Table 19.1 summarizes the frequency distribution of pathogens of non-specific spondylodiscitis according to Nolla et al. [62].

Epidemiology

The incidence of non-specific spondylodiscitis is about 1:250 000 [11, 17, 21], the proportion of spondylodiscitis to osteomyelitis as a whole being about 3–5% [11, 17, 21, 60]. Men are more frequently affected than women by a ratio ranging from 1:1 to 3:1 [9, 20, 21, 32, 41, 49, 50, 60, 66, 73, 83].

Epidemiology of spondylodiscitis following lumbar disc surgery depends on how invasive the procedure has been; for microsurgical procedures or discographies it is reported to be 0.1–0.6%, for macrosurgical procedures 1.4–3% [17, 42, 48, 65]. 10–15% of all vertebragenous infections have been specified as exogenous spondylodiscitis [9, 21, 28, 32, 41, 50]. In principle, patients of all ages can contract specific or non-specific spondylodiscitis, but the 50- to 70-year-olds are most likely to fall ill from it [9, 10, 20, 28, 32, 34, 39, 41, 49, 50, 60, 83]. The peak of disease in HIV-positive patients lies substantially earlier: 10% of them are under 30 years of age when they first contract specific spondylodiscitis.

While specific infections mostly occur in the thoracic spine, approximately 60–100% of unspecific infections affect the lumbar spine and the lower section of the thoracic spine [2, 9 ,17, 20, 21, 32, 41, 46, 50, 69, 83]. In up to 16% of the cases, the cervical vertebrae are sites of infection [9, 17, 20, 21, 28, 32, 46, 83]. In 10–25% a spondylodiscitis with multiple-level involvement is to be found [17, 41, 49, 73].

Predisposition

Immune-suppressed patients run a higher risk of falling ill from spondylodiscitis. Predisposition factors include age, multimorbidity, diabetes mellitus, cardiovascular diseases, kidney insufficiency, chronic hepatitides, rheumatic diseases, chronic steroid ingestion, tumor disorders, immunosuppressive intake, previous infections, previous abdominal surgery, passed tuberculosis, sickle-cell anaemia, obesity, drug abuse, and HIV [4, 9, 17, 21, 28, 32, 34, 50, 60, 73].

Differential diagnoses

Regarding differential diagnoses, erosive osteochondrosis, osteoporotic and pathological fractures, destruction due to tumor, ankylosing spondylitis, and Scheuermann's disease are worth mentioning. Particularly acute inflammatory degeneration is rather difficult to be differentiated clinically and radiologically from spondylodiscitis at its initial stage, as it does not display an increase in inflammation parameters and mostly affects the L4/5 or the L5/S1 segment. Ultimately, patients with spondylodiscitis are on average ten years older than those with degenerative ailments [75].

Diagnostics

Clinical signs

A long history of back pain, not seldom lasting several weeks or even months, is characteristic of spondylodiscitis. Especially at its initial stage, subjective symptoms are rather diffuse. As there are no radiologically visible changes at the onset of the disease, it is often diagnosed belatedly. Two to six months passing by between the appearance of first symptoms and a final diagnosis are not uncommonly found in literature [9, 17, 20, 21, 32, 34, 41, 43, 46, 60, 73]. The troubles being so unspecific, and the fact that back pain has developed into such a widespread disease that it is only diagnosed with certain diffidence, are possible causes of this delay. A patient seeking out a doctor because of back pain is usually treated conservatively at first, as a degenerative disease of the spine is being presumed. Only when a therapy resistance becomes clearly evident, radiological diagnostics is applied. Due to the mostly chronic course of disease, patients suffering from specific spondylodiscitis often have long lasting histories of back pain, whereas, in order to prevent a higher grade of vertebral destruction or the emergence of neurological complications, an early diagnosis would have been of vital prognostic importance [14].

Initially, patients tend to complain of spinal pain on exertion. In the course of the disease, however, the pain begins to appear at night or in rest as well, thus differing from degenerative spinal diseases. Furthermore, non-specific symptoms such as subfebrile or febrile temperatures, night sweat, deterioration of performance, weight loss, inappetency, fatigue, and lassitude have been known to occur. In advanced stages of inflammation, radicular and pseudoradicular pain symptoms have been reported [9, 17, 34, 41, 50, 60].

If the infection spreads dorsally or the abscess breaks into the spinal canal, it can lead to neurological deficits or signs of meningitis, depending on its spinal level localization. Usually this results in complete or incomplete tetraplegic or paraplegic deficits. Dermatome-related neurological deficits, on the other hand, are rare. As the spinal canal is narrower in the thoracic region than in the lumbar region, in case of epidural abscess formation a myelopathy with neurological symptoms is more likely to occur in the thoracic than in the lumbar spine [17, 41, 60]. Frangen et al. examined a collective of 78 patients with spondylodiscitis that had to be treated surgically. 28% of the patients from this group had developed an acute paraplegic syndrome [21]. In other publications, pareses of the lower extremities affecting 11–29% of the total patients' collectives have been reported [9, 32, 34, 50].

If the infection spreads ventrally, the abdominal region can get involved and ileus symptoms can occur, again depending on the spine level the infection is localized at. An involvement of the psoas muscles, e.g. in terms of a psoas abscess or a gravity abscess, can result in pain when the hip is actively flexed or passively overextended, and irritation of the ilioinguinal nerve can be accompanied by a radiation of pain into the inguinal region. An infection of the thoracic region of the spine bears the risk of a pleural empyema. Dysphagia can be a sign of retropharyngeal abscess formation [9, 20, 21, 41, 60].

If the vertebral body is destructed predominantly ventrally, this can lead to a kyphotic malposition, in extreme cases even to gibbus formation, which in turn may cause paraplegia.

13–26% of all cases of spondylodiscitis proceed as a highly acute disease [17], presenting with a septic picture of high-grade fever, chills, even up to septic shock, multiple organ failure and exitus.

Anamnestically, particular attention should therefore be paid to the predisposition factors mentioned above, possible preceding infiltration therapies, or spine surgeries.

Clinical diagnostics

Besides thorough inspection with special regard to local alterations – such as gibbus or inflammatory changes as an aftermath of surgery – clinical examination should comprise an extensive neurological check-up in order to assess if spinal or radicular structures have been affected. Distinct pain on heel strike, compression pain, and pain on percussion are typically present on physical examination, while local pain on palpation is merely slight or non-existent. The patient adopts a relieving posture and tends to avoid bearing weight on the ventral spine segments, describing inclination and the effort to re-attain erect position after inclination (positive pseudo Gowers' sign) as being painful.

Laboratory diagnostics

Laboratory parameters to be determined in spondylodiscitis include leucocytes, C-reactive protein (CRP), erythrocyte sedimentation rate, and thrombocytes. An acute course of disease is characterized by massive elevation of both inflammation parameters and sedimentation rate, while in a chronic disease those parameters may show normal or borderline values. Specific spondylodiscitis tends to be accompanied by merely a slight increase in inflammatory parameters. If tuberculous spondylodiscitis is being suspected, a tine tuberculin test has to be performed. Elevated readings of alkaline phosphatase might point to increased bone metabolic activity and thus serve as an additional indicator.

Leukocytosis is not an obligatory feature, a distinct increase of CRP, on the other hand, seems to be typical [11, 17]. Leukocyte counts show a merely 18% sensitivity, specifity being as high as 90%, while CRP accounts for a sensitivity of 75% and a specifity of 71% [17].

Radiography diagnostics

For in-depth imaging diagnostics, the following techniques are available: conventional X-rays, magnetic resonance imaging, computed tomography, multiphase bone scan, inflammation scintigraphy, and positron emission tomography.

Conventional X-rays

In cases of diffuse pain in the spine, the primary imaging method of choice is conventional two-plane X-rays of the spine segment concerned. Particularly in early phases of spondylodiscitis, there are no native radiological signs present. These often become visible only two to eight weeks after the first appearance of clinical symptoms [11, 34, 50, 60]. Even in the course of the disease it may be that radiological signs remain indistinct and barely distinguishable from degenerative spine diseases. In advanced stages of inflammation, however, with obvious destructions becoming manifest in native X-rays, a clear differentiation from pathological fractures or tumorous change is almost impossible. According to Modic et al., there is an 82% sensitivity of conventional X-rays, compared to its specifity of merely 57% [17, 56].

Diminishment of intervertebral space in stage I (Fig. 19.1) does apparently not originate from a disc reduction but has to be seen as caused by an early destruction of cover and base plates at the onset of the inflammatory event. At the early stages the vertebral discs are rather edematously swollen, which can even bring about an intermittent increase of intervertebral space height [75, 76]. As the disease progresses, prior to the destruction of the endplates by reactive bone growth one can even observe an increased delineation of the endplates [51]. Once destruction sets in, the affected endplates present as diffusely delineated. In stadium II, areas of lysis are already to be seen (Fig. 19.2). With further progression of inflammatory changes and a sub-

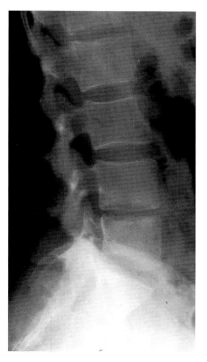

Fig. 19.1. Lateral X-ray of the lumbar spine in a patient with L4/5 spondylodiscitis: diminished intervertebral space, blurred imaging of cover plate and base plate, corresponding to stage I as defined by Eysel and Peters.

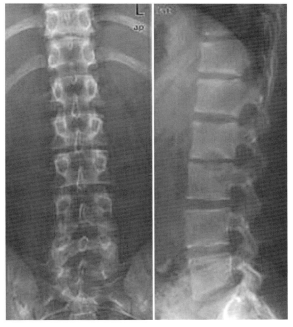

Fig. 19.2. X-rays of the lumbar spine in anteroposterior and lateral projections showing spondylodiscitis at L2/3 and a destruction of base plate and cover plate, corresponding to stadium II of the Eysel-Peters classification.

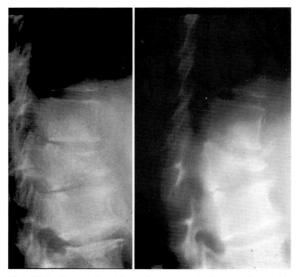

Fig. 19.3. Conventional lateral tomography in a patient with spondylodiscitis at L1/2 and L2/3, revealing kyphotic deformity, corresponding to Eysel and Peters stage III.

Table 19.2. Following Eysel and Peters, conventional imaging of spondylodiscitis can be classified according to four stages [17].

Stage I	Due to an inflammation of the spine, a pressure drop takes place, together with a radiologically visible narrowing of intervertebral space (Fig. 19.1)
Stage II	Progressive inflammation leads to erosions of vertebral body cover and base plates (Fig. 19.2)
Stage III	Inflammatory changes of vertebral bodies result in kyphotic deformity, in rare cases even to scoliotic changes (Fig. 19.3)
Stage IV	Reactive bone growth causes ankylosis and kyphotic malalignment (Fig. 19.4)

stance loss of the ventral parts of the vertebral bodies in stage III, an increasing kyphotic deformity becomes visible (Fig. 19.3). If spondylodiscitis with kyphotic malalignment remains untreated, reactive bone growth and connective tissue fixation will lead to ankylosing of the affected spine segment (Fig. 19.4).

A widened retropharyngeal soft tissue shadow in the lateral view of the cervical spine and a dislocation of the paravertebral soft tissue shadow in the anterioposterior view of the lumbar spine might indicate paravertebral abscess formation. Native X-ray imaging is well suited for follow-up examinations. It enables sound assessment of modifications in spine statics, bony ankylosis following conservative therapy, and consolidation results after operative repair.

Table 19.2 contains the Eysel and Peters classification criteria of spondylodiscitis seen on conventional X-ray examination [17].

Magnetic resonance imaging

If there are well-founded indicators for spondylodiscitis, magnetic resonance imaging (MRI) should be performed, even without explicit support from native X-ray findings. With a sensitivity of 90–100% and a specificity of 85–92%, MRI is the method of choice for diagnosing spondylodiscitis (Fig. 19.5 a, b) [10, 11, 17, 20,

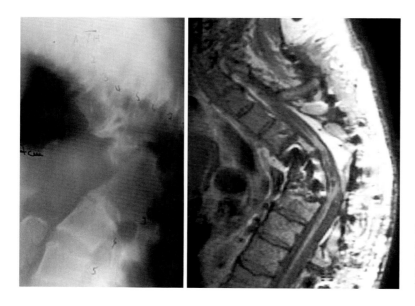

Fig. 19.4. Lateral X-ray and sagittal MRI of the thoracic and lumbar spine in a patient with spondylodyscitis at T8/9 and ankylosis, corresponding to stage IV of the Eysel-Peters classification.

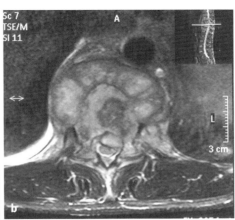
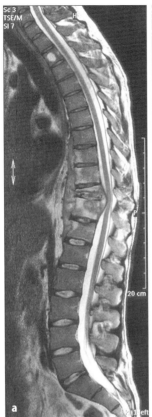

Fig. 19.5 a, b. T2-weighted MRI + contrast medium in sagittal (**a**) and axial (**b**) section planes in a patient with specific spondylodiscitis at T10/11 (atypical mycobacteria: M. xenopi).

24, 42, 50, 71, 80]. It allows imaging the whole length of the spine, so that additional infections of other spine segments can be detected as well. In early stages of spondylodiscitis (stage I and II according to Eysel and Peters [17]) it is often impossible to distinguish spondylodiscitis from erosive osteochondrosis when using X-ray imaging [2, 10, 24, 80]. By analyzing the different weightings, MRI can permit discrimination between the most relevant differential diagnoses. In the acute stage of unspecific spondylodiscitis, the disc and its adjacent vertebral bodies appear hypointense on T1-weighted images, while on T2-weighted, edema-sensitive images high signal intensity is particularly striking, caused by the edema accompanying the infection. In case of degenerative spine disorders, contrast medium administration causes merely a slight accumulation in the marginal areas. Contrary to an infected spinal disc, the disc of a spine segment affected by osteochondrosis does not show increased signal intensity on T2-weighted images [2, 10, 24, 80]. The destruction due to a tumour, an important factor for differential diagnosis, does not primarily concern the intervertebral space but the vertebral body [50]. Apart from that, the high soft-tissue contrast allows for a good presentation of a possible extension of the inflammation process to the paravertebral or the epidural space [10, 24, 50, 80].

In many cases MRI makes it possible to distinguish between specific and unspecific spondylodiscitis [10, 50]. Within a retrospective study, Chang et al. have examined 22 MRI parameters in 66 patients with specific and unspecific spondylodiscitis, exactly one half each. In 17 of these parameters the study group found differences significant for MRI, thus allowing a distinction between specific and unspecific spondylodiscitis. Five of the most characteristic ones, being also workable within everyday clinical settings, are displayed in Table 19.3 [10].

Computer tomography

Computer tomography (CT) is inferior to MRI in sensitivity and specifity when it comes to diagnosing spondylodiscitis or ruling out possible differential diagnoses [2, 10, 24, 50, 80]. Com-

Table 19.3. Five of the most distinctive and feasible MRI findings concerning specific und unspecific spondylodiscitis according to Chang et al. [10].

Unspecific spondylodiscitis	Specific spondylodiscitis
▪ Chiefly destruction of disc	▪ Chiefly destruction of bone
▪ Relatively moderate peridiscal destruction of vertebral body	▪ Disc remains comparatively spared
▪ Diffuse and homogenous enhancement of contrast medium within the vertebral body	▪ Focal and heterogeneous enhancement of contrast medium within the vertebral body
▪ Ill-defined paraspinal area of pathological signal intensity	▪ Well-defined paraspinal area of pathological signal intensity
▪ Peridiscal rim enhancement	▪ Intravertebral rim enhancement in sagittal view

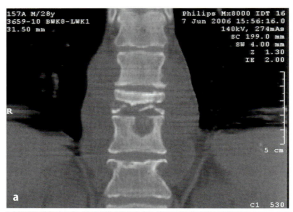
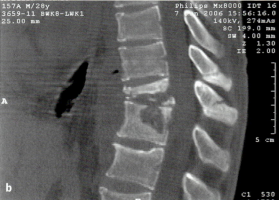

Fig. 19.6 a, b. CT with frontal and sagittal reconstructions in a patient with atypical spondylodiscitis at T10/11 (atypical mycobacteria: M. xenopi).

pared to MRI, in CT-imaging the bony structures are presented in much greater detail – and thus bony destructions as well (Fig. 19.6 a, b). In early phases of spondylodiscitis CT is able to clearly show destructions of endplates or the narrowing of intervertebral space, even if this is not yet visible in conventional imaging [50]. CT is primarily indicated when MRI cannot be performed, e.g. because of a patient's cardiac pacemaker. Furthermore, after contrast medium administration CT is well apt to provide excellent renditions of paravertebral abscess formation [50].

▪ **Multiphase bone scintigraphy**

Modic et al. found a sensitivity of 90% for scintigraphy when used in diagnosing spondylodiscitis, but only a specifity of 78% because it cannot provide a clear differentiation from other metabolically active processes such as activated degenerative diseases or tumour-related changes [56]. It is not possible to distinguish between bone infection and activated osteochondrosis in bone scan. Changes in soft tissue are assessed in the first (perfusion) and the second (blood pool) phase of multiphase bone scintigraphy. The third (delayed) phase detects changes in bone metabolism. Here, determination of localisation and extension of the inflammatory process is much more inaccurate when compared to MRI or CT, due to the lower spatial resolution of the gamma camera. Therefore, bone scan is not a first-choice diagnostic means [70]. On the other hand, a bone scan with no pathological findings excludes the possibility of an osseous inflammation process to a high degree of diagnostic accuracy. In addition, susceptibility artefacts generated by implant materials do not interfere with bone scintigraphy, as they do with CT and MRI.

▪ **Inflammation scintigraphy with labeled leucocytes or by using technetium 99m-labeled antibodies**

In leucocyte scintigraphy, a complement to multiphase bone scanning, the body's own blood cells are radioactively marked (Tc-99m-labeled antigranulocyte antibodies are preferably used today) to help detect inflammatory changes of bone tissue. The procedure is rather time-con-

Table 19.4. Sensitivity and specifity of various imaging techniques.

%	X-Rays	Scintigraphy	Inflammation scintigraphy	F-18 FDG-PET	MRI
■ Sensitivity	82	90	–	100	96–100
■ Specifity	57	78	31–76	–	92

suming, as imaging is usually only completed after 24 or 48 hours. Specifity regarding this method ranges between 31–76% in literature [70]. For diagnosing spondylodiscitis, inflammation scintigraphy with Tc-99m-labeled antigranulocyte antibodies is a technique not very well suited. Antigranulocyte antibodies also label the hematopoietic bone marrow, so that the marrow, and thus the spine as well, show a physiological uptake in the scan. Spondylodiscitis, then, appears as a cold spot within the intense uptake of hematopoietic marrow, but for such a finding various differential diagnoses are possible, e.g. replacement of bone marrow due to degenerative transformation processes. This explains why specifity of this method in diagnosing spondylodiscitis is so low and so fluctuating. Therefore, inflammation scintigraphy with Tc-99m-labeled antigranulocyte antibodies seems more aptly fit for the peripheral skeleton. Extremities, for instance, are physiologically not provided with hematopoietic marrow, so that a peripheral focus of inflammation is detected as a hot spot.

■ **Positron emission tomography with Fluorine-18 fluorodeoxyglucose**

Positron emission tomography (PET) scans using Fluorine-18 fluorodeoxyglucose as tracer (F-18 FDG-PET) have become increasingly important in diagnosing spondylodiscitis. In Germany this technique has meanwhile superseded the Gallium-67 scintigraphy used earlier to decide if a spondylodiscitis is taking place. Gallium-67 as well as F-18 FDG does not physiologically accumulate in bone marrow or in the spine (and if so, then only to a minor degree), so that inflammatory processes appear as hot spots in the scans. The degree of accumulation of F-18 FDG is connected with the increased glucose metabolism in inflammation cells (leucocytes, granulocytes, macrophages). F-18 FDG-PET is regarded as an imaging technique of high diagnostic accuracy with a sensitivity of up to 100% [70, 77].

Advantages of F-18 FDG-PET are fast imaging (images can be acquired as soon as one hour after injection), a relatively low radiation exposure of 3.7–7.4 mSv per patient, and a higher spatial resolution when compared with the gamma camera [70]. PET permits a better differentiation between an osseous process and inflammatory reaction of its encompassing soft tissue than bone scanning [77]. Other than MRI or CT, metal or susceptibility artefacts do not show with this imaging technique. If combined PET/CT scanners with CT-based attenuation corrections are being used, the quality of the images is improved with special algorithms. While a distinction between onset of spondylodiscitis and degenerative changes in vertebral body endplates is easy to make, specifity with regard to malignant processes might be a problem. Inflammation foci and malignant findings alike often show increased accumulation of F-18 FDG, so that a differentiation via PET alone is not possible, even though it can usually be deduced from clinical context. An additional disadvantage of this method is that it still is rather costly [70, 77].

Table 19.4 summarizes the sensitivity and specifity of various imaging techniques.

■ **Pathogen identification**

In order to decide on an effective antimicrobial treatment, one that is targeted against the bacterium and based on the resistance test results, it is of pivotal importance to identify the pathogen involved. Antibiosis must be regarded as one of the pillars in any spondylodiscitis therapy. All in all, identification of the causative organism is successful in 49–83% of the cases, even less likely in a chronic than in an acute progression of spondylodiscitis. A previously administered systemic antibiotic therapy has a negative influence on pathogen identification as well, making it even more important to apply antibiosis only after an attempt at isolating the pathogen [9, 21, 32, 41, 46, 73]. If the course of the disease is rather indistinct, it might be advisable to interrupt antibiotic therapy for a few days while closely monitoring the disease process, until the focus of inflammation has been punctured and an identification of the pathogen has been attempted.

Blood culture

The least complicated method of obtaining material for microbiological diagnosis is to take a blood culture. It is recommended to take at least two to three blood cultures, not only in an acute fever or septic situation, but also in a mild course without fever. In up to 70% of the cases in which the patients are not yet treated with antibiotics, it yields positive results [17, 60, 62].

Biopsy

Another possibility of pathogen identification preceding antibiotic therapy is offered by transpedicular punch biopsy, performed under adequate anaesthetics, or by CT-guided fine-needle aspiration. The latter can at the same time be used therapeutically for placing a CT-guided drainage, should it be necessary to evacuate an abscess. The relatively small tissue sample that is gained from CT-guided aspiration must be regarded as a disadvantage of this technique. Microbiological examination of a biopsy sample yields an unambiguous diagnosis in about 50% of the cases [15, 18, 21, 71], whereas nowadays PCR-based molecular biological methods are increasingly employed. In contrast, Felix and Mitchell found a sensitivity of 91% and a specifity of 100% for CT-guided needle aspiration [18].

Intraoperative incisional biopsy

Because of the relatively big tissue sample, the intrasurgical taking of tissue samples for histopathological as well as microbiological analysis has to be regarded as the most reliable method of pathogen identification [16, 17, 21, 41, 60]. In about 75% of the cases the causative germ is yielded [62]. Figure 19.7 illustrates our stage pattern for pathogen identification.

Histopathology

Unspecific spondylodiscitis

Extensive bone destruction with necrotic bone marrow and osteolysis is typical of unspecific

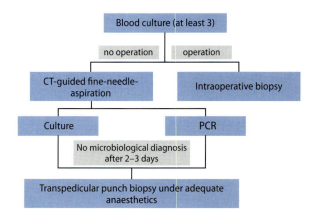

Fig. 19.7. Stage pattern for pathogen identification.

spondylodiscitis. Spread to the adjacent tissue results in unspecific granulation tissue, on microscopic examination containing granulocytes with polymorphous nuclei. Contrary to osteomyelitis of the extremities, spondylodiscitis almost never leads to fistulization [17].

Specific spondylodiscitis

Tuberculous spondylodiscitis mainly occurs in immigrants from underdeveloped or developing countries. It is the most frequent form of specific osteomyelitis. The spine infection with mycobacterium tuberculosis is the most common skeletal manifestation of tuberculosis [60, 78]. Macroscopically, specific spondylodiscitis is characterized by necrotic bone with caseous masses and a narrowed disc space. An extension of the caseous necroses to the adjacent soft tissue may result in a long-segmental paravertebral gravity abscess, in certain circumstances even reaching as far as below the inguinal ligament. In a microscopic examination, it has to be distinguished between the exsudative and the productive form of tuberculous spondylodiscitis. In its exsudative form, the medullary space is completely necrotic, even though some trabecular structures may still be preserved. Destructed trabecula and tuberculous granulation tissue with inclusion of epithelioid cell granuloma and Langhans' giant cells, on the other hand, are typical of the productive form of tuberculous spondylodiscitis. The caseous necroses, mainly found in the ventral segments of the vertebral bodies, can even lead to a collapse of the affected vertebral bodies. Such a destruction results in the formation of an acute angled gibbus [17].

Therapy

Basic principles

Immobilization of the affected spine segments, antibiotic therapy, and, depending on the extent of the disease, debridement and/or decompression are basic requirements for a successful therapy leading to a complete recovery from spondylodiscitis. Immobilization can be achieved via conservative treatment or via surgical intervention. Pathogen-adapted intravenous antibiosis should preferably be started after the pathogen has been identified and a resistogram has been drawn up. If this is not possible because of a septic or highly acute course of the disease, intravenous antibiosis should be aimed at staphylococcus aureus or escherichia coli, the pathogens most common nowadays. A successful antibiotic therapy becomes manifest in a better general condition of the patient with reduced pain symptoms, reduced fever, and declining laboratory infection parameters. No standardized guidelines as to the duration of an intravenous antibiotic treatment are to be found in literature. As a general rule, it is advisable to administer antibiotics intravenously at least for two to four weeks because of better bioavailability. In individual cases parenteral can thus be switched to oral antibiotic therapy earlier, as soon as the patient's general condition has been reliably stabilized and the laboratory inflammation markers have gone back to normal or have at least significantly ameliorated. An oralization of the antibiotic treatment can also take place if bioavailability of the active ingredient is high even when taken enterally, as is e.g. the case with fluorchinolones, clindamycin, or linezolid. Linezolid is mainly used in cases of MRSA infection, although one should be aware of the haematopoetic side effects [47, 62, 74].

Neither are there any consistent recommendations to be found in literature concerning the overall duration of antibiotic therapy. With regards to the treatment of unspecific spondylodiscitis, an antibiotic application of six weeks to up to three months has been recommended [9, 11, 17, 34, 49, 60]. At all events, the length of time depends on the condition of the individual patient. If in doubt, especially high-risk patients (risks being e.g. immunosuppression, diabetes mellitus, drug abuse) should be treated longer. Our own method is to administer antibiotic therapy until inflammation parameters have been at normal range for six consecutive weeks.

If, however, on the basis of anamnestic, clinical, and radiological data a specific spondylodiscitis is suspected, an appropriate antituberculotic therapy should be initiated at once. But normally the course in these cases is not that fulminant, so that one can wait for the microbiological findings.

Especially with atypical mycobacteria chemotherapy poses a serious problem because of frequently occurring resistances [31, 52]. A definite therapy regime regarding chemotherapy of atypical mycobacteria has not established itself yet. The significance of in-vitro test runs seems questionable when compared to results obtained from in-vivo applications [36, 68]. If antituberculous chemotherapy is administered at all, it should be continued for at least 18–24 months to allow for complete healing and prevent a relapse – and even this cannot be backed up by definite, scientifically tenable data [12, 54]. The guidelines of the American Thoracic Society dating from 1997 recommend a combination therapy consisting of isoniacide, rifampicin, and ethambutol, with or without streptomycin or clarithromycin, for the treatment of pulmonary infections [3]. Ongoing studies evaluate macrolides and chinolones as therapy alternatives for the treatment of pulmonary infections caused by atypical mycobacteria [1, 25].

If a mycotic infection has been verified, an adequate antimycotic therapy must be initiated. In case of an infection e.g. caused by aspergillus spp., from the class of azoles, voriconazole is usually implemented as antimycoticum, or, alternatively, amphotericin B derivatives such as liposomal amphotericin B. In spondylodiscitis caused by candida spp., fluconazole is regarded as the preferred medication, unless c. glabrata or c. krusei have been identified as mycotic agents. The significance of recently emerging antimycotica from the class of echinocandins still remains to be clarified [40]. Spondylodiscitis caused by fungi can very well resemble tuberculous spondylodiscitis in MRI [40]. Overall, it is often difficult to identify the fungal agent responsible for spondylodiscitis, and antimycotic therapy meets with many problems. Therefore, Ooij et al. advocate surgical treatment at an early stage of the disease [64].

It goes without saying that sufficient analgesia of the sometimes quite pronounced pain symptoms must be an important part of the basic principles of therapy.

Conservative treatment

Conservative treatment can only be crowned by success if the above-named basic principles have been obeyed. Provided there is no absolute indication for surgical intervention, a conservative approach may be considered when clinical symptoms or bony destructions are only mildly present or the risk of surgical intervention seems too high [41, 73]. As patients suffering from this kind of disease tend to be older and in a less than good general condition, the option of conservative proceeding occurs rather often. The main problem conservative treatment raises, is how to sufficiently immobilize the affected spine segments. For the area reaching from the cervical spine to the middle part of the thoracic spine, a treatment via reclining brace can suffice. The orthesis forces the affected spine segments into a reclining position, thus distributing the weight to the unaffected facet joints and unburdening the infected, ventrally located area [17]. In this orthesis the patient can be fully mobilized. Even when the thoracolumbar or lumbar region is concerned and destruction is not too severe, mobilisation in a reclining brace can be considered [17]. Complete bed rest of at least 6-week duration in order to procure the necessary immobilization is mandatory, however, if the defects featured in the spine are substantial, or if the lower lumbar region or the lumbosacral junction is affected [11, 17]. In the absence of a surgery indication, Flamme et al. primarily recommend a conservative therapy of consistent immobilization of the patient in a reclining plaster shell for six weeks, followed by another six weeks of brace treatment. Through the plaster shell a kyphotic position and therefore fast pain relief can be achieved [20]. But especially with aged patients one has to bear in mind the well-known high co-morbidity of bed rest (deep vein thrombosis, pulmonary embolism, pneumonia, etc.). Only when the onset of osseous consolidation is already radiologically visible, mobilisation and back training of the patient under the guidance of a physical therapist are advised. Follow-up imaging should be performed every six weeks.

Apart from the risk of immobilization the rate of pseudarthrosis and instability, which can both ultimately result in a kyphotic malalignment and a chronic pain syndrome is comparatively high at 16–50% [11, 15, 17, 20, 21, 41]. It is not advisable to continue conservative therapy, if after four to six weeks of treatment there still has been no radiologically verifiable reactive bony fusion, or if destruction has progressed, or if clinical improvement has failed to appear [17, 41, 73]. Generally, it seems that the long-lasting bed rest that was practised in earlier years within the conservative therapy of spondylodiscitis has been abandoned. Our own method is to put the patient on bed rest until the discomfort has subsided, but usually no longer than for two weeks; after that, the patient is mobilized in an orthesis.

Within the context of conservative treatment, abscess formations needing decompression can be treated by CT-guided insertion of a drainage [17]. The drainage should remain in the abscess cavity for at least one week and be only removed after secretion has ceased and the resorption of the abscess has become visible in CT-imaging.

Surgical treatment

Emergency surgical intervention is required in spondylodiscitis at the occurrence of neurological deficits and sepsis. Further indications for surgery are instability, impending or already existing deformities, intraspinal space-occupying lesions, an unclear origin with a suspected tumor occurence, and unresponsiveness to conservative therapy. Relative indications for surgical treatment include uncontrollable pain symptoms and lack of patient compliance with conservative therapy [11, 17, 21, 49, 60]. Aims of surgical procedure are to remove the septic focus and to use the material for pathogen identification as well as to stabilize the infected spine segment, with subsequent bony fusion or a fusion of vertebrae. In comparison with conservative therapy, this approach allows for a safer and faster cure of the inflammation. Also, mobilisation is already possible shortly after surgery [15, 16, 41]. Furthermore, surgery provides an opportunity for decompression of the myelon or the cauda equina and correction of the sagittal spine profile. In 1906, Mueller made public the possibility of transperitoneal approach to spine exposure in tuberculous spondylodiscitis [61]. Five years later, Albee and Hibbs used the interlaminar fusion technique for tuberculous spine deformity [29]. Ito et al. published ten cases of tuberculous spondylodiscitis treated surgically by retroperitoneal approach to the lumbar spine in 1934 [33]. Since the mid-1950s, when Hodgson and Stock published their article on ventral debridement with interbody bone grafting for treating specific spondylodiscitis of the whole spine [30], this procedure became gold standard and remained so until the 1990s [15, 17]. As ventral spondylodesis with bone graft does not bring about primary stability, postsurgical therapy necessitates patient immobilisation for several weeks and consecutive brace treatment of several months duration as well, until firm bone union with the graft has been achieved [41]. Compared to conservative therapy, the fusion rate was thus increased to 90–100% [17, 41, 43]. Especially in cases of multisegmental infestation or longer fusion distances, however, complications such as pseudarthrosis and dislocation of the bone graft with consecutive kyphotic malposture have been described [17, 41]. Therefore, an instrumental stabilization in addition to debridement and graft interposition has established itself as standard procedure, having the advantage of speedy postsurgical mobilization of the patient and a lower risk of pseudarthrosis and kyphotic malposture [21, 41].

By no means indicated is a dorsal decompression via laminectomy without a simultaneously performed instrumentation, as this weakens the intact posterior portions of the affected spine segment, resulting in increased instability and a possible deterioration of the neurological situation [17, 21, 38, 60].

Implanting osteosynthesis material into an infected wound site holds the risk of a persisting infection event, as the metal surface may become colonized by pathogens. This danger can be minimized by extensive debridement with a simultaneous local application of antibiotics carriers. Adding to this, in a well-perfused wound area such as the area of vertebral body spongiosa happens to be, the risk of chronification is again lower [11]. Nowadays, mainly titanium implants are being used, as they do not seem to be associated with a higher relapse rate [46, 57, 63].

Recommendations regarding a surgical approach to spondylodiscitis are still discussed rather controversially [9, 11, 17, 21, 32, 41, 45, 46, 49, 60, 73]. The possibility of agreeing on standardized therapy guidelines is limited due

Table 19.5. Indications for surgery in spondylodiscitis.

- Neurological deficits
- Intraspinal space-occupying lesion
- Sepsis
- Abscess formation (without possibility of percutaneous drainage)
- Instability
- Deformity
- Unresponsiveness to conservative therapy
- Unclear diagnosis (presumed malignancy)

to inhomogeneity of the patient pool and therapeutic variance. Surgical therapy of spondylodiscitis can be performed as one-stage as well as two-stage procedure. If neurological deficits are present, an emergency decompression plus stabilization should be performed, because the prognosis of neurological symptomatology depends on swift surgical intervention [73]. In case of patients with no pathological neurological findings, a two-stage surgical procedure has the advantage of allowing the patient, usually in a reduced general condition anyway, to recover in the interval between surgical stages. The second stage follows one or two weeks after the first, depending on the patient's convalescence.

Recommendations as to the choice of osteosynthetic stabilization are equally diverse: advice for a purely dorsal stabilization can be found as easily as for a purely ventral, a combined dorso-ventral, or a combined ventro-dorsal stabilization [11, 15, 17, 21, 32, 41, 45, 46, 49, 60, 73]. The advantage of primary ventral instrumentation lies in the possibility of cleaning up the infected tissue and ventrally decompressing the spinal canal at the same time. For this, the same instruments are used as in tumor surgery or traumatology. The actual therapy recommendation varies according to the level at which spondylodiscitis has been localized.

Table 19.5 summarizes indications for surgery in spondylodiscitis.

Cervical spine

At cervical level, a purely ventral procedure is usually sufficient, combined with radical debridement and stabilization via bone chips taken from the iliac crest plus plate, or a fusion cage plus plate. For this, the cage is filled with autologous spongiosa. Fixed-angle plate systems are used as well, especially when more than one spine segment is infected [17, 60]. Bi- or polysegmental infestation may necessitate a dorsoventral stabilization [28]. Postoperatively, it is recommended that the patient wears a semi-rigid cervical collar for four to six weeks [28].

∎ Thoracic and lumbar spine

It has to be determined on a case-by-case basis whether to begin dorsally or ventrally, depending on the size of the septic focus.

On a thoracic level, a purely dorsal approach may be sufficient even if ventral destruction is pronounced, because the thoracic spine is additionally stabilized by the rib cage and its mobility is fairly restricted due to physiology [4, 27]. But a solely ventral instrumentation may be just as adequate as an exclusively dorsal stabilization. A thorough debridement down to the vital, well-perfused spongy area is of pivotal importance for a complete cure of the infection [17, 32, 41]. Ventral stabilization of the spine is achieved either by open transthoracic or open postero-lateral approach, or via thoracoscopy. Other than open surgery procedures, the latter is a video-assisted, minimally invasive technique in support of which reduced postoperative pain, better shoulder function, better postoperative lung function, earlier patient mobilization, lesser approach trauma, better cosmetic results, and shorter hospitalization time have been cited as advantageous [59]. By splitting the diaphragm, the incision used for thoracoscopy can be extended as far as L2 [59].

If a ventral approach has been decided on, a plate and a bone graft, or a cage and a plate are used for instrumentation. The cage can be filled with autologous spongiosa, depending on its type (Fig. 19.8). Normally, a tricortical iliac crest bone graft is used for interposition, but in multisegmental defects an autogenous fibula graft (Fig. 19.9) [55] or, especially on thoracic level, an autogenous rib graft can be used as well. In case of insufficient ventral stability, additional dorsal stabilisation should be performed [41].

On a thoracolumbar or lumbar level, if two-stage proceeding has been planned and no emergency ventral debridement is called for, it is advisable to perform dorsal stabilization first. In case of a merely slight ventral destruction, or sufficient stability provided by dorsal instrumentation and increased surgical risk, it might be better to suspend two-stage ventral instrumentation with bone graft interposition, as after stabilization and under antibiosis a spontaneous healing of the infection focus with re-osseointegration and fusion of vertebrae can occur in

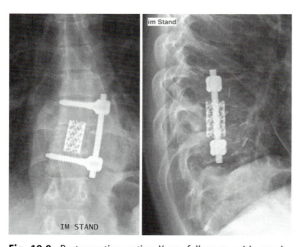

Fig. 19.8. Postoperative native X-ray follow-up with regular position of the hardware after purely anterior procedure with implantation of a cage and anterolateral single-rod system.

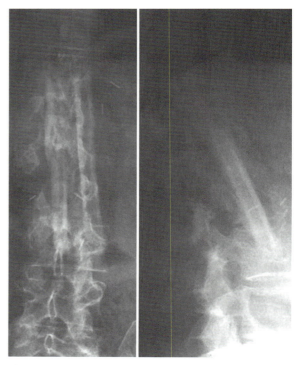

Fig. 19.9. Native X-ray follow-up after ventral interposition of an autogenous pedicled fibula graft and after removal of a fixateur externe.

postoperative course [21]. Likewise, in cases of monosegmental spondylodiscitis with only a minor presurgical kyphotic posture, a solitary ventral bone graft spondylodesis might be considered [6, 41]. By using ventral angle-stable implants, sufficient stabilisation can be achieved [15, 49]. Lee and Juh published a retrospective study on 18 spondylodiscitis patients with only slight bony destruction who were attended to by interposing an autologous iliac crest bone graft in PLIF (posterior lumbar interbody fusion) technique [45]. The advantage of a purely ventral or dorsal over a dorso-ventral proceeding lies in a lesser grade of invasivity and less loss of blood, although especially ventral instrumentation at lumbar spine levels or at the lumbosacral junction holds a higher risk of injuring the large abdominal or pelvic vessels that are often caked together due to inflammation [21]. In a prospective randomized study, Linhardt et al. compared clinical and radiological long-term results of ventro-dorsally versus solely ventrally instrumented thoracic and lumbar spodylodesis in a collective of 22 patients with spondylodiscitis [49]. For both methods, a fusion rate of 100% was ascertained; the mean sagittal loss of correction was 2° for ventro-dorsal fusion, 4° for a purely ventral fusion at thoracic level, and 3° for ventral fusion at lumbar level [49]. The analysis of self-evaluation forms (SF-36, Oswestry low-back pain disability questionnaire, visual pain scales) showed significantly better results of the purely ventral stabilization for the periods two years and 5.4 years after surgery [49]. Similar findings were reported by Eysel et al. who compared primary stable anterior instrumentation (n = 23) with dorso-ventral spondylodesis (n = 32). While both groups featured the same correction loss of 2.8°, the dorso-ventrally fused group showed a surgery duration 50% longer and blood loss 50% higher than the comparison group. Bony fusion was achieved in all patients [16]. In the lower lumbar spine region, with ventral instrumentation there is always the risk of arrosion of the abdominal aorta, the vena cava or the iliac vessels. Other known comorbidities of the ventral approach, apart from the danger of bleeding, are neurological complications, injury of inner organs, intestines and ureter, or cicatrisation [15, 16, 21].

Purely dorsal stabilization of the spine in its thoraco-lumbar and lumbar segments leads to a weight shifting from the ventral spine to the dorsally situated implant. In cases of larger substance defects or destructions due to infection, a bending load might develop that can result in a kyphosis and, in extreme cases, in material fatigue [13]. Leaving aside trauma, spondylodiscitis is considered one of the most frequent causes of kyphotic deformity demanding surgery. Especially under conservative therapy, severe kyphosis and gibbus formation can arise [17, 41]. A kyphotic malposition of the affected vertebral body segment can cause troubles and function loss, because too much weight is shifted to the adjacent spine segments or even further distant areas of the spine. Bearing that in mind, apart from acute therapy of spondylodiscitis, the avoidance of kyphotic malalignment via surgical stabilization of the spine must be another essential goal. Therefore, additional ventral stabilizing basically makes sense when larger ventral substance defects are involved, as a 360° fusion at thoraco-lumbar and lumbar level is the mechanically most stable form of instrumentation with the lowest risk of pseudarthrosis or kyphosis (Fig. 19.10) [11, 41, 46].

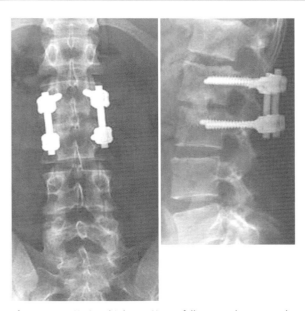

Fig. 19.10. Native biplanar X-ray follow-up three months after two-stage dorso-ventral spondylodesis at L2/3.

In a retrospective study, Lerner et al. evaluated the clinical and radiological results of single-stage dorso-ventral stabilization. The ventral substance defect had been bridged by bone graft interposition in 42 of the cases, by titanium cage in 20 cases. Segmental correction loss after cage insertion turned out to be significantly lower than after bone graft interposition (1° vs 4.1°). In all cases, bony fusion was achieved [46].

Isenberg et al. examined a collective of 37 spondylodiscitis patients in a critically reduced general condition. Therefore, they had to devise a special surgical procedure of short-term duration and with as little blood loss as possible, making allowances for the circulation and ventilation problems caused by sepsis. Was the destruction multisegmental, they first performed a spinal decompression from dorsal, using a fixateur interne for further stabilization. This was then followed by a single-stage ventral debridement and a replenishing of the defect with gentamycin-PMMA chains. Ventral surgery was repeated one or two times ("second look") until macroscopic consolidation and sterility were reached, and completed by a ventrally instrumented spondylodesis [32]. If destruction was monosegmental, the approach was similar, but dorsal surgery was abstained from [32].

Prognosis

Spondylodiscitis can become life-threatening, because it primarily affects older patients in reduced general condition or with risk factors mentioned above. Mean hospital stay has been reported to be 30–49 days, hospital lethality 2–17% [9, 21, 32, 49, 73, 83]. With our own patients we have experienced a mean hospital stay of four weeks with a hospital lethality of 2%.

There often remain residual ailments after conservative therapy as well as after surgical therapy of spondylodiscitis, due to remaining destructions and degenerative concomitants in the adjacent segments after inflammation abated. In a retrospective study, Woertgen et al. researched neurological results and quality of life (SF-36) in 62 spondylodiscitis patients after 16.4 months, 45% of whom had been treated conservatively, 55% surgically. They were able to show that in patients with presurgical neurological deficits, motor deficits persisted in 30%, hypoesthesia in 90%. Furthermore they succeeded in demonstrating that quality of life for those patients is far lower compared to a normal population. Surgically treated patients stated a slightly higher quality of life and a significantly higher level of patient satisfaction [83]. Lerner et al. found in 76% of the 25 spondylodiscitis

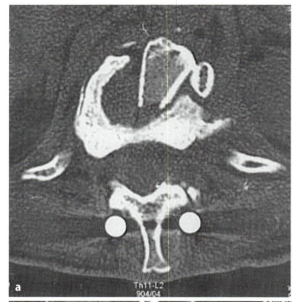

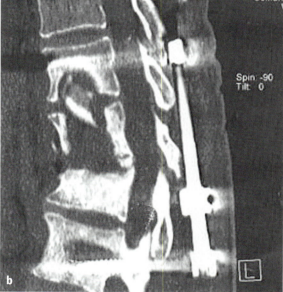

Fig. 19.11 a, b. Axial (**a**) and sagittal (**b**) CT-scans of relapse spondylodiscitis one year after dorso-ventral fusion.

patients with neurological deficits they examined an improvement of their neurological situation after 2.6 years, while 20% showed no change whatsoever. In 75% of patients with acute paraplegia, walking ability could be restored [46]. Similar results can be found in other published studies [21, 28, 45]. Overall, a relapse of spondylodiscitis is unlikely to occur (Fig. 19.11 a, b). In literature, a relapse rate of 0–7% has been recorded [15, 21, 28, 41, 46, 49,

59]. Frangen et al. found five patients with respondylodiscitis in their collective (n = 78) in follow-up examinations after a mean of 5.4 years. Regarding the preceding surgical strategy, the following distribution appeared: two patients had undergone ventral fusion, one ventro-dorsal, one dorsal; one patient had been treated by soft-tissue debridement only [21].

Conclusions for practise

- In cases of non-specific back pain and general illness symptoms, the possibility of spondylodiscitis must be considered.
- MRI is the diagnostic means of first choice for detecting spondylodiscitis. To be able to distinguish between the onset of spondylodiscitis and degenerative changes at the endplates of the vertebral bodies, F-18 FDG-PET can serve as a useful complement.
- Because of exactly monitored conservative therapy via control MRI and primary stable surgical techniques, long-lasting patient immobilisation is no longer necessary today.

References

1. Alangaden GJ, Lerner SA (1997) The clinical use of fluoroquinolones for the treatment of mycobacterial diseases. Clin Infect Dis 25:1213–1221
2. Al-Muhim FA, Ibrahim EM, el Hassan AY (1995) Magnetic resonance imaging of tuberculous spondylitis. Spine 20:2287–2292
3. American Thoracic Society (1997) Diagnosis and treatment of disease caused by nontuberculous mycobacteria. Am J Respir Crit Care Med 156:1–25
4. An HS, Singh K, Vaccaro AR, Wang G, Yoshida H, Eck J, McGrady L, Lim TH (2004) Biomechanical evaluation of contemporary posterior spinal internal fixation configurations in an unstable burst-fracture calf spine model. Spine 29:257–262
5. Arasteh KN, Cordes C, Ewers M (2000) HIV related NTM infection: incidence, survival analysis and associated risk factors. Eur J Med Res 5:424–430
6. Aurich M, Anders J, Wagner A, Bleek J, Wittner B, Holz U (2005) Spondylodiscitis – ventrale oder ventrodorsale Spondylodese? Akt Traumatol 35:274–279
7. Bachmeyer C, Blum L, Stelianides S, Benchaa B, Gruat N, Danne O (2001) Mycobacterium xenopi pulmonary infection in a HIV infected patient under highly active antiretroviral treatment. Thorax 56:978–979
8. Bahloul K, Ghorbel M, Boudouara MZ, Ben Mansour H (2006) Primary vertebral echinococcosis: four case reports and review of literature. Br J Neurosurg 20:320–323
9. Butler JS, Shelly MJ, Timlin M, Powderly WG, O'Byrne JM (2006) Nontuberculous pyogenic spinal infection in adults: a 12-year experience from a tertiary referral centre. Spine 31:2695–2700
10. Chang MC, Wu HTH, Lee CH, Liu CL, Chen TH (2006) Tuberculous spondylitis and pyogenic spondylitis: comparative magnetic resonance imaging features. Spine 31:782–788
11. Cramer J, Haase N, Behre I, Ostermann PAW (2003) Spondylitis und Spondylodiscitis. Trauma und Berufskrankheit 5:336–341
12. Danesh-Clough T, Theis JC, Linden A (2000) Mycobacterium xenopi infection of the spine. Spine 25:626–628
13. Delarmatar RB, Sherman J, Carr JB (1995) Pathophysiology of spinal cord injury. Recovery after immediate and delayed decompression. J Bone Joint Surg 77-A:1042–1049
14. Eismont FJ, Bohlman HH, Soni PL, Goldberg VM, Freehafer AA (1983) Pyogenic and fungal vertebral osteomyelitis with paralysis. J Bone Joint Surg 65-A:19–29
15. Eysel P, Hopf C, Meurer A (1994) Korrektur und Stabilisierung der infektbedingten Wirbelsäulendeformität. Orthop Praxis 11:696–703
16. Eysel P, Hopf C, Vogel I, Rompe JD (1997) Primary stable anterior instrumentation or dorsoventral spondylodesis in spondylodiscitis? Results of a comparative study. Eur Spine J 6:152–157
17. Eysel P, Peters KM (1997) Spondylodiscitis. In: Peters KM, Klosterhalfen B (eds) Bakterielle Infektionen der Knochen und Gelenke. Enke, Stuttgart, S 52–93
18. Felix SC, Mitchell JK (2001) Diagnostic yield of CT-guided percutaneous aspiration procedures in suspected spontaneous infectious discitis. Radiology 218:211–214
19. Flamme CH, Frischalowski T, Gossé F (2000) Möglichkeiten und Grenzen der konservativen Therapie bei Spondylitis und Spondylodiscitis. Z Rheumatol 59:233–239
20. Flamme CH, Lazoviae D, Gossé F, Rühmann O (2001) MRT bei Spondylitis und Spondylodiscitis. Orthopäde 30:514–518
21. Frangen TM, Kälicke T, Gottwald M, Andereya S, Andress HJ, Russe OJ, Müller EJ, Muhr G, Schinkel C (2006) Die operative Therapie der Spondylodiscitis. Eine Analyse von 78 Patienten. Unfallchirurg 109:743–753

22. Frazier DD, Campbell DR, Garvey TA, Wiesel S, Bohlman HH, Eismont FJ (2001) Fungal infections of the spine. J Bone Joint Surg 83-A:560–565
23. Gelfand MS, Cleveland KO (2004) Vancomycin therapy and the progression of Methicillin-resistant staphylococcus aureus vertebral osteomyelitis. South Med J 97:593–597
24. Glaser C, Matzko M, Reiser M (2000) Chronische Infektionen des Skelettsystems. Radiologe 40:547–556
25. Griffith DE, Wallace RJ (1996) New developments in the treatment of nontuberculous mycobacterial disease. Semin Respir Infect 11:301–310
26. Hadjipavlou AG, Mader JT, Necessary JT, Muffoletto AJ (2000) Hematogenous pyogenic spinal infections and their surgical management. Spine 25:1668–1679
27. Hazelrigg SR, Cetindag IB, Fullerton J (2002) Acute and chronic pain syndroms after thoracic surgery. Surg Clin North Am 82:849–865
28. Heyde CE, Boehm H, El Saghir H, Tschöke SK, Kayser R (2006) Surgical treatment of spondylodiscitis in the cervical spine: a minimum 2-year follow-up. Eur Spine J 15:1380–1387
29. Hibbs RH (1911) An operation for progressive spinal deformation. NY State J Med 93:1013
30. Hodgson AR, Stock FE (2006) The Classic: Anterior spinal fusion: a preliminary communication on the radical treatment of Pott's disease and Pott's paraplegia. 1956. Clin Orthop 444:10–15
31. Hoffner SE (1994) Pulmonary infections caused by less frequently encountered slow-growing environmental mycobacteria. Eur J Clin Microbiol Infect Dis 13:937–941
32. Isenberg J, Jubel A, Hahn U, Seifert H, Prokop A (2005) Die mehrzeitige Spondylodese: Behandlungskonzept der destruierenden Spondylodiscitis bei kritisch reduziertem Allgemeinzustand. Orthopäde 34:159–166
33. Ito H, Tsuchiya J, Asami D (1934) A new radical operation for Pott's disease – report of ten cases. J Bone Joint Surg 16:499
34. Jensen AG, Espersen F, Skinhoj P, Frimodt-Moller N (1998) Bacteremic staphylococcus aureus spondylitis. Arch Intern Med 158:509–517
35. Jensen AG, Espersen F, Skinhoj P, Rosdahl VT, Frimodt-Moller N (1997) Increasing frequency of vertebral osteomyelitis following staphylococcus aureus bacteraemia in Denmark 1980–1990. J Infect 34:113–118
36. Juffermans NP, Verbon A, Danner SA, Kuijper EJ, Speelman P (1998) Mycobacterium xenopi in HIV-infected patients: an emerging pathogen. AIDS 12:1661–1666
37. Karabouta Z, Bisbinas I, Davidson A, Goldsworthy LL (2005) Discitis in toddlers: a case series and review. Acta Paediatr 94:1516–1518
38. Kastert J (1969) Knochen- und Gelenktuberkulose. Chirurg 40:533–536
39. Kayser R, Mahlfeld K, Greulich M, Grasshoff H (2005) Spondylodiscitis in childhood: results of a long-term study. Spine 3:318–323
40. Kim CW, Perry A, Currier B, Yaszemski M, Garfin S (2006) Fungal infections of the spine. Clin Orthop 444:92–99
41. Klöckner C, Valencia R, Weber U (2001) Die Einstellung des sagittalen Profils nach operative Therapie der unspezifischen destruierenden Spondylodiscitis: ventrales oder ventrodorsales Vorgehen – ein Ergebnisvergleich. Orthopäde 30:965–967
42. Krämer J (2006) Lumbalsyndrom, Wundinfektion, Spondylodiscitis. In: Krämer J, Hasenbring M, Theodoridis T, Wilke HJ (eds) Bandscheibenbedingte Erkrankungen. Thieme, Stuttgart, S 273
43. Krödel A, Stürz H (1989) Differenzierte operative versus konservative Therapie der Spondylitis und Spondylodiscitis. Z Orthop 127:587–596
44. Kulasegaram R, Richardson D, MacRae B, Ruiter A (2001) Mycobacterium xenopi osteomyelitis in a patient on highly active antiretroviral therapy (HAART). International Journal of STD & AIDS 12:404–406
45. Lee JS, Suh KT (2006) Posterior lumbar interbody fusion with an autogenous iliac crest bone graft in the treatment of pyogenic spondylodiscitis. J Bone Joint Surg 88-B:765–770
46. Lerner T, Hackenberg L, Rösler S, Joosten U, Halm H, Liljenqvist U (2005) Operative Therapie der unspezifischen und spezifischen Spondylodiscitis. Z Orthop 143:204–212
47. Lew DP, Waldvogel FA (2004) Osteomyelitis. Lancet 364:369–379
48. Lindholm TS, Pylkkänen P (1982) Discitis following removal of intravertebral disc. Spine 7:618–622
49. Linhardt O, Matussek J, Refior HJ, Krödel A (2007) Long-term results of ventro-dorsal versus ventral instrumentation fusion in the treatment of spondylitis. Int Orthop 31:113–119
50. Maiuri F, Iaconetta G, Gallicchio B, Manto A, Briganti F (1997) Spondylodiscitis: clinical and magnetic resonance diagnosis. Spine 22:1741–1746
51. Malawski SK, Lukawski S (1991) Pyogenic infection of the spine. Clin Orthop 272:58–66
52. Manfredi R, Nanetti A, Morelli S, Ferri M, Valentini R, Calza L, Chiodo F (2004) A decade surveillance study of mycobacterium xenopi and antimicrobial susceptability levels in a reference teaching hospital of northern italy: HIV-associated versus non-HIV-associated infection. HIV Clin Trials 5:206–215
53. McLean DR, Rusell N, Khan MY (1992) Neurobrucellosis: Clinical and therapeutic features. Clin Infect Dis 15:582–590

54. Meybeck A, Fortin C, Abgrall S, Adle-Biassette H, Hayem G, Ruimy R, Yeni P (2005) Spondylitis due to mycobacterium xenopi in a human immunodeficiency virus type 1-infected patient: case report and review of the literature. J Clin Microbiol 43:1465–1466
55. Michael JWP, Brunkwall J, Fätkenheuer G, Seifert H, Winnekendonk G, Zöller JE, Eysel P (2007) Ein gefäßgestieltes gedoppeltes Fibulatransplantat zur Behandlung der lumbalen Instabilität nach tuberkulöser Spondylodiscitis. Unfallchirurg 110: 86–88
56. Modic MT, Feiglin DH, Piraino DW, Boumphrew F, Weinstein MA, Buchesneau PM, Rehm S (1985) Vertebral osteomyelitis. Assessment using MR. Radiology 157:157–166
57. Moon M, Woo Y, Lee K, Ha K, Kim S, Sun D (1995) Posterior instrumentation and anterior interbody fusion for tuberculous kyphosis of dorsal and lumbar spines. Spine 20:1910–1916
58. Moon MS (1997) Tuberculosis of the spine: controversies and a new challenge. Spine 22:1791–1797
59. Mückley T, Schütz T, Schmidt MH, Potulski M, Bühren V, Beisse R (2004) The role of thoracoscopic spinal surgery in the management of pyogenic vertebral osteomyelitis. Spine 29:227–233
60. Müller EJ, Russe OJ, Muhr G (2004) Osteomyelitis der Wirbelsäule. Orthopäde 33:305–315
61. Müller W (1906) Transperitoneale Freilegung der Wirbelsäule bei tuberkulöser Spondylitis. Deutsche Ztschr S Chir 85:128
62. Nolla JM, Ariza J, Gomez-Vaquero C, Fiter J, Bermejo J, Valverde J, Escofet DR, Gudiol F (2002) Spontaneous pyogenic vertebral osteomyelitis in nondrug users. Semin Arthritis Rheum 31:271–278
63. Oga M, Arizono T, Takasita M, Sugioka Y (1993) Evaluation of the risk of instrumentation as a foreign body in spinal tuberculosis. Spine 18:1890–1894
64. Ooij A, Beckers JM, Herpers MJ, Walenkamp GH (2000) Surgical treatment of aspergillus spondylodiscitis. Eur Spine J 9:75–79
65. Osti OL, Frazer RD, Roberts B, Vernon-Roberts B (1990) Discitis after discography. The role of prophylactic antibiotics. J Bone Joint Surg 72-B:271–274
66. Peronne C, Saba J, Behlouhl D, Salmon-Ceron D, Leprot C, Wilde JL, Kahn MF (1994) Pyogenic and tuberculous spondylodiscitis (vertebral osteomyelitis) in 80 adult patients. Clin Infect Dis 19:746–750
67. Pina MA, Modrego PJ, Uroz JJ, Cobeta JC, Lerin FJ (2000) Brucellar spinal epidural abscess of cervical location: report of four cases. Eur Neurol 45:249–253
68. Research Committee of the British Thoracic Society (2001) First randomised trial of treatments for pulmonary disease caused by M. avium intracellulare, M. malmoense, and M. xenopi in HIV negative patients: rifampicin, ethambutol, and isoniazid versus rifampicin and ethambutol. Thorax 56:167–172
69. Ridley N, Shaikh MI, Remedios D (1998) Radiology of skeletal tuberculosis. Orthopaedics 21: 1213–1220
70. Risse JH, Grünwald F, Gassel F, Biersack HJ, Schmitt O (2001) Fluorine-18 fluorodeoxyglucose positron emission tomography findings in spondylodiscitis: preliminary results. Eur Spine J 10: 534–539
71. Ruffer MA (1918) Arthritis deformans and spondylitis in ancient Egypt. J Pathol Bacteriol 22: 212–226
72. Sapico FL, Montgomerie JZ (1990) Vertebral Osteomyelitis. Infect Dis Clin North Am 4:539–550
73. Schinkel C, Gottwald M, Andress HJ (2003) Surgical treatment of spondylodiscitis. Surgical Infections 4:387–391
74. Shuford JA, Steckelberg JM (2003) Role of oral antimicrobial therapy in the management of osteomyelitis. Curr Opin Infect Dis 16:515–519
75. Stäbler A, Baur A, Kruger A, Weiss M, Helmberger T, Reiser M (1998) Differentialdiagnose der erosiven Osteochondrose und bakteriellen Spondylitis in der Magnetresonanztomographie. Fortschr Röntgenstr 168:421–428
76. Stäbler A, Reiser MF (2001) Imaging of spinal infection. Radiol Clin North Am 39:115–135
77. Stumpe KDM, Zanetti M, Weishaupt D, Hodler J, Boos N, von Schulthess GK (2002) FDG positron emission tomography for differentiation of degenerative and infectious endplate abnormalities in the lumbar spine detected on MR imaging. AJR 179:1151–1157
78. Tuli SM (2002) General principles of osteoarticular tuberculosis. Clin Orthop 398:11–19
79. Wiley AM, Trueta J (1959) The vascular anatomy of the spine and its relationship to pyogenic vertebral osteomyelitis. J Bone Joint Surg 41-B:796–809
80. Wilkström M, Vogel J, Rilinger N (1997) Die infektiöse Spondylitis. Radiologe 37:139–144
81. William RL, Fukui MB, Meltzer CC, Swarnkar A, Johnson DW, Welch W (1999) Fungal spinal osteomyelitis in the immunocompromised patient: MR findings in three cases. Am J Neuroradiol 20:381–385
82. Willis TA (1949) Nutrient arteries of the vertebral bodies. J Bone Joint Surg 31-A:538–540
83. Woertgen C, Rothoerl RD, Englert C, Neumann C (2006) Pyogenic spinal infections according to the 36-Item Short Form Health Survey. J Neurosurg Spine 4:441–446

Non-fusion technology

20 Biomechanical characteristics of different non-fusion implants

Hans-Joachim Wilke

Introduction

In the 1980s and 1990s spinal surgery often had the goal to fuse motion segments in order to treat different spinal pathologies, such as fractures, instabilities or degeneration. Although the outcome of these surgical interventions was quite good in many cases it was found that degeneration in the adjacent segments could occur [11, 23]. It is still not proven [21] but it was quickly hypothesized that the fusion is responsible for this "adjacent level syndrome" because the stiff region in the spine leads to an overload in their segments above and below [4].

Therefore non-fusion technologies in spinal surgery gain more and more popularity [12]. Constantly new ideas are created and turned into new products. Each idea has its own philosophy with the principle goal to maintain the motion in the treated segment and to preserve as many spinal structures as possible. Furthermore, the implants shall restore and maintain the disc height and/or original mobility. Some of these changes result from the injury or the degeneration but some of them result from the surgical intervention, e.g. from the decompression or from the nucleotomy, or from the removal of the facet joints.

These non-fusion technologies can be divided in posterior or anterior devices. The posterior devices either unload or replace the facet joints or stabilize the treated segments but preserve the discs. Some of the most important representatives are flexible stabilisation systems like the dynamic fixator Dynesys, interspinous implants, which are just placed between the spinous processes, or implants to replace just facet joints or the entire posterior complex. The anterior technologies are total disc prostheses or nucleus replacement devices.

Different representatives of these implants have been tested in own in-vitro experiments to determine their biomechanical characteristics. The most important results will be summarized in this article. Details about these studies can be read in original publications, which are already published or in preparation.

Methods of the performed in-vitro tests

All tests were performed at room temperature in our specially designed spine tester [28] with at least six human cadaver spine specimens per experiment or per implant. Until testing the specimens were kept frozen in triple sealed plastic bags at $-20°C$. Before testing they were thawed at $6°C$ and all soft tissue was dissected, keeping the capsules, ligaments and supporting structures intact. For the fixation in the spine tester the most cranial and caudal vertebrae were embedded in PMMA cement (Technovit 3040, Heraeus Kulzer, Wehrheim/Ts, Germany) in such manner, that the middle disc was oriented in the horizontal plane.

For testing the specimens were always fixed rigidly with the caudal end to the loading frame of the spine tester and the cranial flange was mounted to a gimbal, which allowed rotation around all three coordinate axes as well as vertical translation. A travelling gantry and a second slide enabled translation in the remaining two planes. The specimens were loaded with pure moments of ± 7.5 Nm or ± 10 Nm (experiment with Dynesys) but without preload in all the three principal motion planes flexion-extension, left-right lateral bending, left-right axial rotation, respecting internationally accepted recommendations for in-vitro testing of spinal implants [32].

The moments were applied continuously in a quasi-static manner so that one cycle lasted

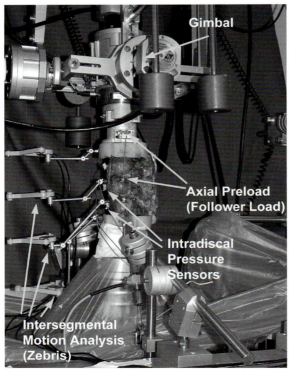

Fig. 20.1. For in-vitro testing the specimens are fixed in a spine tester and motion and intradiscal pressure can be measured.

about 20 seconds. The specimens were allowed to move unconstrained in the five uncontrolled degrees of freedom. During loading the motion of the segments was recorded by a three-dimensional ultra sound based motion analysis system (Zebris, WinBioMechanics v.1.2, Isny, Germany) and range of motion (ROM) and neutral zone (NZ) for the segments of interest and sometimes the adjacent segments were evaluated (Fig. 20.1). In some studies also the intradiscal pressure was continuously measured to estimate the load sharing between discs and implants. For each test three loading cycles were applied to precondition the specimens and the third was evaluated.

Generally, the tests were started with the intact specimens to create a base line. Then the tests were repeated with defined defects that should simulate injuries or degenerations or a specific clinical scenario. Finally the postoperative stability was determined after implantation.

Dynamic stabilization system (Dynesys) versus rigid fixators

Internal fixators are generally used as adjunct to fusion, where in many instances the disc is replaced by either intervertebral cages, allografts or autologous bone grafts. From the clinical point of view, to sacrifice a moderately degenerated disc and – in case of the use of autologous bone graft – donor site morbidity may not be desirable. Only few surgeons use the internal fixator and at the same time try to preserve the disc [22] because this may lead to a possible fatigue failure of the implant system [7, 13] when a bony fusion cannot be achieved with the internal fixator. This problem may be overcome with dynamic fixators, which connect the screws with flexible longitudinal elements instead of rigid rods.

The Dynesys Spinal System (Zimmer Spine, Warsaw, IN, USA) is indicated to provide spinal alignment and dynamic re-stabilization in skeletally mature patients up to five contiguous levels from L1–S1 while preserving the disc as well as the facet joints (dynamic neutralisation). The selection criterions for the procedure include patients with neurogenic pain, radicular pain and/or chronic low back pain resistant to conservative treatment, presenting some form of instability, where stabilization is judged beneficial [5].

The system is composed of pedicle screws, PET cords and PCU spacers. The spacers are placed bilaterally between the pedicle screw heads to withstand compressive loads. The cords are running through the hollow core of the spacers and stabilize the construct by a tensile preload.

The aim of this in-vitro study was to compare the stabilizing effect with the dynamic stabilization system and an internal fixator. This study was performed with six L2–5 lumbar spines with an age range from 33 to 59 years and a mean age of 43 years. The specimens were destabilized in the L3–4 segment by dissection of the lig. supraspinous, lig. interspinous, lig. flavum, tenotomy of facet joint capsules and a nucleotomy. Afterwards this segment was stabilized with the Dynesys system and an internal fixator, respectively.

Important to note is, that the temperature dependency of the polymeric spacers of the Dynesys system may influence the results. There-

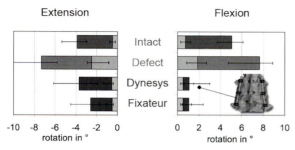

Fig. 20.2. Range of motion (entire bars) and neutral zone (light part of the bars) in flexion and extension of the Dynesys and an internal fixator in comparison to intact and defect states (for further details please read [24, 25]).

fore the manufacturer made these spacers for this experiment with another material, which had the same stiffness at room temperature (21 °C) as at body temperature (37 °C).

The chosen defect strongly destabilized the segment and could be stabilized again with both implants in most directions [24, 25] (Fig. 20.2). The Dynesys stabilized the spine significantly but was more flexible than the internal fixator, most pronounced in extension. In flexion, however, the Dynesys provided the same stiffness as the internal fixator, because both implants act as a tension band posteriorly of the spine. Similarly, in lateral bending the Dynesys led to a stiffer situation than may be expected. In contrast, in axial rotation there was a big difference between the implants. The internal fixator was able to restrict the range of motion, which was even below values of the intact spine, whereas the Dynesys still allowed larger motions, i.e. it was not able to restore normal values, probably because it unlocks the facet joints. The stability in this direction was found in another study to be a function of the spacer length [16].

Overall our results suggest that the Dynesys provides substantial stability in case of degenerative spinal pathologies and may therefore rather be considered as an alternative to fusion for these indications, while the motion segment is preserved.

Interspinous implants (X-Stop, Coflex, Wallis, Diam)

Interspinous implants are used for motion-preserving stabilization of primarily posterior lumbar spinal pathologies like spinal stenosis or facet joint arthritis. The goal is to unload the facet joints, to restore foraminal height and to provide sufficient stability especially in extension whilst still allowing motion in the treated segment.

This technology is still in an early stage of development and the indications are not yet clearly defined because scientific evidence is lacking [3, 27]. However, there are already several interspinous implants on the market today.

The purpose of this biomechanical in-vitro study was to investigate the segmental stability and intradiscal pressure achieved with the following various types of such implants: Coflex, Wallis, Diam, and X-Stop (Fig. 20.3).

For this study the different implants could not be tested in the same specimens. Therefore 24 human lumbar spine specimens were divided into four equal groups. Again the specimens were first tested in the intact state before a defect was created, which was a bilateral hemifacetectomy and the resection of flaval ligaments. Then they were again tested directly after implantation.

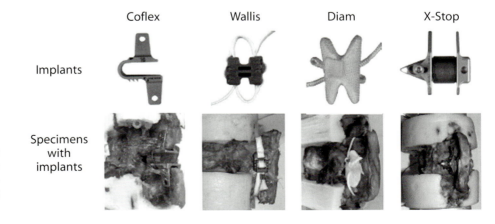

Fig. 20.3. Interspinous implants and their recommended implantation (for further details please read [6]).

The Coflex implant (Paradigm Spine, New York, NY, USA) is a "U" shaped interspinous spacer with lateral wings. These wings are crimped to the spinous processes to secure the implant in place. Additionally to the defect the interspinous and supraspinous ligament had to be resected in our study.

The Wallis implant (Abbott Laboratories, Abbott Park, IL, USA) is an interspinous spacer, which is composed of polyetheretherketone. Additionally to the defect the interspinous and supraspinous ligaments were transected. The implant was secured in place with two ligatures. They were wrapped around the two adjacent spinous processes. After implantation the supraspinous ligament was refixed in place with stitches.

The Diam implant (Medtronic Sofamor Danek, Minneapolis, MN, USA) is a silicone interspinous spacer, which is covered by a polyethylene coat. Two ligatures secure it in place. For this implant only the interspinous space had to be prepared while the supraspinous ligament could be left untouched.

The X-Stop implant (St. Francis Medical Technologies, Alameda, CA, USA) is an oval titanium interspinous implant, which is – similary to the Coflex – secured in place with two lateral wings. However, these wings are not crimped to the spinous processes. In order to implant the X-Stop, the interspinous ligament had to be pierced only.

In each implant-group the defect caused an increase in range of motion by about 8% in lateral bending to 18% in axial rotation [6]. Coflex, Wallis, Diam, and X-Stop led to a similar effect. They all compensated the destabilizing effect in extension and allowed about 50% of the range of motion of the intact state. In all other planes and especially in lateral bending and axial rotation the values of the range of motion were pretty much equal to the values of the defect state. The intradiscal pressure after implantation was similar to that of the intact specimens in flexion, lateral bending and axial rotation but much smaller during extension.

In conclusion, Coflex, Wallis, Diam and X-Stop had a similar effect on the three-dimensional flexibility of the treated segments: they significantly stabilized in extension, but had almost no effect in flexion, lateral bending and axial rotation.

Total posterior-element replacement system (TOPS)

The posterior systems are of interest because in a spinal segment not only the disc but also the facet joints may degenerate independently from each other.

The TOPS system, a mobile spinal implant for total posterior arthroplasty, addresses a range of posterior pathologies including facet joint arthrosis, spinal stenosis, and spondylolisthesis.

The TOPS device is a unitary implant comprised of two titanium plates with an interlocking flexible articulating core, surrounded by a polyurethane elastomer cover; its metal arms connect horizontally to the pedicles via four polyaxial pedicle screws [31]. The device is implanted after decompression by removal of the lamina and the medial facets, and provides mobility in flexion, extension, and lateral bending while stabilizing in axial rotation and shear directions.

In this in-vitro study, TOPS implants were available in two heights, normal and low profile. They are designed to bridge the segment L4–5, because that level will be probably the most common level where this implant will be applied.

The aim of this study was to investigate whether the TOPS implant is suitable for posterior stabilization of the lumbar spine and whether the implant is capable of restoring the physiological motion of the intact segment. Additionally the characteristics of stability with the TOPS implant during axial rotation in different flexion/extension angle positions were analyzed.

Six human cadaver specimens (L3–S1) (median age 61 years, range 47 to 74 years) were used for this in-vitro experiment. Before implantation at the level L4–5 a laminectomy (including facetectomy of the descending facets) at L4 was performed.

This defect increased significantly the range of motion in all directions, in flexion/extension from 8.1° to 12.1°, in lateral bending right plus left from 7.6° to 8.5°, and in axial rotation right plus left from 3.6° to 8.5°. After implantation of TOPS the range of motion was reduced to 6.8°, 7.8°, and 3.8°, respectively. In a flexed posture, axial rotation was slightly increased compared to the neutral position (Fig. 20.4). With increas-

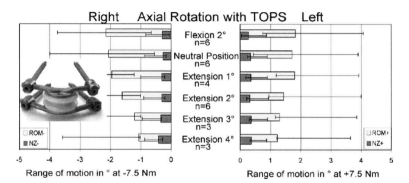

Fig. 20.4. Median and ranges for the range of motion (ROM) and neutral zone (NZ) in axial rotation with different flexion/extension angles in the instrumented segment L4–5 with the TOPS implant (for further details please read [31]).

ing extension, axial rotation decreased linearly from 3.7° in neutral position to 2.3° in 4° extension in the segment L4–5. The characteristic of the intradiscal pressure with the implant was similar to that of the intact specimen.

Overall, the TOPS implant almost ideally restored range of motion in lateral bending and axial rotation compared to the intact specimen. In the sagittal plane 85% of the initial range of motion could be obtained. The range of motion in axial rotation as a function of the flexion and extension angle also mimics the biomechanical behavior of the posterior complex of the lumbar spine. This relationship between range of motion and posture, however, emphasizes the importance of a proper implantation.

Total disc prostheses

The current concept of total disc prosthesis reminds at the first glance of replacement system in other joints. They consist of two endplates mostly made of metal with direct contact to the cranial and caudal vertebrae [2]. They either articulate directly with each other or have a swimming inlay, often made of polyethylene, in between. The influence of the prosthesis design on the segmental biomechanics after total disc replacement (TDR) is still unclear. The two main design philosophies of TDR can be summarized with unconstrained and constrained implant types. In both types the center of rotation seems to be of special interest. As TDR results also in a distraction of the ligamentous structures, the resulting height of the disc space theoretically has also an influence on segmental motion.

The purpose of this study was to evaluate the influence of different design philosophies and

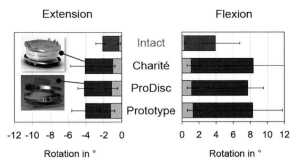

Fig. 20.5. Range of motion (entire bars) and neutral zone (light part of the bars) in flexion and extension of different disc prostheses in comparison to the intact state (n=6, level of implantation: L3–4).

the prosthesis height on the biomechanics of the treated segment. We compared the unconstrained Charité TDR (DePuy Spine, Raynham, MA, USA), the constrained ProDisc TDR (Synthes, Solothurn, CH) and a constrained TDR prototype with a more posteriorly located center of rotation compared to the ProDisc. All prostheses were implanted at the level L3–4 in lumbar spine specimens L2–5. Since some manufacturers recommend maintaining the posterior longitudinal ligament and others rather suggest sacrificing it, this effect was also investigated.

All types of prosthesis resulted in a significant increase of segmental lordosis compared with the intact status. Furthermore, implantation of disc prosthesis increased the range of motion (Fig. 20.5). The resection of the posterior longitudinal ligament even increased this effect. In flexion/extension this almost doubled the flexibility in the treated segment with respect to the intact state; changes in rotation were even more pronounced. The smallest increase was found for lateral bending. The axial rotation with the unconstrained implants (Charité) was higher than for the two constrained ones. In flexion/extension and lateral bending the differences were not significant between the three implants tested. These changes, however, can be influenced by the implant height. The higher interface (12 mm) led to more stability than the lower interface (10 mm).

Overall, it can be summarized that an unconstrained prosthesis increases the segmental lordosis more than a constrained TDR. Resection of the posterior longitudinal ligament further aggravates this increase, however, this effect can be avoided by using a higher implant. The prosthesis height seems more crucial than the preservation of the posterior longitudinal ligament in terms of stability. The location of the center of rotation in a constrained prosthesis did not alter the magnitude of range of motion. However, this cannot be extrapolated to a change in position, which probably has a strong influence.

Prosthetic disc nucleus (PDN)

Alternatively to a total disc replacement nucleus implants may be used [19]. One advantage of such a concept is the preservation of the existing anatomical structures, which include the annulus, the endplates of the vertebral bodies and the ligaments, presuming that they show only slight signs of degeneration. In theory, besides maintaining the mobility, a nucleus replacement has the potential to re-establish the intact disc height and thereby restoring the nominal stresses and strains of the collagen fibres in the annulus. Such a nucleus replacement, which provides probably most clinical data, is the prosthetic disc nucleus device PDN.

The PDN (Raymedica, Minneapolis, MN, USA) is composed of a structural polymeric hydrophilic hydrogel that is constrained in a woven polyethylene fabric jacket. The hydrogel component is a block co-polymer of polyacrylamide-polyacrylonitrile. The jacket is a maximally dense woven circular tube fabricated from a highly orientated polyethylene fiber. The weave is made from bundles of individual fibers, which are meshed in a particular pattern. Once the weave is formed it behaves as a flexible inelastic jacket. The device consists of an anterior and posterior implant, which are both oriented in a transverse position within the disc

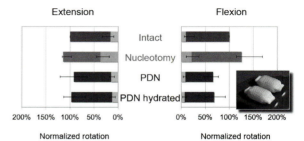

Fig. 20.6. Range of motion (entire bars) and neutral zone (light part of the bars) in flexion and extension of the dehydrated and hydrated PDN in comparison to the intact state or after nucleotomy (for further details please read [30]).

cavity. In order to accommodate the variation in shape of the intervertebral disc space (anterior to posterior and also between the endplates) and the differences in patient's anatomy, a range of implants has been developed. The current version is a single but bigger implant called PDN-SOLO. In order to minimize the access through the annulus the device is implanted in a dehydrated state, which has a reduced volume and profile. Once implanted, the hydrophilic hydrogel will absorb fluid and increase in volume until the dimensions of the polyethylene jacket restrict it.

The purpose of this study was to determine if the original flexibility and disc height of a denucleated L4–5 motion segment is restored post device implantation and whether the degree of hydration effects these results.

Compared to the intact state (100%), nucleotomy increased the ROM in flexion/extension to 118%, lateral bending to 112%, and axial rotation to 121% [30]. Device implantation reduced the ROM slightly compared with the state before nucleotomy (Fig. 20.6). The neutral zone increased to values of 210%, 173%, 107% after nucleotomy, and 146%, 149%, 44% after device implantation. The original disc height was restored after implantation of the device. However, an effect from the hydration could not be measured.

Tissue engineered collagen matrix nucleus replacement

The PDN and other artificial nucleus implants have already been clinically applied but their success was not optimal yet [1, 5, 9, 10, 20, 26, 30].

Therefore, more and more biological solutions are discussed. Recently, it has been shown that seeding or reinserting cells inside the intervertebral disc may preserve disc structures by slowing down the degeneration process [17, 18]. It was also hypothesized that cell insertion might restore the annulus and nucleus tissue [8, 14]. These methods, however, may not be suitable to restore disc height.

The idea of such implants is to seed cells in a three-dimensional collagen matrix. This matrix may serve as a scaffold to provide more mechanical stiffness compared to pure biological solutions. The requirements therefore are to provide a scaffold with adequate mechanical properties, which allows to culture suitable cells in it, for example intervertebral disc cells or mesenchymal progenitor cells (MPCs). A recent study showed that a three-dimensional collagen matrix might be suitable to serve as scaffold for cell seeding, which might be used as a nucleus replacement [15]. It could be shown that the cells were able to proliferate and that cell viability was still 92% after four weeks. The cell morphology showed spindle-shaped and rounded cells and a tissue specific gene expression pattern [15].

The success of such an implant, however, does not depend on its biological performance only, but also on the biomechanical requirements and its reliability. Further important requirements are appropriate implantation techniques and adequate biomechanical performance after implantation.

This in-vitro study was performed with six bovine lumbar functional spinal units, aging between five and six months. An oblique incision was performed to remove the nucleus and to replace it by an implant made of a collagen-type-I matrix.

It could be shown that removal of the nucleus significantly reduced disc height by 0.84 mm in respect to the intact state and caused an instability in the segment [29]. By implantation of the tissue engineered nucleus it was possible to compensate the loss of stability and to restore disc height with even a slight increase of disc height of 0.07 mm compared to the intact state. There was no statistical difference between the stability provided by the implant and initial stability. Results of movements in lateral bending and axial rotation showed the same trend compared to flexion/extension. However, implant extrusions have been observed in three of six cases during the flexibility assessment.

This experiment showed that such collagen implants are able to restore the biomechanical characteristic of an intervertebral disc but do have a high risk of extrusion. Interestingly this happened during the standard flexibility testing at ±7.5 Nm and not even after a few thousand cycles. Therefore it is important to search for possibilities to seal the annulus or to prevent extrusion in another way. A solution to this problem therefore is one of the most important biomechanical prerequisites if such a tissue engineered implant shall have a chance for clinical application.

Summary

This article describes a series of in-vitro tests to investigate the biomechanical performance of the currently discussed implant types for motion preservation in spine surgery. The results of these biomechanical tests showed the following:

The Dynesys system is capable to sufficiently stabilize a degenerated segment, allowing more motion than an internal fixator. However, it is stiffer then one might expect.

The interspinous implants Coflex, Wallis, Diam and X-Stop have shown that they have in general a similar behaviour: they restrict motion in extension without being able to restore the motion in flexion, lateral bending and axial rotation.

The total posterior-element replacement system TOPS almost ideally restored the ROM in lateral bending and axial rotation compared to that of the intact specimen. In the current version flexion/extension was 85% of the intact ROM. The ROM in axial rotation as a function of flexion and extension angle also mimics the biomechanical behavior of the posterior complex of a lumbar spine.

The tests with the total disc replacement showed that an unconstrained design increases the segmental lordosis more than a constrained prosthesis. A posterior center of rotation in a constrained prosthesis relieves an unphysiological increase of segmental lordosis after TDR. Unconstrained prostheses have a tendency towards higher ROM for axial rotation and lateral bending, but towards smaller ROM for flexion/extension compared to constrained prostheses.

The location of the center of rotation in a constrained prosthesis did not alter the magnitude of ROM.

Prosthetic disc nucleus implants (PDN) can potentially restore ROM, NZ and disc height after a nucleotomy. The same is potentially true for vital tissue engineered nucleus implants. Both implant types, however, have the risk of being extruded. Therefore it remains the challenge to find an appropriate annulus fibrosus sealing method, which is capable to keep the nucleus implants in place over a long-time period.

The adjacent segments for all implant types were not significantly affected by the instrumentations.

Limitations and conclusion

In this paper all described data were obtained without axial preload or muscle forces. However they respect internationally accepted recommendations for the standardized testing of spinal implants [32] and therefore the results can be compared directly. If additional loads are applied they can lead to an uncontrolled buckling of the specimens and thus provoke unrealistic motion behaviour of the specimens. In some studies we did simulate a preload, a follower load or muscle forces in additional test runs. They are reported elsewhere, but in general the results showed the same trends.

There might also be more problems with this kind of implants such as loosening of screws or the implant itself or sintering of implants into the vertebral bodies. Such problems may question the outcome of these treatment modalities. This chapter only summarizes the most important parts of a series of flexibility studies. More details may be found in the cited original papers.

In-vitro tests provide fundamental information concerning the biomechanical performance of spinal implants. However, biological effects cannot be explored with such studies. Therefore, animal studies and clinical trials are of utmost importance and therefore should be considered as well when discussing the biomechanical efficacy of spinal implants.

Despite of these limitations such biomechanical in-vitro tests and also complementary finite-element-calculation may provide interesting results for the clinical discussion. Sometimes this kind of tests demonstrates that implants behave as suggested or that they can be optimized, and sometimes specific features do not lead to significant differences as well as sometimes the results do not support the promised behaviour. Therefore pre-clinical tests should be warranted.

Acknowlegement

This paper summarizes a series of different in-vitro studies, which were carried out by different teams. Therefore I would like to acknowledge all co-workers of these studies: Werner Schmölz, Jörg Huber, and Thomas Nydegger in the Dynesys study; Jörg Drumm, Kim Häussler, Annette Kettler, and Karin Werner in the study about interspinous implants; Werner Schmölz, Hendrik Schmidt, Karin Werner, Michael Tauber, and Lutz Claes in the TOPS study; Balkan Cakir, Werner Schmölz, René Schmidt, Wolfhart Puhl, and Marcus Richter investigated the total disc protheses; Annette Kettler, Marcus Mohr, Sinead Kavanagh, Allison Bain, and Britt Norton evaluated the prosthetic disc nucleus; and Frank Heuer and Cornelia Neidlinger-Wilke supported the study with the tissue engineered nucleus.

The studies were supported financially by the following companies: DePuy Spine, Impliant Ltd., Raymedica, Paradigm Spine, Synos Foundation, Ulrich medical, and ARS Arthro.

References

1. Allen MJ, Schoonmaker JE, Bauer TW, Williams PF, Higham PA, Yuan HA (2004) Preclinical evaluation of a poly (vinyl alcohol) hydrogel implant as a replacement for the nucleus pulposus. Spine 29:515–523
2. Büttner-Janz K, Schellnack K, Zippel H (1987) Eine alternative Behandlungsstrategie beim lumbalen Bandscheibenschaden mit der Bandscheibenendoprothese Modulartyp SB Charite. Z Orthop 125:1–6
3. Christie SD, Song JK, Fessler RG (2005) Dynamic interspinous process technology. Spine 30 (Suppl):73–78
4. Cunningham BW, Kotani Y, McNulty PS, Cappuccino A, McAfee PC (1997) The effect of spinal destabilization and instrumentation on lumbar intradiscal pressure: an in vitro biomechanical analysis. Spine 22:2655–2663

5. Di Martino A, Vaccaro AR, Lee JY, Denaro V, Lim MR (2005) Nucleus pulposus replacement: basic science and indications for clinical use. Spine 30 (Suppl):16–22
6. Drumm J, Kettler A, Häussler K, Mack C, Steudel WI, Claes L, Wilke HJ (submitted) Biomechanical effect of different lumbar interspinous implants on flexibility and intradiscal pressure. Spine
7. Esses SI, Sachs BL, Dreyzin V (1993) Complications associated with the technique of pedicle screw fixation. A selected survey of ABS members. Spine 18:2231–2238
8. Ganey T, Libera J, Moos V, Alasevic O, Fritsch KG, Meisel HJ, Hutton WC (2003) Disc chondrocyte transplantation in a canine model: a treatment for degenerated or damaged intervertebral disc. Spine 28:2609–2620
9. Husson JL, Korge A, Polard JL, Nydegger T, Kneubühler S, Mayer HM (2003) A memory coiling spiral as nucleus pulposus prosthesis: concept, specifications, bench testing, and first clinical results. J Spinal Disord Tech 16:405–411
10. Korge A, Nydegger T, Polard JL, Mayer HM, Husson JL (2002) A spiral implant as nucleus prosthesis in the lumbar spine. Eur Spine J 11 (Suppl 2): 149–153
11. Lee CK (1988) Accelerated degeneration of the segment adjacent to a lumbar fusion. Spine 13: 375–377
12. Mayer HM, Korge A (2002) Non-fusion technology in degenerative lumbar spinal disorders: facts, questions, challenges. Eur Spine J 11 (Suppl 2): 85–91
13. McAfee PC, Weiland DJ, Carlow JJ (1991) Survivorship analysis of pedicle spinal instrumentation. Spine 16(Suppl):422–427
14. Meisel HJ, Ganey T, Hutton WC, Libera J, Minkus Y, Alasevic O (2006) Clinical experience in cell-based therapeutics: intervention and outcome. Eur Spine J 15(Suppl 3):397–405
15. Neidlinger-Wilke C, Wurtz K, Liedert A, Schmidt C, Borm W, Ignatius A, Wilke HJ, Claes L (2005) A three-dimensional collagen matrix as a suitable culture system for the comparison of cyclic strain and hydrostatic pressure effects on intervertebral disc cells. J Neurosurg Spine 2:457–465
16. Niosi CA, Zhu QA, Wilson DC, Keynan O, Wilson DR, Oxland TR (2006) Biomechanical characterization of the three-dimensional kinematic behaviour of the Dynesys dynamic stabilization system: an in vitro study. Eur Spine J 15:913–922
17. Nishimura K, Mochida J (1998) Percutaneous reinsertion of the nucleus pulposus. An experimental study. Spine 23:1531–1538
18. Okuma M, Mochida J, Nishimura K, Sakabe K, Seiki K (2000) Reinsertion of stimulated nucleus pulposus cells retards intervertebral disc degeneration: an in vitro and in vivo experimental study. J Orthop Res 18:988–997
19. Ray CD (1992) The artificial disc. In: Weinstein JN (ed) Clinical efficacy and outcome in the diagnosis and treatment of low back pain. Raven Press, New York, p 205–225
20. Ray CD (2002) The PDN prosthetic disc-nucleus device. Eur Spine J 11 (Suppl 2):137–142
21. Rohlmann A, Neller S, Bergmann G, Graichen F, Claes L, Wilke HJ (2001) Effect of an internal fixator and a bone graft on intersegmental spinal motion and intradiscal pressure in the adjacent regions. Eur Spine J 10:301–308
22. Rudig L, Runkel M, Kreitner KF, Seidel T, Degreif J (1997) Kernspintomographische Untersuchung thorakolumbaler Wirbelfrakturen nach Fixateur-interne-Stabilisierung. Unfallchirurg 100:524–530
23. Schlegel JD, Smith JA, Schleusener RL (1996) Lumbar motion segment pathology adjacent to thoracolumbar, lumbar, and lumbosacral fusions. Spine 21:970–981
24. Schmölz W, Huber JF, Nydegger T, Claes L, Wilke HJ (2006) Influence of a dynamic stabilisation system on load bearing of a bridged disc: an in vitro study of intradiscal pressure. Eur Spine J 15:1–10
25. Schmölz W, Huber JF, Nydegger T, Dipl I, Claes L, Wilke HJ (2003) Dynamic stabilization of the lumbar spine and its effects on adjacent segments: an in vitro experiment. J Spinal Disord Tech 16:418–423
26. Schönmayr R, Buch C, Lotz C (1999) Prosthetic disc nucleus implants: the Wiesbaden feasibility study. 2 years follow up in ten patients. Riv Neuroradiol 12(Suppl 1):163–170
27. Whitesides TE Jr (2003) The effect of an interspinous implant on intervertebral disc pressures. Spine 28:1906–1907
28. Wilke HJ, Claes L, Schmitt H, Wolf S (1994) A universal spine tester for in vitro experiments with muscle force simulation. Eur Spine J 3:91–97
29. Wilke HJ, Heuer F, Neidlinger-Wilke C, Claes L (2006) Is a collagen scaffold for a tissue engineered nucleus replacement capable of restoring disc height and stability in an animal model? Eur Spine J 15 (Suppl 3):433–438
30. Wilke HJ, Kavanagh S, Neller S, Haid C, Claes LE (2001) Effect of a prosthetic disc nucleus on the mobility and disc height of the L4–5 intervertebral disc postnucleotomy. J Neurosurg 95(Suppl 2): 208–214
31. Wilke HJ, Schmidt H, Werner K, Schmölz W, Drumm J (2006) Biomechanical evaluation of a new total posterior-element replacement system. Spine 31:2790–2796
32. Wilke HJ, Wenger K, Claes L (1998) Testing criteria for spinal implants: recommendations for the standardization of in vitro stability testing of spinal implants. Eur Spine J 7:148–154

21 Interspinous devices – implants, indications and results

RENÉ SCHMIDT and BALKAN CAKIR

Introduction

After the "fusion era" which made spinal fusion a "gold standard" for different spinal pathologies, some surgeons now herald the era of dynamic stabilization. One reason therefore is that despite significantly enhanced fusion rates by better implants and "fusion additives" (such as BMP) the clinical outcome did not improve in the same way. Furthermore late sequelae of fusion, especially adjacent segment degeneration, become apparent. The philosophy of dynamic stabilization is mainly based on the principle to alter movement and load transmission so that adjacent segment degeneration can be prevented. The dynamic systems can be divided in anterior and posterior devices. Anterior devices comprise e.g. nucleus replacement or total disc replacement. Posterior devices can further be divided in pedicle screw-based systems such as the dynamic neutralization system (Dynesys) [13] or the Fulcrum Assisted Soft Stabilization System (FASS) [11] and floating devices. The difference here is simply the type of fixation to the spine. Interspinous devices are attributed to the floating group and although the name dynamic stabilization is new, these implants are not. Probably one of the first documented interspinous devices is from the 1950's by Fred L. Knowles [18]. Some more devices followed such as the Minns device [6], which was supposed to be the first "soft" interspinous implant. These implants never came to a broad use and were outdated by the increasing application of fusions. Since the renaissance of dynamic stabilization many different interspinous devices came on the market, some of them are presented below. This choice does not intend to give any rating or preference and is solely based on the fact that these implants are quite known and clinical data exists on a limited scale.

Implants

Implants actually in clinical use are, amongst others, the X-Stop (Fig. 21.1 a, b, St. Francis Medical Technologies, USA), the Coflex (Fig. 21.2 a, b, Paradigm Spine, USA), the Wallis (Abbott Spine, USA), and the DIAM (Medtronic, USA). The X-Stop consists of a titanium alloy body and a PEEK spacer. Coflex is also made of titanium alloy, whereas the Wallis consists of PEEK spacer in addition with a flat polyester band. The core of the DIAM is made of silicone

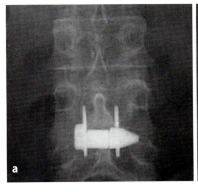 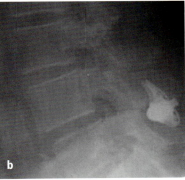

Fig. 21.1 a, b. AP (**a**) and lateral (**b**) x-ray of the X-Stop implanted at level L4/5 (image with permission of St. Francis Medical).

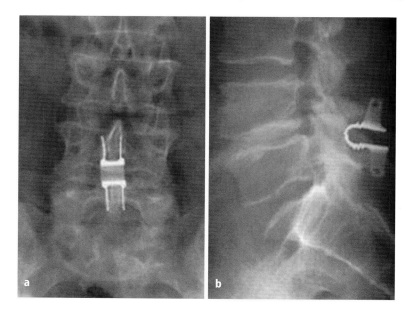

Fig. 21.2 a, b. AP (**a**) and lateral (**b**) x-ray of the Coflex implanted at level L4/5 (image with permission of Paradigm Spine).

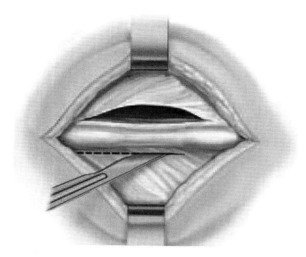

Fig. 21.3. Fascia incision (image with permission of St. Francis Medical).

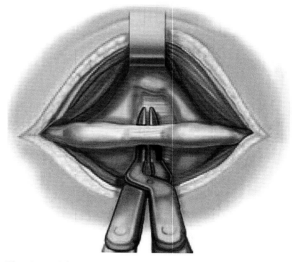

Fig. 21.4. Dilation of interspinous ligament during implantation of the X-Stop (image with permission of St. Francis Medical).

with an outer mesh and tethers of medical-grade polyester. Based on the design these implants can further be divided in "total free floating" like the Coflex or X-Stop and "partially free floating" as the Wallis or DIAM, where a fixation to the adjacent spinous processes by the ligaments/bands exists.

Surgery can be performed in general, but also in local anaesthesia. The implantation technique is quite similar in all devices. Patients are usually placed in a prone position, except for the X-Stop, where a right lateral decubitus position is recommended. After location of the segment(s) by image intensifier, a short median incision is performed. The fascia is incised (Fig. 21.3) and the paraspinous muscles are dissected. The supraspinous ligament is either retracted laterally or detached. Different recommendations are given for an additional direct decompression. If an additional direct decompression is performed, it is important from a biomechanical point to assure enough remaining stability of the facet joints [2]. Then the interspinous ligament is resected or dilated (Fig. 21.4) depending on the chosen device. Implant size is determined by trial spacers or special instruments. Correct implant size and position is confirmed fluoroscopically. Implant fixation is achieved by attachable or firm wings or tightening of ligaments/bands around the adjacent spinous processes, depending on implant type. A detached supraspinous ligament is reinserted and wound closure is carried out. Usually free functional mobilisation of the patients is possible, although a graded increase of physical activity over the first weeks is often recommended to prevent early fractures of the spinous processes.

Mode of action

The development of interspinous spacers is mainly based on the perception that neurogenic claudication due to lumbar spinal stenosis is exacerbated by extension of the lumbar spine, at least in mild to moderate stenosis. This leads to the design of implants capable to block or limit extension (Fig. 21.5 a, b). Lindsey et al. found in an in-vitro study that only flexion/extension was limited by the spacers, whereas other motions were unrestricted [5]. Furthermore they found no difference for the adjacent segments. Rohlmann et al. in contrast calculated with an finite element study that motion at adjacent levels was increased due to the restriction of motion at the implanted level [9]. The main difference between the studies is that Lindsey chose a load-controlled design, whereas Rohlmann favored a motion-controlled design. It is clear that presuming an unchanged overall motion, range of motion (ROM) at adjacent levels must increase in a motion-controlled test setting. It is until now unclear which approach best simulates the in-vivo situation. This means that although theoretically there is the possibility that interspinous spacers might avoid adjacent segment degeneration, this cannot be conclusively predicted. Proof is only possible by long-term clinical follow-up. For neurogenic intermittent claudication the proposed clinical effect by restricted motion in extension is the prevention of buckling of the ligamentum flavum. Theoretically this results in greater canal and foramen diameter. Richards et al. evaluated this effect in-vitro and found at treated levels enhanced diameters in extension without affection of adjacent segments [8]. In-vivo, Siddiqui et al. found corresponding results for the spinal canal and foramen, although they saw no differences for the posterior disc height [12]. In another in-vitro study Swanson et al. found no increase for adjacent disc pressures [14], which is in line with Rohlmann et al. [9]. This could support the hypothesis of avoidance of adjacent segment degeneration. For the instrumented segment, Swanson et al. saw a decreased disc pressure in extension [14], whereas Rohlmann et al. found an increase of disc pressure for extension in the degenerated disc, but a strong decrease in comparison to a healthy disc [9]. For walking, which reached higher disc stresses than extension nearly no difference was calculated between instrumented and uninstrumented segments. The pressures in the vertebral arch were much higher for extension than for walking and dependent of implant size. This could lead to failure of the spinous process, which is a concern raised by some authors. Studies concerning the long-term failure are missing, only one in-

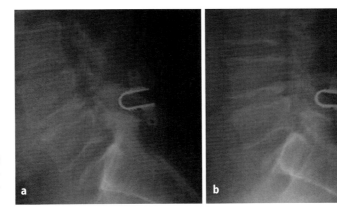

Fig. 21.5 a, b. Lateral x-rays of the Coflex implanted at level L4/5, (**a**) in neutral position, (**b**) in extension (image with permission of Paradigm Spine).

vitro study comparing insertion loads of the X-Stop is available. Talwar et al. came to the conclusion that the insertion technique provides a sufficient margin of safety against spinous process failure, however a significant relationship between the bone mineral density (BMD) and spinous process strength was found which exposes patients with lower BMD to a higher risk [16]. Concerning the facet joints one in-vitro study dealt with that topic. Wiseman et al. saw a decreased facet joint pressure in the implanted segment, with unaltered loads in adjacent levels [19]. Other biomechanical studies focused on the ability of interspinous devices to stabilize degenerated segments. Fuchs et al. suggested that the X-Stop may be used in conjunction with a unilateral medial or unilateral total facetectomy, but not a bilateral total facetectomy [2]. Tsai et al. concludes that the Coflex is able to return a partially destabilized segment to the intact condition [17]. The DIAM showed biomechanically the ability to reduce increased flexion/extension and lateral bending after discectomy, but not the increased axial rotation [7]. Based on these, mainly in-vitro studies, the indications proposed for the interspinous devices vary greatly.

Indications

The main indication for interspinous devices is the neurogenic intermittent claudication due to central or lateral spinal stenosis of the lumbar spine, with pain relief in flexion. Implantation is usually limited to bilevel at the moment according to the manufacturers recommendations, but enlarged implantation is possible (Fig. 21.6). Due to the size of the spinous process of S1, implantation comprises usually the region of L1 to L5, although some implants try to overcome this restriction (Fig. 21.7 a, b). Referring to the in-vitro studies about potential unloading of the discs and/or facets and potential stabilizing effects, some devices include further indications:

- contained or large voluminous disc herniations,
- recurrent disc herniation,
- primary disc degeneration up to varying grades of degeneration,
- post-discectomy syndrome,
- axial load-induced back pain, chronic low back pain with Modic I changes,
- facet syndrome,
- "Kissing Spine" (Baastrup's syndrome),

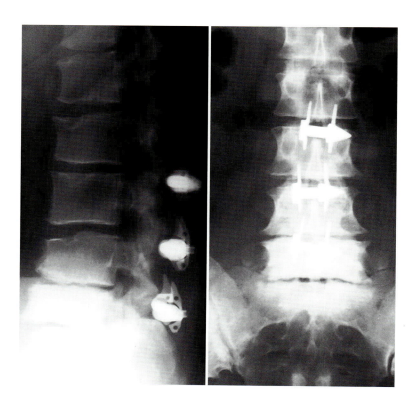

Fig. 21.6. Biplanar x-rays of a trilevel implantation of the X-Stop at the levels L2/3, L3/4, and L4/5 (image with permission of St. Francis Medical).

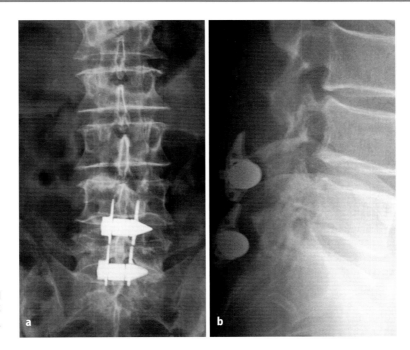

Fig. 21.7 a, b. Biplanar x-rays of a bilevel implantation of the X-Stop at levels L4/5 and L5/S1 (image with permission of St. Francis Medical).

- primary or secondary unloading of segments adjacent to fusions ("topping off").

Possible indications in the future could include the combination with anterior dynamic devices, such as nucleus replacement or total lumbar disc replacement. Contraindications are of general nature, e.g. tumor or infection. Specific contraindications comprise, amongst others, severe osteoporosis, non-specific back pain, severe spinal stenosis without pain relief in any position, high grade disc degeneration, morbid obesity, conus/cauda syndrome or significant scoliotic deformity. Traumatic instabilities are also contraindications, whereas some see an indication for degenerative listhesis up to a grade of 1–1.5 of 4.

Results

Most of the currently available clinical data is for the "classic" indication of neurogenic claudication by lumbar stenosis. Most of the studies are by the group of Zucherman et al. who presented the data of their approval trials of the X-Stop for one, two and four years. In the four year unrandomized trial they reported about 78% successful outcomes [3]. For the two year results they concluded a satisfaction rate of 73.1% in the X-Stop group compared to 35.9% in the non-operative group [20]. Lee et al. found after a minimum follow-up of nine months that 70% of the patients were at least somewhat satisfied (5/10 very satisfied; 2/10 somewhat satisfied) [4]. Anderson et al. reported about similar results after two years (clinical success 63.4% X-Stop vs. 12.9% controls) for the X-Stop in patients with lumbar stenosis and additional spondylolisthesis up to 25% [1]. For the DIAM and Wallis current data is mainly for lumbar degeneration. Schiavone and Pasquale had 16 excellent and four good outcomes in 22 patients with segmental degeneration after ten months [10]. Sénégas reported 74% improvement in low back pain in 40 patients treated with discectomy and Wallis for recurrent disc herniation L4/5, compared to 52% improvement in patients treated by discectomy alone [15]. In this study one directly device-related complication occurred, as one of the patients had revision surgery due to failure of the ligament fixation. Zucherman et al. reported about three device-related complications after two years, one dislodgement after a fall, one asymptomatic spinous process fracture and one recurrent pain after one year which was possibly attributed to a mal-positioned device [20].

Conclusion

There is some evidence for a potential effect of interspinous devices for the "classic" indication of neurogenic intermittent claudication, although these clinical data are mainly for one implant (X-Stop). Open questions are here especially up to which extent of stenosis these implants are useful and whether the clinical results could be enhanced in some cases by additional decompression. Further on, as the motion is at least partially preserved, the underlying process of progressive stenosis, e.g. by increasing arthrosis of the facet joints, continues. This could lead to deterioration over time. As always in the case of new implants, this question cannot be answered actually due to missing long-term follow-up. Regarding the indication of unloading and/or stabilizing instrumented segments, clinical data is even more rare. Although biomechanical studies give hints of possible indications, clinical indications are quite unclear. Another question to be answered is whether differences in implant design ("total floating" vs. "partial floating" devices) have an impact on clinical outcome and if so for which indications. Also the materials of the devices could have a possible impact. Does e.g. a total titanium device lead to higher erosion and loosening than a PEEK coated? Is silicone or PEEK better for the spacer or is there no impact at all? This shows that besides the need for general clinical outcome data for interspinous devices also the different implant types have to be studied closely. It seems therefore of indispensable importance to study these implants in selected patient cohorts for every possible indication. Otherwise it seems impossible to set up clear indication criteria. Although these devices are promising, it seems unlikely that they will be the universal tool for all types of lumbar spinal pathology as one might feel when reading the suggested indication lists. The rapid expansion of indications in combination with inappropriate patient selection by mixed indications, bears the possibility that the true value of these implants will never be known. Clear advantages of the interspinous devices, which allow further evaluation, are the easy application, less invasive surgery even for older patients or such with severe co-morbidity, short term acceptable implant-related complications and the preservation of all surgical alternatives after failure. Summarizing, the interspinous implants are interesting and promising devices, which should be carefully studied for clearly defined indications to identify their true value in the field of spinal surgery.

References

1. Anderson PA, Tribus CB, Kitchel SH (2006) Treatment of neurogenic claudication by interspinous decompression: application of the X-Stop device in patients with lumbar degenerative spondylolisthesis. J Neurosurg Spine 4:463–471
2. Fuchs PD, Lindsey DP, Hsu KY, Zucherman JF, Yerby SA (2005) The use of an interspinous implant in conjunction with a graded facetectomy procedure. Spine 30:1266–1272
3. Kondrashov DG, Hannibal M, Hsu KY, Zucherman JF (2006) Interspinous process decompression with the X-Stop device for lumbar spinal stenosis. A 4-year follow-up study. J Spinal Disord Tech 19:323–327
4. Lee J, Hida K, Seki T, Iwasaki Y, Minoru A (2004) An interspinous process distractor (X-Stop) for lumbar spinal stenosis in elderly patients. Preliminary experience in 10 consecutive cases. J Spinal Disord Tech 17:72–77
5. Lindsey DP, Swanson KE, Fuchs PD, Hsu KY, Zucherman JF, Yerby SA (2003) The effects of an interspinous implant on the kinematics of the instrumented and adjacent levels in the lumbar spine. Spine 28:2192–2197
6. Minns RJ, Walsh WK (1997) Preliminary design and experimental studies of a novel soft implant for correcting sagittal plane instability in the lumbar spine. Spine 22:1819–1825
7. Phillips FM, Voronov LI, Gaitanis IN, Carandang G, Havey RM, Patwardhan AG (2006) Biomechanics of posterior dynamic stabilizing device (Diam) after facetectomy and discectomy. Spine J 6:714–722
8. Richards JC, Majumdar S, Lindsey DP, Beaupré GS, Yerby SA (2005) The treatment mechanism of an interspinous process implant for lumbar neurogenic intermittent claudication. Spine 30:744–749
9. Rohlmann A, Zander T, Burra NK, Bergmann G (2005) Effect of an interspinous implant on loads in the lumbar spine. Biomed Technik 50:343–347
10. Schiavone AM, Pasquale G (2003) The use of disc assistance prostheses (Diam) in degenerative lumbar pathology: Indications, technique and results. Ital J Spinal Disord 3:213–220
11. Sengupta DK, Mulholland RC (2005) Fulcrum assisted soft stabilization system. A new concept in the surgical treatment of degenerative low back pain. Spine 30:1019–1029

12. Siddiqui M, Nicol M, Karadimas E, Smith F, Wardlaw D (2005) The positional magnetic resonance imaging changes in the lumbar spine following insertion of a novel interspinous process distraction device. Spine 30:2677–2682
13. Stoll TM, Dubois G, Schwarzenbach O (2002) The dynamic neutralization system for the spine: a multi-center study of a novel non-fusion system. Eur Spine J 11:170–178
14. Swanson KE, Lindsey DP, Hsu KY, Zucherman JF, Yerby SA (2003) The effects of an interspinous implant on intervertebral disc pressures. Spine 28:26–32
15. Sénégas J (2002) Mechanical supplementation by non-rigid fixation in degenerative intervertebral segments: the Wallis system. Eur Spine J 11:164–169
16. Talwar V, Lindsey DP, Fredrick A, Hsu KY, Zucherman JF, Yerby SA (2006) Insertion loads of the X-stop interspinous process distraction system designed to treat neurogenic intermittent claudication. Eur Spine J 15:908–912
17. Tsai KJ, Murakami H, Lowery GL, Hutton WC (2006) A biomechanical evaluation of an interspinous device (Coflex) used to stabilize the lumbar spine. J Surg Orthop Adv 15:167–172
18. Whitesides TEJ (2003) Letters to the Editor: The effect of an interspinous implant on intervertebral disc pressures. Spine 28:1906–1907
19. Wiseman CM, Lindsey DP, Fredrick A, Yerby SA (2005) The effect of an interspinous process implant on facet loading during extension. Spine 30:903–907
20. Zucherman JF, Hsu KY, Hartjen CA, Mehalic TF, Implicito DA, Martin MJ, Johnson II DR, Skidmore GA, Vessa PP, Dwyer JW, Puccio ST, Cauthen JC, Ozuna RM (2005) A multicenter, prospective, randomized trial evaluating the X-Stop interspinous process decompression system for the treatment of neurogenic intermittent claudication: Two year follow-up results. Spine 30:1351–1358

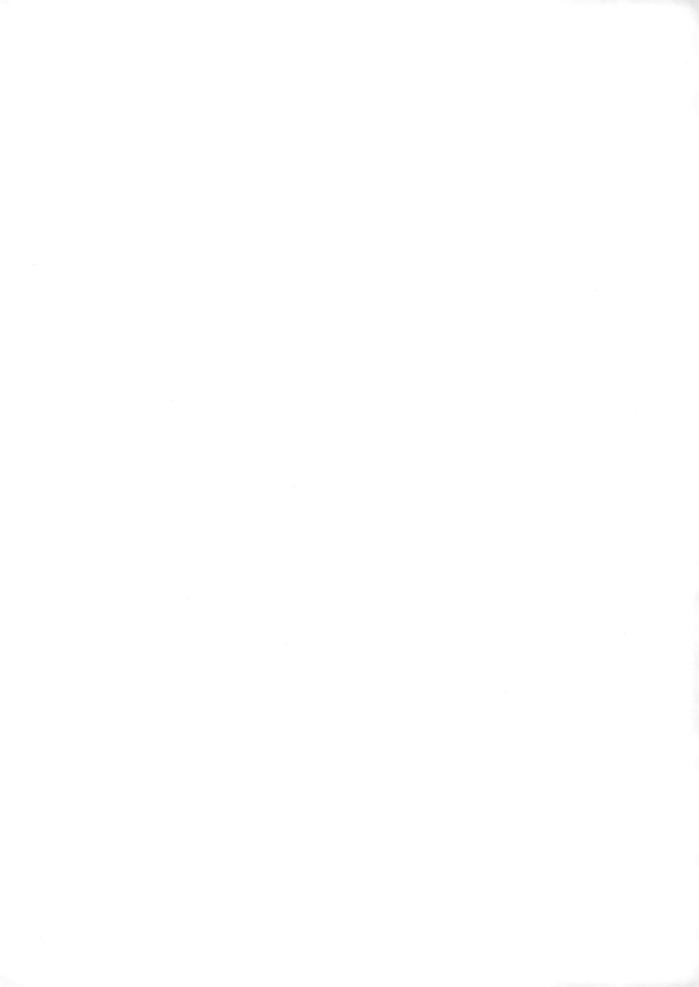

22 Lumbar total disc replacement – implants, indications, and results

Balkan Cakir, René Schmidt, Wolfram Käfer, and Heiko Reichel

Background

Spinal fusion has gained the status as therapeutical "gold standard" for a variety of deformities and instabilities unresponsive to conservative treatment. Despite advances in surgical techniques and implants since the beginning of the "fusion area" in the early 20th century, fusion still has to face negative side-effects such as pseudarthrosis, donor-site pain, and collateral damage to soft tissue [14, 21]. Moreover, some investigators believe that fusion may induce accelerated degenerative changes in the neighboring segments due to the loss of motion, often necessitating additional fusion surgery [8]. To preserve segmental mobility and thereby avoiding the cascade of adjacent segment degeneration (ASD), the development of dynamic implants already started in the early 1950's [7]. A survey of these implants was published recently by Szapalski et al. [22]. Besides other implants such as posterior dynamic stabilization, nucleus replacement and interspinous devices, the device which best represents the philosophy of spine arthroplasty is the total lumbar disc replacement (TDR). The enormous clinical but also economical role of these new devices in the next years is emphasized by the fact that
- every spine surgeon probably will be forced to offer some kind of spine arthroplasty to his patients [15] and that
- the estimated overall turnover of the spine arthroplasty industry will rise from 9.2 Mio. $ in 2003 up to 1 Bil. $ in 2007 [24].

With these prospects in mind and the fact that no evidence-based data are available at the moment it will be a challenge for each physician in the field of spine surgery to deal critically with this new technology.

Postulated goals of TDR

The postulated mode of action of disc prosthesis includes
1. resection of the pain generating degenerated disc,
2. restoration of the disc height thereby restoring foraminal height and unloading the facet joints,
3. restoration of segmental lordosis, providing a physiological sagittal alignment, and
4. preservation of mobility.

Arguments 1–3, which propagate TDR as a possible solution for degenerative disc disease can be achieved also with a fusion operation. Therefore the main postulated advantage of TDR compared to fusion, beside possible advantages in approach-related and donor-site related morbidities [17], is motion preservation (Fig. 22.1 a–f). The preservation of mobility together with the restoration of the physiological sagittal balance of the spine should result in pain relief and lead to a reduced number of adjacent segment degeneration.

Implants and biomechanical concepts

Only two out of the five TDR designs available for the lumbar spine have already been approved by the Food and Drug Adminstration (FDA) in 2004 (SB Charité III, DePuy Spine, Raynham, USA) and in 2006 (Prodisc-L, Synthes, Paoli, USA). Beside other differences, the prostheses can mainly be divided in subgroups by means of
- biomechanical concept,
- their interface, and
- the fixation technique to the vertebral body (Table 22.1).

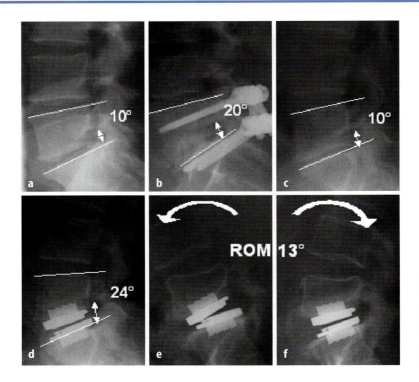

Fig. 22.1 a–f. Sufficient restoration of disc height and segmental lordosis both after 360° fusion (**a, b**) and total lumbar total disc replacement (TDR) with a Prodisc prosthesis (**c, d**) at level L5–S1; additional preservation of range of motion (ROM) following TDR (**e, f**).

Table 22.1. Comparison of lumbar total disc prostheses with regard to concept, interface and special features.

Prosthesis	Concept	Interface	Feature
■ SB Charité III (Depuy Spine, Raynham, USA)	Unconstrained	Metal on PE	Floating COR due to rotating core
■ Prodisc-L (Synthes, Paoli, USA)	Semi-constrained	Metal on PE	Fixed COR below endplate, unconstrained for rotation
■ Maverick (Medtronic, Minneapolis, USA)	Semi-constrained	Metal on metal	Fixed, posterior COR below endplate, unconstrained for rotation
■ Flexicore (Stryker Corp., Kalamazoo, USA)	Semi-constrained	Metal on metal	Fixed COR at the level of disc space, constrained for rotation
■ Mobidisc (LDR Médical, Troyes, France)	Unconstrained	Metal on PE	Floating COR due to sliding core in ap and lateral direction

COR: center of rotation; PE: polyethylen

From a biomechanical point of view the design concept has the biggest impact on the resulting qualitative segmental movement. The most striking difference between an unconstrained and semiconstrained prosthesis is the ability of an unconstrained prosthesis to carry out a translational movement without rotation (Fig. 22.2 a, b). Although some authors believe that an unconstrained prosthesis will have a greater range of motion (ROM) there is no evidence at the moment for this statement. Moreover the authors of this article could not find any significant differences in-vitro when comparing the ROM of the Charité and the Prodisc prosthesis [19]. The postulated effect of the design concept on the facet joint load and shear forces [13] are still speculative at the moment and have to be evaluated in further clinical and biomechanical studies.

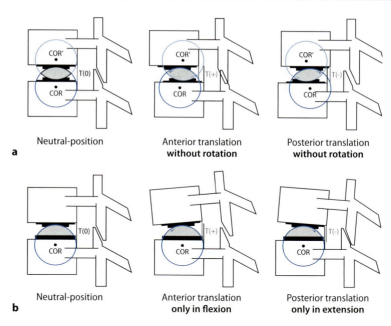

Fig. 22.2 a, b. Translational movement of an unconstrained prosthesis (e.g. Charité prosthesis) and a semi-constrained prosthesis (e.g. Prodisc-L prosthesis): anterior and posterior translation without rotational movement is only achieved with an unconstrained prosthesis (**a**); in a semi-constrained prosthesis anterior translation is only possible in flexion and posterior translation only in extension (**b**) (COR = center of rotation; T(0) = no translation; T(+) = anterior translation; T(–) = posterior translation).

Inclusion and exclusion criteria for TDR

Currently, there is no evidence-based consensus on indications/contraindications for TDR. Nevertheless, based on the short-term results, some inclusion/exclusion criteria have been established and are accepted in the spine society (Table 22.2). As the indication for TDR remains still a matter of debate and long-term results are still missing, TDR should not be taken into consideration for "extended indications" as proposed by some authors [1].

Table 22.2. Inclusion and exclusion criteria currently proposed for total lumbar disc replacement.

Inclusion criteria	Exclusion criteria
▪ Symptomatic degenerative disc disease at one or two levels (L3–S1)	▪ More than two levels with symptomatic DDD
▪ Age 18–60 years	▪ Allergy to the constituents of prosthesis
▪ At least six months of unsuccessful conservative therapy	▪ Infection, malignancy
▪ Low back pain without signs of root compression	▪ Facet joint degeneration, spinal stenosis, spondylolysis, degenerative listhesis > 1°
▪ Most studies request an Oswestry score of > 40%	▪ Autoimmune or systemic-metabolic disease, osteoporosis
▪ Postdiscectomy without intraspinal scar tissue formation (controversial!)	▪ Curvature deviations (e.g. scoliosis)
	▪ Pregnancy
	▪ Small vertebral body size
	▪ Morbid obesity (BMI > 40)

BMI: body mass index; DDD: degenerative disc disease

Diagnostics

There is no general consensus with regard to compulsory diagnostics before the implantation of a TDR, beside plain radiographs and magnetic resonance imaging (MRI), which have to prove the disc degeneration. Additional non-invasive diagnostic tools comprise dynamic X-rays for exclusion of translational instability and computed tomography (CT)-scans for preoperative planning of the prosthesis size and to rule out an advanced stage of facet joint degeneration. Invasive diagnostic tools like facet blocks, nerve root blocks, epidural injections and sacroiliac joint-blocks seems to have no predicative value for the results of surgery, but are still often used to preclude other sources of low back pain. One of the most discussed invasive diagnostic tools is discography. Although the specifity and sensitivity to visualize disc degeneration and annulus ruptures is high, the attributed capability to verify a "discogenic pain" (also called memory pain) is still in debate [20].

Operative technique

Surgery is performed through an anterior retroperitoneal approach. Compared to the standardized anterior lumbar interbody fusion procedure (ALIF) the whole anterior portion of the disc space has to be accessed, which requires a significant mobilization of the major retroperitoneal vessels in case of level L4–L5 and higher. After access to the disc space the anterior longitudinal ligament (ALL) is removed while preserving the lateral annulus. The TDR is inserted after removal of disc material and preparation of the endplates to ensure a proper alignment and contact surface of the prosthesis and vertebral endplate. Although most steps of TDR implantation are already standardized, there is still ambiguity with regard to the ALL and posterior longitudinal ligament (PLL). Although David [5] describes suturing of the ALL, this seems to be hard to achieve due to the huge distraction of the disc space by the implant. This observation is also supported with regard to the literature since a referral for ALL suturing is uncommon. In general the recommendations for the PLL are more consistent with advice for preservation if possible. However, in case of a concomitant disc herniation [11] or in cases with insufficient vertical mobilization of the disc space resection is considered by some authors [1]. Irrespective of these recommendations, actually there is no clear evidence about a relevant impact of PLL resection on segmental biomechanics after TDR [4].

Clinical and radiological results

Most of the peer-reviewed literature favor disc replacement with good or very good short to mid-term results [3, 10, 20, 25]. From a methodological point of view the most valuable data are from the FDA-controlled investigational device exemption studies for the Charité and Prodisc prosthesis. For the Charité prosthesis an overall success rate of 63% was reported compared to a success rate of 53% for fusion 24 months after index surgery [10]. Similar preliminary results were presented for the Prodisc prosthesis [25]. Indeed, not all results are encouraging. Van Oiij et al. published unsatisfactory results in a series of 27 patients with the Charité prosthesis [23]. Most of the problems resulted from degeneration of adjacent discs, facet joint arthrosis at the same or other levels and subsidence of the prosthesis. Putzier et al. presented the longest currently available follow-up of 53 patients operated on with the Charité prosthesis [18]. After an average follow-up of 17 years 60% of the patients demonstrated a spontaneous ankylosis. Although no adjacent segment degeneration was observed in the few mobile implants (17%), these patients had a worse outcome than patients without motion.

When looking at the radiological results after TDR, the proposed goals of TDR are not always achieved and the published results are sometimes inconsistent. We could demonstrate that TDR implantation results in most of the cases in over-distraction of the disc space [3]. Although the clinical relevance of this finding is not clarified at the moment, some authors advice to use the smallest disc height in cases with previous disc surgery [20]. This could avoid a consecutive nerve root traction due to postoperative fibrosis [6]. With regard to the sagittal balance a significant increase of the segmental lordosis angles with only minor changes in the total lumbar lordosis could be observed,

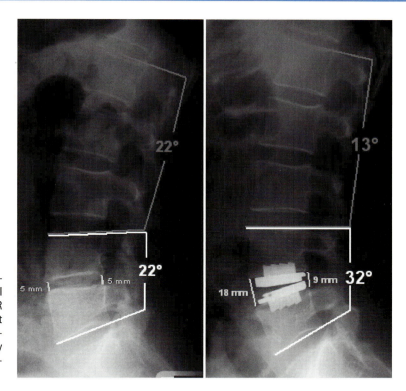

Fig. 22.3. Segmental and total lumbar lordosis and disc height before and after total disc replacement (TDR) at level L4–L5: TDR results in a decrease of lumbar lordosis at the adjacent levels as well as a huge increase in segmental lordosis postoperatively and in a remarkable, non-physiologic increase of disc height postoperatively.

which implies an compensatory hypolordosis in the adjacent segments [2] (Fig. 22.3). Mayer already mentioned that potential benefits of TDR are only valid if a preoperatively balanced spine is not forced to compensate for a TDR induced disturbance of sagittal balance [16]. With regard to ROM it seems that TDR is capable of maintaining mobility in the operated segment. But the results are inconsistent with regard to the quantity of movement. Bertagnoli et al. could observe an improvement of mobility in all patients after implantation of a Prodisc-L prosthesis [1]. In contrast, we could not notice a significant improvement of ROM after Prodisc implantation [3] and Huang et al. recognized a movement more than 2° only in 66% of their patients [12]. There is also no evidence that the unconstrained Charité prosthesis has a greater ROM than the semi-constrained Prodisc prosthesis in-vivo.

Reported complication rates after TDR range from 1% to 40% [1, 9], which reflects the inconsistency of the published results. The reported complications are often related to the surgical access and are rarely implant-related (laceration of vessels, hematoma, wound infection, postoperatively ileus, retrograde ejaculation, malpositioning of the prosthesis, nerve root irritation, fracture of vertebral bodies). Prosthesis-related complications compromise polyethylene dislocation/wear and prosthesis subsidence.

Summary

At the moment the popularity and therefore the widespread use of TDR is mainly based on studies with small patient cohorts. Although promising clinical mid-term results are presented on every occasion and in most of the peer reviewed literature caution should be given not to overstrain the capability of a new technology by using it for various indications, before successful results are scientifically proven in clearly defined pathological conditions. TDR may open a new era in spinal surgery in the future but not at the moment as the evidence that long-term results are as good or even better than fusion is still missing.

References

1. Bertagnoli R, Kumar S (2002) Indications for full prosthetic disc arthroplasty: A correlation of clinical outcome against a variety of indications. Eur Spine J 11(Suppl):131–136
2. Cakir B, Richter M, Käfer W, Puhl W, Schmidt R (2005) The impact of total lumbar disc replacement on segmental and total lumbar lordosis. Clin Biomech 20:357–364
3. Cakir B, Schmidt R, Huch K, Puhl W, Richter M (2004) Sagittales Alignement und segmentale Beweglichkeit nach endoprothetischer Versorgung lumbaler Bewegungssegmente. Z Orthop 142:159–165
4. Cakir B, Schmoelz W, Schmidt R, Wilke HJ, Puhl W, Richter M (2005) Resect or not to resect – the role of posterior longitudinal ligament in total disc replacement. 5th Annual Global Symposium Spine Arthroplasty Society, New York
5. David T (2005) Revision of a Charite artificial disc 9.5 years in vivo to a new Charite artificial disc: Case report and explant analysis. Eur Spine J 14:507–511
6. Dickerman R, Zigler JE, Sachs BL, Matt B, Rashbaum R (2005) Stretch neuropraxia after anterior lumbar interbody fusion or artificial disc replacement: Incidence and prevention. 5th Annual Global Symposium Spine Arthroplasty Society, New York
7. Fernström U (1966) Arthroplasty with intercorporal endoprothesis in herniated disc and in painful disc. Acta Chir Scand 357(Suppl):154–159
8. Gillet P (2003) The fate of the adjacent motion segments after lumbar fusion. J Spinal Disord Tech 16:338–345
9. Griffith SL, Shelokov AP, Buttner Janz K, LeMaire JP, Zeegers WS (1994) A multicenter retrospective study of the clinical results of the LINK SB Charite intervertebral prosthesis. The initial European experience. Spine 19:1842–1849
10. Hochschuler SH, Ohnmeiss DD, Guyer RD, Blumenthal SL (2002) Artificial disc: preliminary results of a prospective study in the United States. Eur Spine J 11(Suppl):106–110
11. Hopf C, Heeckt H, Beske C (2002) Der Bandscheibenersatz mit der SB Charite-Bandscheibenendoprothese – Erfahrungen, Frühergebnisse und Feststellungen nach 35 prospektiv durchgeführten Operationen. Z Orthop 140:485–491
12. Huang RC, Girardi FP, Cammisa Jr FP, Tropiano P, Marnay T (2003) Long-term flexion-extension range of motion of the prodisc total disc replacement. J Spinal Disord Tech 16:435–440
13. Huang RC, Girardi FP, Cammisa FP Jr, Wright TM (2003) The implications of constraint in lumbar total disc replacement. J Spinal Disord Tech 16:412–417
14. Lee C, Dorcil J, Radomisli TE (2004) Nonunion of the spine: A review. Clin Orthop 419:71–75
15. Mayer HM (2005) Degenerative Erkrankungen der Lendenwirbelsaule: Bandscheibenersatz als Alternative zur Spondylodese? Orthopäde 34:1007–1014
16. Mayer HM (2005) Total lumbar disc replacement. J Bone and Joint Surg Br 87:1029–1037
17. Mayer HM, Korge A (2002) Non-fusion technology in degenerative lumbar spinal disorders: Facts, questions, challenges. Eur Spine J 11(Suppl):85–91
18. Putzier M, Funk JF, Schneider SV, Gross C, Tohtz SW, Khodadadyan-Klostermann C, Perka C, Kandziora F (2006) Charite total disc replacement-clinical and radiographical results after an average follow-up of 17 years. Eur Spine J 15:183–195
19. Richter M, Wilke HJ, Schmidt R, Schmoelz W, Puhl W, Cakir B (2005) Constrained versus unconstrained and anterior versus posterior center of rotation – The role of prosthesis design on segmental biomechanics. 5th Annual Global Symposium Spine Arthroplasty Society, New York
20. Siepe CJ, Mayer M, Wiechert K, Korge A (2006) Clinical results of total lumbar disc replacement. Spine 31:1923–1932
21. Summers BN, Eisenstein SM (1989) Donor site pain from the ilium. A complication of lumbar spine fusion. J Bone Joint Surg Br 71:677–680
22. Szpalski M, Gunzburg R, Mayer M (2002) Spine arthroplasty: A historical review. Eur Spine J 11(Suppl):65–84
23. Van Ooij A, Oner FC, Verbout AJ (2003) Complications of artificial disc replacement: a report of 27 patients with the SB Charite disc. J Spinal Disord Tech 16:369–383
24. Vicogliosi Bros LLC (2003) "Beyond total disc" – The future of spine surgery. Spine industry analysis series, New York
25. Zigler JE, Burd TA, Vialle EN, Sachs BL, Rashbaum RF, Ohnmeiss DD (2003) Lumbar spine arthroplasty: Early results using the ProDisc II: A prospective randomized trial of arthroplasty versus fusion. J Spinal Disord Tech 16:352–361

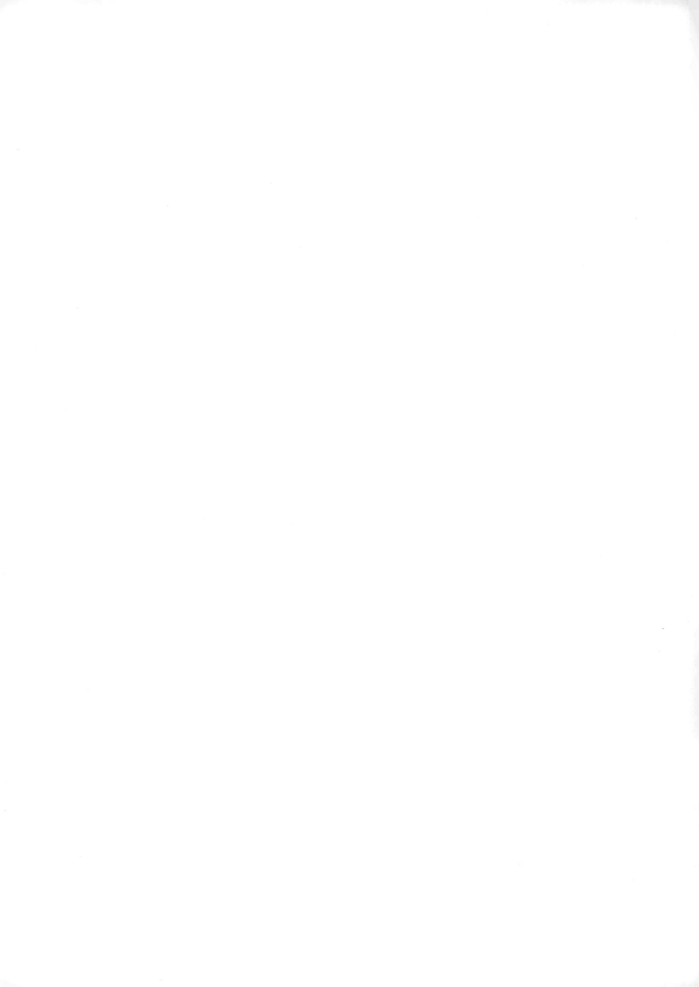